Assessment in Psychiatric and Mental Health Nursing

IN SEARCH OF THE WHOLE PERSON

Philip Barker

Professor of Psychiatric Nursing Practice,
University of Newcastle upon Tyne

Stanley Thornes (Publishers) Ltd

First published in 1997 by:
Stanley Thornes (Publishers) Ltd
Ellenborough House
Wellington Street
CHELTENHAM
GL50 1YW
United Kingdom

97 98 99 00 01 / 10 9 8 7 6 5 4 3 2 1

A catalogue record for this book is available from the British Library

ISBN 0-7487-3174-1

Distributed in the USA and Canada by Singular Publishing Group Inc., 4284 41st Street, San Diego, California 92105

Typeset by WestKey Limited, Falmouth, Cornwall
Printed in Great Britain by TJ International, Padstow, Cornwall

Dedication

This book is dedicated to the memory of my late colleague –
Dr Phil Hearne.

Assessment in Psychiatric and Mental Health Nursing

Contents

Foreword

Assessment in psychiatric and mental health nursing is a straightforward process in which nurses use specialized knowledge and technical skills to identify and document psychopathology. These are the myths shattered forever in this completely revised edition of Phil Barker's well known *Patient Assessment in Psychiatric Nursing*, first published by Croom Helm in 1985. Assessment is neither a straightforward process nor the mere application of specialized knowledge and technical skills, and its purposes are a great deal more constructive than finding out what is wrong with a person. The questions of whether diagnosis or assessment is the appropriate term and of whether assessment is concerned with normal or abnormal behaviour are considered as well as the human values appropriate to the practice of assessment. When all these issues have been taken into account, it becomes clear that assessment is a process for making educated guesses. This is not to say that assessment is a wholly subjective process, but to acknowledge that all forms of assessment are fallible because they rely on human judgement. Such judgements are important because they confer an implicit status on the person who is assessed, from that of a person dehumanized by a psychiatric diagnosis to that of a person who has the right to participate as an equal partner in their assessment. Mindful of these implications for mental health nursing practice, Professor Barker examines assessment in the broadest sense and considers the procedures it. may involve as well as issues of methodology. He proceeds by demonstrating the ordinariness of assessment and encourages mental health nurses to think beyond formal psychiatric categories to the needs of the person who lies behind the presenting problem.

The language Professor Barker uses is chosen with meticulous care and will assist mental health nurses to think more carefully about assessment. The word *patient* no longer appears in the title of his book and there are frequent references in the new edition to the *person-in-care*. This change in terminology makes an ontological point about the way of *being-in-the-world* of the person who is assessed. Such questions of ontology owe much to the writings of RD Laing and point beyond Laing to the hermeneutic phenomenology of Martin Heidegger and the existential philosophy of Kierkegaard and Sartre. Readers will not find such theorizing arid because it enables Professor Barker to make a practical point – the assessment process needs to be adapted to suit the needs of the person-in-care by taking into account appropriate factors such as age, gender and cultural background. However, taking such factors into account is insufficient unless the nurse and the person-in-care can collaborate to control the interview in a spirit of reciprocity in which neither partner is dominant. Professor Barker shows how the nurse can facilitate this sharing of control by remaining unbiased, by avoiding preconceptions and by putting aside personal prejudices. The empathy required involves accepting the value system of the person in care and engaging with their vantage point to perceive the world from their unique perspective. The use of the life history in assessment can assist this process and may enable the nurse to understand the experiences that have shaped the identity of the person.

Equal stress is placed on the range of other assessment techniques that are available to the nurse, their uses, advantages, disadvantages and limitations. Readers are encouraged to think about these methods not as a collection of recipes for unreflective application, but as techniques for particular purposes. Professor Barker makes the point that methods of assessment can be no less complex than the complexity of the person. Thus, what it means to be a person with emotional, cognitive, behavioural, social and spiritual dimensions rules out anything other than the assembly of an 'assessment battery' appropriate to the purposes at hand and agreed to by the person-in-care.

The general principles and possibilities of assessment that Professor Barker discusses take on added significance when he applies them to the assessment of people with particular needs. The assessment of people with anxiety and people with altered experiences of mood are considered along with the even more widespread experience of problems in interpersonal relationships. All the changes Professor Barker has made to his book are for the better, but I regret the passing of the former title of his chapter, 'Here Comes Everybody: The Assessment of Relationship Problems'. I may be alone in my attachment to the phrase 'here comes everybody', but it sums up for me our willingness to attribute to ourselves, or more commonly to others, problems in relationships, from the quarrels that sometimes occur in families to the misunderstandings that can arise among colleagues. However, Professor Barker has avoided these and other contentious issues such as what he refers to, tongue in cheek, as the 'magical interaction' that takes place between the nurse and the person. The aptness of his approach is demonstrated by his insight that even when someone is different from us, there is still one thing that we have in common with them – 'a difficulty in maintaining ... social competence'.

The assessment of people who experience psychosis is treated with equal sensitivity. The insidious tendency to dehumanize people through the application of a 'master status' or a 'within-group deindividuation', to use Professor Barker's preferred term, is discussed openly along with his reminder that it is not the classification of people that is the intention of psychiatric diagnosis, but the classification of the disorders that people have. This insight leads Professor Barker to reflect further on the role of assessment in the care of people who experience psychosis and, while not criticizing approaches that seek to quantify their experience, he argues the need to clarify exactly what it is that seems to be 'going on' within their unique experience. Professor Barker goes on to discuss ways in which assessment of the experience of psychosis can be used by the nurse to empower people in care.

What emerges from Professor Barker's book is an insightful perspective on assessment in mental health nursing practice. It turns out that the complexity of mental health assessment lies not in the specialized knowledge and technical skills required to conduct an assessment, but in the insights needed to remain open to the person in care, in the patience necessary to collaborate with the person in the assessment process, and in the ability to mistrust one's judgement. Professor Barker's reflections on these and related issues will inspire a generation of nurses whatever their specialization. His lucid style, sense of humour and superb scholarship make this book a joy to read. *Assessment in Psychiatric and Mental Health Nursing* is among the best written books on mental health nursing practice and will remain so for a very long time.

Michael Clinton
Brisbane
11 November 1996

Preface

I entered nursing 25 years ago. Little of what I learned in my training and within my early experience appears of use to me now. Or rather, I should say that everything I learned then has been of some *value* to me down the years: prompting my exploration of alternative ways of thinking about the **people** who are our 'patients', 'clients', 'users', 'consumers' or 'residents'. Those formative experiences continue to prompt me to think about how we ought to respond to the people in our care.

I learned little about assessment when I was a student. Or I should say that I learned little about the kind of assessment that will be discussed in this book. We were encouraged to use our senses, in an effort to collect observations about the patient's 'state'. These observations tended to be used only to lend support to the doctor's diagnosis. On some occasions they served a real function, however limited, as a guide to the management of the person-in-care. However, nurses did not talk readily about their 'assessments', which were little more than a scaled-down version of the psychiatric diagnosis. Having learned all the major diagnostic criteria, we waited for 'patients' who had been labelled in a particular way to behave in a particular way. It was the nurse's task to monitor the 'patient's' condition. The idea that they were people did not have the philosophical credibility it has today. For this reason, we paid scant attention to studying the person who was sheltered by his towering label.

Assessment is the most important thing that any nurse can do in her interactions with people-in-care. Historically speaking, it is the thing she does least well. We are getting better – albeit slowly. One worrying trend – at least in the UK – is for nurses to develop sophisticated assessment skills but to use these to complete diagnostic measures indistinguishable from those used by their psychiatrist colleagues. If nursing is to become better at assessing the people who are our patients, then we must be able to overlap with other disciplines (like psychiatric medicine) where appropriate. We need also to be able to *complement* other forms of assessment by supplying our unique forms of information.

Psychiatric nursing has been slow to develop its own tradition of assessment: the nursing textbooks seem to support this unfortunate conclusion.

Hildergard E. Peplau observed recently that, in the USA, psychiatric nursing textbooks often did no more than 're-frame' the knowledge base of psychiatric medicine. She expressed a hope that psychiatric nurses would publish more about the *proper focus* of psychiatric nursing: the phenomena that people-in-care present to nurses; and to which nurses respond [1]. I hope that the focus of this text will be understood as a move in the direction recommended by Dr Peplau.

Nurses in the United Kingdom have over two decades of experience of the development of a *formal* assessment methodology – especially through the medium of the 'nursing process'. However, there is a difference between 'doing' assessment and doing it properly. Observing people through their behaviour; forming hypotheses about what those patterns of behaviour might mean; collecting data on, for example, the strength, weakness and severity of those behaviour patterns are things which – in principle – anyone can do. This is much the same as saying that anyone can give massage or draw a house. What people-in-care should expect, by right, is sophisticated assessment; something which does justice to the problem under review.

To continue my analogy, people-in-care deserve an assessment that is more like the sensitive manipulation of a physiotherapist or the precise accuracy of a draughtsman. I am under no illusions about the scope and potential of this book. I shall not show you how to achieve the symbolic peak of reliable, sensitive, clinical judgement. Instead, I hope to introduce you to some of the principles and practices of assessment. Neither do I intend to offer the reader a **manual** of assessment. I have spent almost two decades trying to learn about assessment and have had the good fortune to have worked with, met or studied the work of some very good 'tutors'. As I sit down to write, however, the enormity of the assessment task still seems overwhelming. If we are to offer people-in-care a 'quality' nursing service, based on 'high quality' assessment, we need to recognize that there may well be no short cuts to such a goal.

I need here to acknowledge that perhaps I wrote this book for myself. I have been a lifelong doubter of my own ability to make reasonable judgements. Recently, someone asked me what exactly a professor *did*. Almost without a moment's reservation I suggested that a professor 'professes doubt'. In this book I shall share with you my own ideas about assessment, as well as a few observations on the subject from some of the great thinkers. Much of the time my conversation with the reader will allow me to reconsider some of my doubts and anxieties concerning the whole business of assessment.

I shall also discuss the main methods briefly and shall finish by describing the use of several of these methods in the exploration of one or two of the more outstanding 'populations' in psychiatry: I refrain from saying the **most** outstanding populations. All the assessment approaches and illustrated methods are psychosocial in form and function. I have excluded assessment methods that do not involve the person's experience of himself, his relationship with his mental distress, others or the world in general. This focus is intentional, given my assumption that psychiatric nursing possesses, primarily, an interpersonal focus.

A few of the assessment instruments that are used as examples are restricted for use by professionals who have completed special forms of training. However, most of the methods illustrated or acknowledged can be used by any professional, but carry no guarantee of success. Just as we would not dream of restricting the use of pocket calculators, or even measuring tapes, to the mathematicians who developed them, it seems foolish to restrict the use of psychosocial assessments.

I intend this book to be stimulating and informative. I hope that it will give the reader an idea about the kinds of assessment method that my colleagues and I have practised, with great satisfaction, over the past two decades. I do not know whether these methods have made us better 'carers' or not, but we have enjoyed the reassurance these methods gave us.

I wish also to interest the reader in the philosophy of assessment – as distinct from diagnosis. I hope to illustrate which kinds of method might be helpful in exploring which kinds of problem. I also want to communicate something of the thinking that needs to lie behind the selection of these methods. I have resisted the temptation to publish a catalogue of assessment methods and hope that the reader will consult the original sources to find out how to use the standardized methods in the correct manner. I have also tried to suggest how nurses might construct their own simple methods of assessment, using principles that are very much 'tried and tested'.

All the people-in-care illustrated in the book are real. The methods discussed are examples of the kinds of approach we have adopted to try to understand the person called 'patient'. Assessment of the whole person in psychiatric nursing is a very wide remit. Such a range of problems and people is embraced by the term 'psychiatric' and 'mental health' that I can do justice to some of these areas only by the exclusion of others.

In Part One I have tried to look at assessment in its most general sense and consider which principles or actual methods have widespread applicability. Part Two looks at specific problem areas that are of common concern to psychiatric nurses, whether working in hospital or community settings. I have tried to ignore discussing psychiatric disorders as such. Instead, I have favoured looking at problems of living, which are common to a variety of disorders.

I have chosen to deal exclusively with adults. Children and older people are missing from my coverage. Although both groups are very important I have excluded them for a number of good reasons. Children present with very special problems – whether they are physically or psychologically disturbed. They are not simply immature adults. The world of the child is a special place that demands special consideration. Children do not think like adults: as a result their behaviour, although similar in appearance, does not always follow the same rules as that of adults. Although many of the principles of assessment covered in the book can be adapted to suit children, I did not think that I could do this group justice within the space of a short chapter, or even two. Given the pressure on space I thought that it would be more realistic to omit them altogether in the hope that the reader would be stimulated to pursue the subject of assessment in a specialist childhood text.

My views on older people are similar. Although aspects of the assessment of older people are touched upon in later chapters, they are not dealt with in any detail. People who are changing, both physically and mentally, present special problems. I hope that by omitting any detailed consideration of this group I have conveyed – albeit obliquely – my feeling that older people are a very special case. They cannot, indeed should not, be seen as just another subgroup of the psychiatric scene.

In a similar vein I have excluded completely from consideration people with an unambiguous organic disorder. I think that this omission is justified on the grounds that nurses have been well prepared to assess aspects of organic disorder: detecting and gauging muscular weakness, tremors, dyskinesia, paresis and paralysis, etc. I do not wish to suggest by my omission that these organic problems have no place in psychiatric nursing assessment. However, they may represent a group of problems that involve the presentation of mental symptoms based upon underlying physical disorder. In many senses they are qualitatively and quantitatively different from the disorders reviewed here, where the problem is largely a psychosocial one with no obvious underlying physical explanation.

Despite these exclusions I am confident that many of the general principles of assessment covered in the early chapters and some of the background issues that thread their way through the remaining chapters will be of some relevance to adults, children, older people and those with an organic disorder. In the sense that all are people first and groups of 'patients' second, this book was written with all of them in mind, whether they are specifically dealt with or not.

Throughout the book I have retained the use of the female gender (she) for the role of the nurse, and the male (he) for the person-in-care. I have done so partly to reverse the unfortunate tradition in many texts where the active 'helper' is usually defined as a man, and the unfortunate person on the receiving end is invariably seen as a woman. My depiction of the nurse as female reflects, also, the typical care scenario in psychiatric nursing. Within the gender context, I have included also some reference to the effect that sexism has had within the field of psychiatry. In attempting to give women their place in the text I hope that I have made a small contribution to the demise of the patriarchal attitudes, which limit men almost as much as they have attempted to limit women.

I hope that I shall be forgiven for speaking directly to the reader, and for involving her in my reflections on my experience. It is a common practice in academic writing to adopt the third person, even where this creates a clumsy writing style or, more importantly, the impression that the author is not really speaking for her or himself. I regard all my writing as a personal affair. I am telling the reader what I think, at least at this point in time. It seems inappropriate, if not foolish, to try to cover my tracks, so to speak, by distancing myself from the personal nature of my communication with the reader. I hope that the reader will interpret my directness as a signal for my respect for the relationship between reader and author.

In an earlier version of this text [2] I concluded the preface by acknowledging that I was not sufficiently sure of my identity to argue that what followed (in that book) was undeniably 'nursing'. Some 10 years on I am no less beleaguered by doubts in general. I am fairly confident that what follows, however, is undeniably about nursing, if not representative of what has been called 'the proper focus of nursing' [3, 4]. This shift in my confidence is largely a function of the time I have spent, listening, discussing and debating the notion of what is or is not the proper focus of the psychiatric nurse, with my 'significant others'. These 'others' range around the globe – from established authorities from the USA through some of my more valued colleagues at home in the UK to some of the more emergent nursing thinkers in Australia. To each of them I extend a special and silent 'thank you'.

Finally, I need to acknowledge the specific support of some people without whom this text might not have been possible.

- A special acknowledgement is due to my editor, Rosemary Morris, who has shown the patience and understanding which is characteristic of nursing at its best.
- Like many of my contemporaries I owe much to two *grandes dames* of psychiatric nursing: Annie T. Altschul in the UK and Hildegard E. Peplau in the USA. Both have shown the generosity of spirit which one associates with those blessed by talent and experience. Their mentoring was priceless and, in the spirit of the finest gifts, given freely. I hope to repay their mentoring by attempting to emulate their example with my own peers and students.

I should like to acknowledge the ongoing stimulation which I have received from three colleagues whom I can also call friends: Dr Bill Reynolds, Senior Lecturer, University of Stirling Highland Campus, Inverness; Kenneth Larson, formerly Director of the Payne Whitney Clinic at the Cornell Medical School, New York Hospital; and Dr Shirley Smoyak, Professor of Planning at the Institute for Health, Health Care and Ageing Research, at Rutgers University, New Jersey. These three have offered me their own insights into psychiatric nursing while helping me gain further insight into my own view of my chosen discipline.

Finally, I acknowledge the people who have helped me 'hold the dream' of developing the proper focus of psychiatric and mental health nursing: at the University of Newcastle upon Tyne: my academic colleagues Dr Chris

Stevenson, Shaun Parsons and the late Dr Phil Hearne; and at Newcastle City Health Trust my clinical colleagues Ann McKenzie, Mike Davison, Elsa Conway, Steven Michael, Brendan Hill, Alan Steele, Bill Bell and Dick Maugham.

Phil Barker, Newcastle upon Tyne, August 1996

NOTES

1. Peplau, H. E. (1994) Another look at schizophrenia from a nursing standpoint, in *Psychiatric Nursing 1946–94: A Report on the State of the Art*, (ed. C. A. Anderson), C. V. Mosby/Yearbook, St Louis, MO.
2. Barker, P. (1985) *Patient Assessment in Psychiatric Nursing*, Croom Helm, London.
3. Barker, P. and Reynolds, B. (1994) A critique of Watson's caring ideology: the proper focus of psychiatric nursing. *Journal of Psychosocial Nursing and Mental Health Services*, **32**, 17–22.
4. Barker, P., Reynolds, W. and Ward, T. (1995) The proper focus of nursing: a critique of the 'caring' ideology. *International Journal of Nursing Studies*, **32**, 386–97.

A note on language

It was intended that when Newspeak had been adopted once and for all and Oldspeak forgotten, a heretical thought should be literally unthinkable, at least so far as thought is dependent on words.

George Orwell, *1984*

One significant social development in Britain of the past decade was the insidious introduction of political correctness. 'PC' has by now lost much of its original attraction and has become almost wholly the subject of conceit or the object of ridicule. It retains some status, however, within the health and social services, where the naming of the people who receive services remains a provocative subject area.

It is important to show respect for the people who are the subject matter of this book: those who receive psychiatric and mental health nursing. I have chosen to avoid taking sides in the *'patient'*-or-*'client'*-or-*'user'*-or-*'consumer'*-or-*'service-recipient'* debate. The construction and production of such synonyms seems foolhardy when we can simply refer to the people in our care as *'people'*. I have tried to observe this simple convention throughout the text.

Where there might be a risk of confusion with any other 'people' I have used the clumsy but accurate term *'people-in-care'*. This may emphasize that *people* remain the subject of nurses' attention and *care* remains the universal term for how nurses attend to the needs of such people. I hope that this simple gesture may also be interpreted as an acknowledgement of the fundamental *human* nature of nursing practice.

PART ONE

The principles of nursing assessment

The first rule of assessment is 'begin at the beginning'. Although this rule – like most rules – may on occasions be broken, I shall adhere to the rule here. Nursing assessment involves the exercise – in practice – of a wide range of theoretical principles. The various methods of assessment all depend for their success on the use, as appropriate, of these principles. In this first part of the book I shall discuss and illustrate the main principles that underpin the practice of assessment in psychiatric and mental health nursing.

The philosophical and theoretical principles that define psychiatric and mental health nursing assessment are explored first. Their origins and their interdependent relationship with other forms of 'human enquiry' are reviewed and discussed in Chapter 1.

Many forms of assessment rely heavily on asking questions. This can be the simplest, yet often the most complex, form of assessment. Some approaches to interviewing and aspects of the structure of interpersonal enquiry are reviewed in Chapter 2.

Although nurses aim to address the whole person, the sheer scale and inherent complexity of people – and their life experiences – make this largely impossible. How we attempt to address the complexity of the people in our care is discussed in Chapter 3.

The final chapter in Part One provides an overview of assessment methods, their construction and application. Not all of the assessment 'tools' at nurses' disposal belong to nursing. However, like many other tools in everyday life, a range of assessment instruments and approaches can be used profitably by nurses. The relative value of and practical problems in using different methods of assessment are discussed in Chapter 4.

He who merely knows right principles is not equal to him who loves them.

Confucius

An overview of the assessment process: bringing life into the light

Men are not to be judged by their looks, habits and appearances; but by the character of their lives and conversations and by their works. It is better to be praised by one's own works than by the words of another.

L'Etrange

It requires a very unusual mind to undertake the analysis of the obvious.

A. N. Whitehead

Everyone complains of his memory; nobody of his judgement.

La Rochefoucauld

THE MEANING OF ASSESSMENT

As I write the British winter bites hard for the first time this year. Overnight, my neighbours and I seem to have become keen meteorologists. We discuss at length today's conditions and make various predictions about the likelihood of further snow or the chance of a thaw. In a few short months our present concern will be transformed into an equally anxious search for signs of 'good weather' for our summer vacation. And so it goes throughout the seasons. Each day, men and women everywhere assess the weather, each one judging the role it might play in the fabric of her/his life.

My neighbours and I do not talk about **assessing** the weather. Yet, this is what we do, day in and day out. It is part of the set of routines we use to make sense of our lives and our selves. Our 'weather assessment' differs little from the way we judge the value of a second-hand car, how we review our social calendar or how we evaluate our children's performance at school. In each case, having collected some information about the situation, we are then in a position to comment upon what we have observed: we can make judgements or pronouncements. Is the car worth the asking price? Are we going to be busy in the months ahead? How is our daughter progressing with her maths? Each example shares an important feature – the hallmark of all assessments. They are rarely, if ever, done for their own sake.

Assessments are usually undertaken with a view to taking some action in the future. My weather assessment helps me to decide whether I should take an umbrella or sunglasses. The assessment of our daughter's school report helps us decide whether or not to offer her some extra help with her homework. In health care a small proportion of assessments are done mainly for statistical purposes: for instance, how many people with a diagnosis of depression pass through a hospital service in 1 year? However, even here such an audit may indicate a need to change the nature or organization of the service. When we turn our attention to the concept of nursing assessment we can safely assume that the aims are similar to the simple examples already quoted. In a small number of cases we collect information on people-in-care to help to study the service offered. However, in the majority of cases assessment is undertaken with a view to planning and then evaluating a specific pattern of nursing care.

In this chapter I shall discuss the meaning of the term 'assessment'. I shall try to say what role assessment might fulfil in the care of people with what used to be called a mental illness but is increasingly described as 'mental health problems'. I shall suggest also why assessment lies at the core of the nurse's function. I shall take the line that nurses cannot offer valid and reliable forms of nursing care without valid and effective assessment. Given the emphasis placed upon the 'process' – or various 'models' – of nursing, it might be assumed that nursing care is always based upon valid and reliable forms of assessment. It would be more accurate to say that most nurses take considerable care in their assessment of the people in their care. Such care is not always synonymous with the kind of rigorous assessment described in the following chapters. People may present with a wide range of mental health problems, many of which require highly individual forms of attention. Consequently, the notion of 'scientific assessment' may be an inappropriate concept. This does not mean that nursing assessment cannot involve the attribution of a numerical measure, using a standardized instrument.

Assessment can measure the characteristics that different people have in common (see Appendices A and B). It also plays an important role in telling us how one person differs from another: what makes the person unique. The emphasis given to theory-building and the use of models in nursing in recent years confirms the view that nursing is becoming more methodical and systematic. One consequence of these developments is that we are beginning to develop a common language of assessment, where different nurses can describe and attempt to measure the phenomena with which the person-in-care presents and can expect other nurses to understand exactly what is being communicated.

In an earlier book on assessment I suggested that the text was written with tomorrow in mind [1]. The developments in psychiatric and mental health nursing in the decade which has elapsed since I wrote that book suggest that we may already have entered a 'brave new world' of mental health care, in which nursing is playing an increasingly important role. The challenges presented by this new world of mental distress and mental health care require that we sharpen not only the focus of nursing assessment but also the tools of assessment, which might address the new agenda. In this sense, the assessment of the **whole person** in mental health nursing is coming of age.

THE NATURE OF ASSESSMENT

Most English dictionaries offer a fairly restrictive definition of 'assessment', referring to taxation, where an 'assessor' fixes the value of something. This seems to be the traditional meaning of the word. More recently we have come to understand the term as having something to do with **estimating the character** of something or someone. This definition seems to be more relevant to psychiatric and mental health nursing, where we are interested in estimating the people in our care in terms of who and what they might be. This meaning appears to have been popularized first by psychologists, who believed that assessment should be concerned with the worth of a person [2]. This view contrasted with traditional medical diagnosis, which tried to identify the nature of the pathology of the patient: looking for what was wrong with him. Among the important characteristics of professional nursing, Hildegard Peplau recognized the importance of theory as a support to assessment: 'Every nurse in all nursing situations uses three principal operations: observation, interpretation and observation. What is observed or noticed must be interpreted; that is, the raw data must be transformed into **some meaningful explanation**' [3].

In search of the whole person

Over the past two decades in the UK – and over almost four decades in the USA – nurses have begun to move away from the strict use of a medical–diagnostic model in favour of an assessment of the worth of the individual. The voice of the nursing process movement [4] urged all nurses to show concern for the person behind the patient label, reminding us to look for 'worth' amid what might seem like insurmountable problems. Although nurses may still be working towards the attainment of this ideal there are many indications that each day brings us closer to dealing with the 'whole person', rather than simply the sum of his parts. Nurses are gradually beginning to appreciate that assessment involves looking at the person-in-care from the broadest possible viewpoint. By implication, this will mean studying his strengths as well as his weaknesses.

Many traditional forms of assessment in psychiatric nursing involved derivations of the diagnostic methods used by psychiatrists. In common with the practice of physical medicine, 'psychological medicine' also emphasized the search for a class of disorder. Unfortunately, experience has shown that 'people-in-care' often do not fit the rather tidy definitions of disorder covered by the diagnostic system [5]. Some psychiatrists have even suggested that psychiatric disorder should perhaps be seen as 'states' where different kinds of problem may be evident to varying degrees in the same person, rather than assuming that the person-in-care can have only 'one kind of psychiatric disease' that excludes the possibility of any other kind of psychological disorder [6]. In the United States especially this sort of philosophy has led to a broadening of traditional medical diagnostic categories. Increasingly, it is suggested that people might suffer from any one of a wide range of (for example) psychotic disorders rather than the restricted number of narrow definitions to which we have grown accustomed.

A definition of assessment

The value of 'pigeon-holing' people within different diagnostic categories has been questioned considerably over the past 30 years. Some critics have favoured, instead, looking at 'patients' as people who have certain problems of living – which can range from severely disabling to mildly inconvenient. Such people also have strengths or assets, which might play a part in helping them to resolve these problems of living. This approach distinguishes traditional diagnosis from the emerging tradition of assessment. In this sense a definition of assessment might be 'the decision-making process, based upon the collection of relevant information, using a formal set of ethical criteria, which contributes to an overall evaluation of a person and his circumstances'.

Although assessment may involve a wide range of functions, in nursing the assessment may seek an answer to the question 'what does it mean to be this person?'

Human responses: the proper focus of nursing

Psychiatric nurses from the USA have long been interested in the phenomena that people-in-care present to nurses. Such phenomena – or 'things shown' – might be described as the proper focus of nursing [7]. What the person-in-care 'shows' to the nurse is, inevitably, what nurses focus on.

Robinson noted that as soon as the patient (*sic*) entered the health care system the nurse begins to make evaluations of his needs. She defined such needs as 'what brings him [the patient] to nursing's attention' [8]. She noted that the assessment stage of the nursing process always began with naming or otherwise identifying the person's problems: 'The best source of data (information) about the patient is always the patient. Likewise. the most efficient way of obtaining information is to ask direct questions: "What brings you to the clinic?" "How can I help you?"'

It is obvious that the person's needs (or problems) cannot be met or resolved until they are identified or named. Although it may be difficult to obtain such definitions of the problem or need from the person-in-care, clearly the person is the most obvious starting point.

Robinson noted also that nursing assessment differed from medical assessment since it focused on the person's need for help in relating to himself or others. Nursing focuses on the person's thoughts, feelings and behaviour, which are assumed to be human responses to life problems. This concept of 'human responses' derives from the work of the American Nurses' Association (ANA) [9], which also defined nursing by identifying the focus of nursing practice: 'the phenomena of concern to nurses are human responses to actual or potential health problems. Any observable manifestation, need, concern, event, dilemma, difficulty, occurrence or fact that can be described or scientifically explained and is **within the target area of nursing practice** is of interest to nurses [emphasis added].'

The ANA identified two kinds of 'human response' which it saw as the object of nursing action: an individual's or group's reaction to actual health problems; and concerns of individuals or groups about potential health problems. The difficulty in defining clearly what exactly is meant by human responses has been noted by several authorities [10]. Ward, however, offered a definition which appears disarmingly simple. Nurses do not try to solve the problem of, for example, a hallucination. Rather, nurses attempt to deal with the problems that the hallucination creates for the person who experiences it [11].

Likewise, if a person has become increasingly detached from his or her surroundings and the people in it, if he or she feels threatened by the reality of life, and if perceptual and thought processes are distorted, the problem is that he or she cannot satisfy the need to live a meaningful existence, free of fear and confrontation. The nurse needs to identify how those changes in behaviour inhibit the client's ability to lead his or her own life and then construct care that will help the person tackle them [12].

Ward noted that by so doing the nurse was considering the consequences of illness, not the illness itself, as the source for the intervention. This focus on the person's experience was noted recently by Peplau. She observed that nurses increasingly claim that:

consideration of (the patients') their needs and interests as persons having dignity and worth, are primary values inherent in the design and execution of nursing services. These values should be implicit in a nursing approach for the care of patients having a diagnosis of schizophrenia. In keeping with these claims, it would behove nurses to give up the notion of a disease, such as schizophrenia, and to think exclusively of patients as persons [13].

The separate views of Peplau, Robinson and Ward share a similar view of psychiatric nursing: that it is concerned to address the person's human response to problems involving his relationship to himself or others. We might distinguish this approach from that of physicians, who see and assess: 'the atypical, socially unacceptable behaviours which are called symptoms, and view them as indicators of disease [14]'.

Given this distinction between the focus of medicine and nursing, Peplau suggested that nurses: 'ought to recognize such behaviours as problem-solving actions and emblematic of difficulties arising within interpersonal relationships [15]'. At various points in this book I shall emphasize the central nature of this 'interpersonal' view of mental health problems, for nursing assessment and practice. For the moment we need only note that if nursing assessment involves valuing anything, it is the person's human responses to general or specific mental health problems.

FORMAL AND INFORMAL METHODS OF ASSESSMENT

Most assessments have similar aims. However, the processes by which assessments are conducted can vary enormously. Such differences are highly significant. They can influence greatly the value of the information that is produced. The way that an assessment is carried out can make the exercise very worth while or largely a waste of time. The main differences between assessment methods relate to the manner in which the information is collected. In general, this means that the process can be 'formal' or 'informal'.

In a formal assessment some kind of structure is emphasized. Usually, this is one which has been planned and studied carefully, usually through research. In an informal assessment the information is collected by less structured, perhaps even haphazard, methods.

Although formal and informal methods appear to have much in common, this similarity is often only superficial. For instance, an interview can be formal or informal; structured or unstructured. In both cases the person-in-care is asked questions and his replies are noted. However, in a formal interview the questions will be prepared out carefully in advance. They are likely to be worded in a particular way. The informal interview lacks this structure. The nurse merely asks the questions she considers important at that time and words them in the way she thinks appropriate. Although both kinds of assessment are in common use, we should be aware that any formal system has important advantages over less structured ways of looking at persons-in-care. The rules, guidelines and specific procedures that are established in a formal system may help us to study different people-in-care in more or less the same way. As a result, our own prejudices and idiosyncrasies are reduced, if not cancelled out entirely. The outcome of the assessment should be the same irrespective of who completes it. The same cannot be said of more informal methods. Here our biases, opinions and other 'value judgements' influence the conduct of the assessment. Such factors can have a big influence on the kind of information collected.

We should emphasize the distinction between formal and informal methods when considering how nurses plan nursing care. In general, a nursing assessment calls for information about the nature and scale of the person-in-care's problems. What is his problem and how big is it? These questions should be as detailed and unambiguous as possible, especially where we hope to evaluate the effects of different forms of care or treatment. However, the way such information is collected often depends on the problem involved, and can even be influenced by the personality of the person-in-care himself. Traditionally, nurses have concentrated on assessing the person's biophysical state. Here the nurse uses highly formalized methods of assessment. Even routine measures – such as taking a pulse or testing the reaction of pupils to light – require the use of a precise, controlled procedure. Nurses are taught such procedures in a systematic manner. They are expected to use them with the minimum of adaptations in an equally systematic manner. The reason for this is simple: information about the person-in-care's biophysical state needs to be as accurate as possible. The method used to collect this information reflects the need for reliability and precision. It must not be influenced by the attitudes or mood of the person carrying out the assessment.

When we consider the nurse's assessment of the person's non-physical state – his psychological, social or otherwise 'human' functioning – the picture is quite different. The procedures a nurse uses to gauge the person's core temperature or the various functions of his heart are orderly and fairly unreliable. The assessment of the person's relationship with himself or the world around him, however, appears almost casual by comparison. Without doubt such 'psychosocial' targets are less clearly defined, and as such are more difficult to assess. Increasingly, the nursing literature suggests that nurses assess all aspects of the person – including the spiritual dimension. The reader needs to ask: 'What do I understand by the term "spiritual"?' I suspect that there will be a wide range of answers to this simple question. This variation illustrates the difficulty in asking fairly basic questions about what it means to be human.

However, if we want to understand the 'whole person' in our care we must strive to use the best methods of assessment available – methods that will help clear away some of the mist of confusion and mystery which surrounds the person. In this sense assessment may be formal or informal, but should always be rigorous.

In some situations the choice between formal and informal methods is determined by the person-in-care himself. Where the person is talkative, intelligent and anxious to communicate, the nurse may get most of her information from open-ended conversations. Where the person is less articulate or rarely speaks, the assessment is likely to favour more specific measures of behaviour. This might involve the use of standardized rating scales, rather than casual interviewing, and will be more formal as a result. There appears to be a strong tradition in nursing for use of formal methods when studying the person's physical state and more informal methods when studying the person 'psychosocially'. We must ask ourselves whether it is time to discontinue this tradition. We need to ask: 'Should the method be determined by the person, and his situation?'

WHAT DO WE NEED TO ASSESS?

So far I have talked about studying the person's functioning. But what do I mean by the term 'functioning'? What do we pay attention to when we say we are trying to study the 'whole person'?

Levels of living

Everyone functions – or lives – on a number of levels at once (Figure 1.1).

- We live within our **physiological self**. Although we are not sensitive to this level of functioning, the biochemical level of existence is of crucial importance to the stability of our lives. This molecular or biochemical level of functioning is clearly the most basic level of our lives.
- At a level slightly removed from this lies our **biological self**. Here, our various organs work constantly to maintain the outward appearance of 'life', supported by our complex muscular and skeletal system, of which we have only the crudest awareness. Usually, we are only aware of this level of experience when we experience pain on exertion.
- At a third level lies our **behavioural self**: how we think, feel and act – each changing from moment to moment; from one situation to the next. How we think and what we feel appear to have a major effect on how we behave.
- At another stage removed lies our **social self**: our relationships with the many people who make up our world. Some are close to us, such as family and friends. Others are simply the rest of 'humanity'.
- Finally, we have a level which might be called our **spiritual self**. Here we live in the world of our hopes, dreams and – perhaps most of all – our beliefs. Here we experience views of ourselves and our world that are often obscure, symbolic and ill-defined. The very nature of our spiritual self might suggest that it is impossible to define.

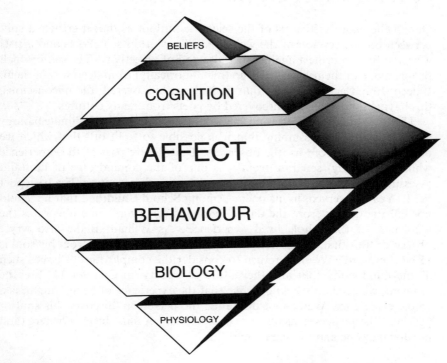

Figure 1.1   Levels of living.

We have developed a wide range of metaphors for both the 'molecular' and 'spiritual' aspects of human experience. Such definitions are metaphorical for the simple reason that both 'ends' of the human condition are abstract and unobservable. The extent to which our observation of our biological, behavioural and social selves is any less metaphorical is open to question. Most of us are either ignorant of or take for granted our experience at these different levels of living. This is very true of our molecular existence and is probably true of our 'spiritual self': either we rarely consider it or we have developed a language and grammar – such as religion – that allows us to take that too for granted.

Most of us accept that our molecular or biochemical life is important – and that we have some kind of spiritual identity. We know that these aspects of ourselves are there; but we do not fully understand what exactly this involves, far less how it functions.

However, the distinction between our different 'selves' or 'levels' of living is inherently false. Our **whole lived experience** [16] is just that: an experience that is whole and complete in itself. We can only isolate these different aspects of our 'whole self' in our imaginings.

OBJECTIVITY: THE FALSE GOD OF SCIENCE?

One of the major criticisms of the scientific outlook is that it creates a split between our perception of the world, and the world itself. Poets and artists were the first to protest against the false god of objectivity. The sense which people make of themselves wells up (metaphorically) from deep within them. Indeed, Freud acknowledged that he had not 'discovered' the unconscious, this having long ago been discovered by poets from many cultures.

The Newtonian and Cartesian views of reality still tend to dominate biology and medicine, both assuming that it is possible to 'split off' that which we observe (reality) from us, the observers. That we are part of the experience while (apparently) separate from it is one of the conundrums of life (and assessment), which we might best deal with by merely accepting. The Irish poet W. B. Yeats observed, in his poem 'Among School Children', that he 'could not tell the dancer from the dance'. Perhaps this simple line illustrates the wholeness of the 'whole lived experience'. As William Blake also wryly observed: 'But first, the notion that man has a body distinct from his soul is to be expunged'. We shall return to consider the complexities of issues such as the mind–body split and the nature of 'reality' in Chapter 11. For the moment, we need only acknowledge that the experience of being human is a whole experience. We cannot dismantle the person to 'discover' his soul or psyche. If he possesses such a core characteristic it must be everywhere (and nowhere) at one and the same time.

People: story-telling animals

The state of being human involves a complex interaction of different things; some which we can name and understand; others which are a virtual mystery to us. Most of us are only aware of how we live on a psychological and social level. Even then, we are often confused about these 'open' – or surface – aspects of our lives. It should be apparent that each of us lives on all these levels of experience all the time, whether we are aware of it or not. Often we only become aware of these levels when we begin to 'malfunction': when some aspect of our chemistry, biology, thoughts, emotions, habits, relationships or our symbolic view of 'ourselves' goes awry.

This is also true of the person-in-care. He needs help because some aspect of his functioning is 'dysfunctional'. Or rather we should say that the person experiences 'problems' on one level, and this experience is 'relayed' – like a message – to other parts of his whole self. People often know that they have a problem of living, but not where it comes from or what part of 'themselves' it is affecting.

Although we can study how the person-in-care functions, one level at a time, there may be disadvantages in such an approach. We should be aware of how one problem area – such as disturbed biochemistry – can influence how the person-in-care thinks and feels. We should also be aware that such influences might also operate in the opposite direction – how we think and feel – influencing even our cellular structure. Given that the person **feels** whole, we should always try to respect this by addressing them wholly. This is no more or less than we would ask for ourselves.

People know who they are and become more knowledgeable about themselves, their lives, and their problems by talking about themselves. In Hilda Peplau's insightful words: 'people make themselves up as they talk' [17]. This illustrates the story-telling characteristic of people. This quality of humans probably is our major distinction from all other species. Empirical philosophers, like John Locke and David Hume, tried to give an account of personal identity solely in terms of psychological states or events. Such accounts failed to take account of the background to personal identity: the stories that people are born into, and become part of, by the telling of their own story.

Just as history is not a simple catalogue of events, or a list of characters, so the story of our lives involves more than the events which we (as persons) experience. The American philosopher Alasdair MacIntyre suggested that:

> it is through hearing stories about wicked stepmothers, lost children, good but misguided kings, wolves that suckle twin boys, youngest sons who receive no inheritance but must make their own way in the world and eldest sons who waste their inheritance on riotous living and go into exile to live with the swine, that children learn or mislearn both what a child and what a parent is, what the cast of characters may be in the drama into which they have been born and what the ways of the world are [18].

When nurses sit down to assess the person-in-care, they are obliged to ask: Who is this person? In so doing, they cannot divorce that individual (and his story) from all the stories that helped him become who he is. As MacIntyre observed, should we deprive children of stories we may: 'leave them unscripted, anxious stutterers in their actions as in their words' [19].

MacIntyre's philosophy seems to carry a profound message, which also appears relevant to the objective of this book. If we are to understand who **are** the people in our care, we need to listen to the stories of their lives. That we are the stories we tell – or sometimes that are told about us – is as true for us as it is for those in our care. In MacIntyre's words:

> I am the **subject** of a history that is my own and no one else's, that has its own peculiar meaning. When someone complains – as do some of those who attempt or commit suicide – that his or her life is meaningless, he or she is often and perhaps characteristically complaining that the narrative of their life has become unintelligible to them, that it lacks any point, any movement toward a climax or **telos** [20].

If psychiatric and mental health nursing assessment leads anywhere, it might lead to the nurse and person-in-care considering further the story of the person's life, and to re-authoring that story, through the therapeutic process of nurse's relationship with the person [21].

HOW LONG IS A PIECE OF STRING?

Each time we set out to find out something, we embark upon an assessment. Each time we ask about what is happening now, what happened in the past or what might happen in the future, we are involved in the curious business of assessment. I say 'curious', for we are inquisitive and anxious to learn. Also, the way we go about finding out can often appear strange or in some way extraordinary. As I noted at the start of this chapter, looking out of the window just now, making mental notes on cloud formation, the colour of the sky, how the wind bends the trees; all are aspects of the assessment process. How can I describe today's weather to you, or make a prediction about tomorrow's, if I do not make some observation of the 'elements': how they appear and how they behave? Assessment of the person-in-care differs only in kind from assessments of the weather, of educational progress, or the worth of a painting or piece of pottery. They all share the same principle: that a reliable judgement can be made only if reliable information is available. If we do not scrutinize the painting carefully, we may judge it to be more or less valuable than it really is. The same is true of people. If we do not study people carefully, methodically, with the minimum of bias (using an appropriate ethical framework), how can we reliably judge their 'worth'?

Presentation and performance

There is a difference between a nursing assessment and judgements we might make about the weather, cars or objects. The judgement of the person that results from our assessment will, in most cases, be of crucial importance. In some cases a nursing assessment, combined with other forms of medical or psychological assessment, might make the difference between life and death. This could be said of the person who is a suicide risk or the disturbed or disoriented person who might unwittingly be a danger to himself. Having said that, we cannot afford to be glib about the potential value of assessment information. Neither should we complain too much about the work required to collect such information.

It is difficult to say anything concrete about psychiatric nursing assessment except to say that it is in its infancy and is often gravely misunderstood. I opened this chapter from a rather oblique angle. I tried to show how assessment is a part of everyday life. It becomes assessment – the professional tool – only when we standardize or make more formal the things we do each day, and which we take very much for granted.

We must accept that 'assessment' is a word with a broad range of meanings.

I am aware that here I am simply adding my own interpretation of the word. However, each definition of assessment, including my own, emphasizes the collection of information with the intention of making a judgement. These two actions are the very heart of assessment.

Although nurses aim to address and understand the whole person, they can assess people-in-care in much the same way as mechanics might diagnose faults in a car engine. Indeed, in some situations this highly focused form of assessment may be the most appropriate. The mechanic is not diagnosing in the same way that a doctor would. Yet there are similarities. The mechanic monitors, for example, the functions of the engine, comparing these with some ideal – what she would call 'normal' engine running. When a doctor studies a person's cardiovascular system and diagnoses some malfunction she uses the self-same process. I make this analogy merely to reinforce the point that nurses can embrace the idea of assessment in much the same way that a mechanic embraces diagnosis.

Assessment involves looking at the person-in-care with a view to gaining a picture that will help us see him as a unique human being. This process involves developing a working model of the person. This model should show, in a simplified manner, how he functions in relation to himself and the world around him. But before we set this process in motion we must decide what we are going to observe. Any assessment involves collecting information about performance and presentation.

If you were invited to assess a teapot or a car, you would make various notes on its **appearance**: size, colour, shape, etc. You would then try to relate these to the way in which it **works**: does the teapot pour easily? Is the handle easy to grip? What is the car's top speed? What is its average fuel consumption? Answers to these questions will give you information about presentation and performance: or, to continue our earlier discussion, **form** and **function**. The appearance and the performance of things are not always related. The colour of a teapot has no relationship with how it pours. However, the shape of the spout or the contours of the car will have a relationship with 'pouring' or 'fuel consumption'. This analogy illustrates how the 'design' of something is related to its function: how it works in practice.

We are often required to look for similar kinds of 'connection' – between presentation and performance – in the people in our care. The blushing (presentation) of a young man's cheeks and the stammering (performance) of his voice may have a relationship, one to the other. In assessment, we collect information about the appearance of the person (presentation) and how he behaves (performance); and then try to see if we can understand the person better by combining these two viewpoints.

Fishing for clues

Any assessment may be broad or narrow. However, some kinds of assessment are concerned only with a narrow focus. These are usually called 'diagnostic

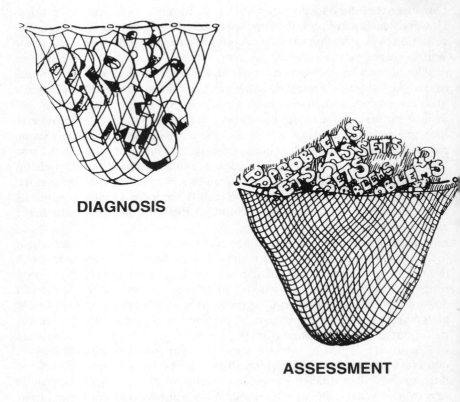

DIAGNOSIS

ASSESSMENT

Figure 1.2 The difference between diagnosis and assessment.

assessments'. Some confusion seems to exist between the terms 'diagnosis' and 'assessment'. Before going further perhaps we should clarify the difference – illustrated in Figure 1.2.

This shows the difference between assessment and diagnostic functions in a symbolic manner. In a **diagnosis** the 'assessor' sets out to identify the presence of certain problems, dysfunctions or abnormalities. If these are not found the person is given 'a clean bill of health'. Indeed, whether we are looking at a person's heart or a car engine, a diagnosis involves the detection of faults. The diagnostician rarely, if ever, looks for things that are right with the person, or are in good working order. A diagnostic report describes only those aspects of functioning that are abnormal. This is true of a doctor's diagnosis of a patient, a mechanic's diagnosis of a car or an engineer's diagnosis of the structure of a bridge. The common denominator is the search for, and ultimate detection of, **problems**.

The diagnostic 'net' is designed to catch only a certain size and shape of problem. All other aspects of the person's functioning will pass through this net. This is the symbolic representation of the 'screening' or diagnostic process.

Assessment, in its purest sense, might be seen as involving looking at people in a more general sense. Assessment tries to gain an **overall picture**: one that describes positive characteristics as well as problems. A full assessment describes the skills, assets and other positive features of a person. On the flip side of the coin can be seen his list of handicaps, disabilities or other dysfunctions. To use a sporting analogy, we often talk about cricketers 'assessing' the field of play. On the positive side the batsman studies the positioning of the fielders and tries to judge where to direct the ball to score maximum runs. On the negative side, he looks for possible problems: how he might be caught out. The assessment net shown on the right side of the illustration is designed to screen as many aspects of the person as possible. The weave of the net, which represents the format of the assessment, is much finer. As a result the person is subjected to a different kind of analysis. Aspects of the person's performance and presentation, which might be ignored or overlooked in a diagnosis, will be 'caught' under this broader form of assessment.

Objectivity and the search for meaning

So far I have discussed the concept of assessment by describing what we should look at and how we might organize our study of the person-in-care. This is usually called the assessment process: suggesting that the activities involved in assessment can be isolated and defined. I have tried to show how some of our observations assume that they are objective where we use standardized methods, but that – philosophically – there are problems with this idea. In other cases assessment is highly subjective, such as when we interview the person informally. I have emphasized that there is a need to at least attempt to be as objective as possible, knowing that all the time we are part of the 'dance' which is our relationship with the person.

The importance of our assessment can never be overstated. Can we ever afford to make casual observations or snap judgements when the quality of people's lives is at stake? Although we try to collect information on the person-in-care objectively, in the final analysis we must judge the significance of the information. Asking ourselves the question 'What does all this mean?' requires some subjectivity.

Critics of the trend towards a more rigorous approach to care and treatment in psychiatry have said that 'dealing with human problems' and 'trying to be rigorous' do not mix. Certainly, this would be true if we tried to assess people in exactly the same way that we studied atoms or chemical elements. It goes without saying that it would hardly be possible either. However, that does not mean that we cannot try to abide by the spirit of a more objective approach: become more aware of our biases and prejudices. In most of the chapters in this book I have included philosophical – or even literary – insights concerning human nature. These have helped me to appreciate the nature and function of my own prejudices about the state of being human. I include them as alternatives to the many insights that will have already helped readers become aware of their own prejudices and the effect they may have upon the assessment process.

Judgements – does a problem exist?

There may be some value in comparing the assessment of people-in-care with the judicial system. The assessment system used in courts is not far removed from the assessment process of psychiatric nursing. Evidence is collected, presented and reviewed, to allow a judgement to be made. This judgement is often made by someone in a 'learned' position: a person of high status whose impartiality is taken for granted. Where the judge is instructed by the jury, these laypersons are expected to make an impartial judgement of the facts. Obviously, their judgement will rely on their own subjective viewpoint. However, they are encouraged by the judge to try to prevent their own prejudices and opinions from influencing their final decision.

Judgements of this sort are found in almost all forms of health care. They are, however, more in evidence in some than in others. Even where we use highly objective means of recording or measuring the person-in-care's state – as in temperature readings or electrocardiogram print-outs – we end up using our own subjective judgements. Objective measures are, by definition, free of meaning: they tell us about something, but cannot make us any wiser as to the significance of this information.

- What does the height of mercury tell us about the person-in-care?
- What do these traces on the ECG paper mean?

Most often we ask 'is this normal or abnormal?' We can ask this question about every level of the person's life.

- Are these ESR levels normal?
- Is his heart rate normal?
- Is this level of anxiety normal?
- Is this kind of behaviour normal?
- Are these beliefs normal?

These are rarely the straightforward questions they seem. When we use the term 'normal', do we mean 'average' or 'healthy'? Do we mean normal by comparison with ourselves; by comparison with most people in this hospital, in this town, this country or the whole world? Or are we talking about normality as it relates to this one individual? We shall return to a discussion of the important concept of **personal norms** later. Even if the person's problems are abnormal by most standards we must still judge whether or not they represent a serious threat to the person or those around him. Virtually everyone, ourselves included, has some problem that others might consider in need of resolution. A key aspect of our assessment involves deciding whether or not the person-in-care 'needs' help or treatment, or do we 'need' to be more tolerant, accepting or understanding?

A high temperature or lapses of consciousness might signify a biological or physiological problem for most of us. The 'life problems' of the person receiving psychiatric care are rarely so clear-cut. The range of so-called 'normal behaviour' is so wide that what is seen as disturbed by one person may be an acceptable way of life to another. The axiom that 'one man's meat is another man's poison' appears to extend to behavioural conventions also. So how do we judge the seriousness of a person-in-care's problems? If we accept that we have a duty to make such a judgement, it is apparent that we need some help to arrive at such an important decision.

We often take for granted the biological knowledge that helps us decide that a certain temperature reading may suggest the presence of an infection or that lapses of consciousness might signify cardiovascular or central nervous system disorders. In such cases the person may even look ill. This 'fact' may even be evident to the layperson. However, we always take our 'layperson's hunch' a stage further, by applying more rigorous forms of assessment. As professionals, we make our judgement only after certain formal examinations have been made. In principle, the assessment of the person-in-care's psychosocial problems should be no different.

The person-in-care may complain of certain problems – such as anxiety or hearing voices – which disturb him. Alternatively, these patterns of behaviour may be reported by family or friends. Neither the person nor the family need any specialist knowledge to identify these problems. They rely upon their senses and their intuitive judgements. This means that their observations will be highly informal or imprecise. Our professional responsibility is to follow up these casual observations by introducing more formal examination of the phenomena presented. This might be seen as the psychosocial equivalent of the biological and physiological examinations mentioned already. These methods should be more reliable and objective and less arbitrary and subjective in nature. They should help us to clarify the nature and significance of the person-in-care's problems. If there is indeed something wrong with this person, our assessment should tell us what that might be and how serious it is. However, our assessment should mainly be concerned with asking 'What does the problem mean for the person concerned?'

THE ASSESSMENT PROCESS

On a technical level any assessment involves choosing some method of observation which will allow us to collect information which we analyse and interpret, allowing us to produce some kind of 'picture' of the person-in-care. Finally, we make predictions about how the person might function under a

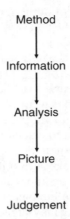

Method

↓

Information

↓

Analysis

↓

Picture

↓

Judgement

Figure 1.3 The assessment process.

different set of circumstances: under treatment or 'therapeutic' conditions (Figure 1.3).

This definition of assessment suggests that we need to collect fairly precise measures of the person's functioning. We need this precise information to make some hypothesis about why the person-in-care functions in this way. This represents our understanding of who he is as an individual. Then we test out our hypothesis under the conditions of caring, continuing to monitor the person's performance throughout. This might be described as a 'quasi-scientific' model of nursing assessment. This model would, I hope, take account of 'human science': all that we know and can discover about the experience of being human.

The six honest serving men

To establish and follow through the assessment process, we need to ask ourselves a series of simple, yet far-reaching, questions. These are built around the 'six honest serving men' who taught Rudyard Kipling 'all he knew'. Their names were 'What and Why and When and How and Where and Who' [22]. Kipling's 'serving men' can be used as the basis for any kind of assessment. Here I select some of these questions to illustrate the process of enquiry.

- **Why am I doing this assessment?** The simple answer to 'why' we do anything is 'I don't know!' We ask questions about life when we are uncertain of what, exactly, is going on. When it comes to the person-in-care, it seems obvious that we have little idea of what exactly is going on. This is why we undertake an assessment.
- **What is the aim of the assessment?** What do I want to know or find out

about the person-in-care? Am I studying him with a view to discharge? transfer to another ward? suitability for employment or resolution of specific distresses? In answering this question we give the assessment a necessary 'slant'. We are deciding what kind of assessment we are planning: one that will assess the extent to which the person is distressed, misunderstood, wrongly placed, understimulated, overworked or otherwise in 'need' of some help.

- **When should I assess?** If you want to take a snapshot portrait of someone you must stand close enough and must focus the camera, so that the person's features can be caught clearly on the photograph. Capturing the 'person' requires timing – among other things. An assessment also tries to capture the person-in-care's important features. To do this requires some selection. You must decide what to focus upon and, by implication, what you are going to ignore or allow to merge into the background.

- **How will I get the information I need?** Various options are open to you when it comes to deciding how to tackle the assessment. You might interview the person-in-care, gaining an insight on his view of the problem. You might observe the person-in-care, building up a picture from your own viewpoint. In other cases information might be supplied by family or friends, or through the observations of other members of the care team. Within each of these general approaches lies a range of variations: from highly structured through to informal interviewing and from self-observation using rating scales through to methods using direct recording techniques. The cardinal rule is to use the method that gives you the most valid information for the least amount of effort.

- **How will I judge what this information means?** The 'meaning' of the information we collect about the person can be looked at from several angles. We could ask, 'How big a problem does this represent?' This would involve evaluating the problem in terms of scale or quantity. However, before we can do this we have to find a standard, or norm, against which to compare the person. Our question then becomes, 'To what extent is the person's behaviour or experience abnormal?' As we shall discuss later, a single norm or standard is rarely available. Instead we use a variety of norms – determined by factors such as class or cultural affiliations, educational background, occupation, religion or political persuasion. These different influences determine how something I might consider 'normal' might be viewed by someone else as 'deviant'.

We should also try to remember that much of our behaviour is 'expressive': through our behaviour we say something about ourselves, about our situation and our relationship with the world in general. The behaviour we show to the world often acts as a signal or symbol for what we experience on other levels of our functioning. In trying to understand what the person-in-care's behaviour means we should try to judge what it might be saying about the person-in-care and his life. What does it signify about other, more hidden, aspects of his life experience? Even should we conclude that, in some sense the behaviour or experience is 'abnormal', we need to ask: 'Does it really matter?'

- **How might the person function under different conditions?** By this stage you should have arrived at a fairly objective assessment of the person-in-care's present functioning. You have described how he functions, on as many levels as is appropriate. You have also described the conditions under which this functioning takes place. Your final task is to consider how the person might function if any of these conditions were altered. This is the last stage of the assessment, and may well be the first stage of the treatment plan.

The product of the assessment

These six questions will help us to decide upon the general aim of the assessment and the major objectives that might achieve that aim, and will help us to decide what to do in the name of care or treatment. The general aim of assessment might be to measure the person-in-care's level of anxiety, level of independence or level of social interaction. Our objectives in carrying out the assessment again involve the use of Kipling's 'honest serving men'.

- **Measurement**: What does the person-in-care do? How often does he do it? For how long does he do it? All these questions will help yield quantitative measures which will help judge the **scale** or **size** of the problem.
- **Clarification**: How does the person-in-care perform these behaviours? On his own? With others? Where does the person show these patterns of behaviour and when? People do not live in a vacuum. All our behaviour and experience exists within some context. Answers to these questions will help us understand the **context** – or **conditions** – under which these things happen.
- **Explanation**: What is the effect of the person's behaviour? How do others react? Can the person explain why he does this, rather than that? Answers to these questions will help us to appreciate the possible **purpose** or **function** of the person's behaviour.
- **Variation:** How does the person-in-care's behaviour change from day to day, from week to week or from one situation to another? Information of this sort helps us to appreciate the **scale** of the person-in-care's problems: their '**seriousness**'. It also helps us to see how they may vary from time to time, or from one situation to another.

I suggested earlier that our assessment might be described as 'quasi-scientific'. In this sense this kind of overview also helps us to form hypotheses. In more simple terms, it helps us make up 'hunches' about why the problem exists at all. It is to this last area that we turn first when we start to think about using our assessment to design care or treatment. Information about the size, the nature and the variations in the problem can be used to monitor any changes that occur during care or treatment. This monitoring function helps us to decide whether treatment has been successful or unsuccessful.

Focus

Before we leave the process of assessment let us consider how closely we should study the person-in-care. How many questions should we ask? How detailed should our enquiries be?

The question of focus is of crucial relevance. We can study a single flower by looking at it with the naked eye, against the background of the whole garden. Alternatively, we could take the flower apart, putting each petal under the microscope. This analogy holds true for the assessment of people. We can study people in fairly general terms, making notes and observations upon what is audible or visible, within the general context (or story) of their lives. We can also study the person in much closer detail, examining every aspect of his functioning, embracing the many layers of his life mentioned earlier. For example, a person who complains of 'anxiety' might be asked to rate his anxiety: to describe how he feels (an internal account). At the same time we could observe how the person behaves when he says he is anxious (an external account). This is the simplest kind of assessment possible. It might also, in some cases, be the best.

Yet we could also undertake a much finer-grained analysis of the problem. We might use biofeedback equipment to monitor the person's sweating, pulse, blood pressure and muscle tension, assessing these biological 'behaviours' across different situations. This sort of analysis would not only describe very precisely the variations in the person's anxiety, but would also indicate any possible 'trigger situations'. This kind of fine-grain analysis is appealing, especially to those nurses who feel the need to demonstrate the scientific status of their 'art'. However, a number of considerations need to be taken into account before we decide to undertake such an in-depth study.

- Do we have the time to devote to such a detailed assessment?
- Do we have access to such sophisticated equipment?
- Would we know how to operate it?

These involve professional costs – time, resources and expertise. There are also possible costs to the person-in-care.

- How will the person feel if he is wired up to all this equipment?
- How realistic is it to expect the person to move from one situation to another carrying such equipment?
- To what extent will the presence of all this 'hardware' influence the measures we are taking?

These considerations involve balancing out the costs of the assessment, for staff and person-in-care, against the advantages of gaining certain kinds of information. It should be apparent that the advantages of a system should always outweigh the disadvantages involved in taking the measure. However, there is an additional consideration. On occasions, we may believe that information can be obtained by relatively simple means. For example, we may believe that we can find out all we need to know by asking the person-in-care a few simple questions. In such a case there is no need to look any further.

However, such a simple form of assessment is rarely adequate. More often than not we are obliged to add additional layers of enquiry. We may need to undertake various physiological measures, such as blood or urine analysis. We may also need to collect information about aspects of biological functioning, such as thyroid function tests. We may also need to study the person's behaviour closely: how he interacts with others and what his reactions are to everyday situations. Finally, we may need to ask much more carefully prepared questions in order to unravel the mysteries of the person's thoughts and beliefs.

These aspects of the person's life may be as much a mystery to him as they are to us. However, we should not assume that this kind of 'global analysis' is needed for every person-in-care. In some cases a simple 'enquiry' may suffice, while for others something bridging a simple enquiry and this kind of global analysis is required. In general, however, if a useful picture of the person-in-care can be achieved by simple means, why use something more complex? This is the nurse's application of the law of parsimony [23]. We should always aim to use as little information as is necessary to arrive at an understanding of the person's problems. This should also involve doing only what we need to do in terms of assessment.

PERSON-CENTRED ASSESSMENT

It is taken for granted that no two people are alike. Yet traditional psychiatry, in its aspiration to become a science, has often tried to deny this – searching for the similarities between patients with similar diagnoses, looking for the 'disease' that can explain their disorder or the syndrome that unites them. In our search to understand the mysteries of mental disorder we have often reduced people to the level of one stereotype or another. The world seems to be populated by a host of 'types': a plethora of neurotics and psychotics; hypochondriacs and exhibitionists; introverts and extroverts; men with mother fixations, women with father fixations; hysterical women, but rarely, if ever, hysterical men. (In this male-dominated world they are usually referred to as 'inadequate psychopaths'. Increasingly, people who are difficult to understand are described as 'borderline personalities'.)

I do not wish to discuss the value of such typecasting or the schools of thought that gave them birth. I wish only to remind the reader that this is the traditional face of psychiatry, but one which is increasingly challenged. Perhaps this 'face' masks the underlying anxiety of the field: if we cannot understand, we can at least label. Much of what follows in this book takes the line that such stereotyping may be convenient – for example in finding out how many 'schizophrenics' have been diagnosed in Britain. However, such typecasting may be less than helpful to those nurses who want to help Tom, Dick or Harriet who happen to be so labelled. I say 'much of what follows' since on occasions I find myself lapsing into the unfortunate professional vernacular and talking about 'patients' as though they were plants or some other species of life that attracts our interest.

Yet, it is clear that on a few occasions it is helpful to emphasize the similarities between one person and another – when, for example, writing a book like this. It is also appropriate to consider Harry Stack Sullivan's dictum that all people are 'more alike than different' [24]: to what extent do all people share similar characteristics which are exaggerated through the experience of mental distress of one form or another?

In most cases assessment discovers that many problems are shared by a whole host of people. Traditionally, we have assumed that only people with a psychosis hear voices. Professor Marius Romme, from the University of Limburg, in Holland, has shown how many members of the 'ordinary public' report hearing voices [25]. This finding suggests that the distinction between who is or is not a 'patient' is subtler or more complex than we think.

The methods which are discussed in detail later in the book may help us discover something of the uniqueness of the individual person-in-care. Most nurses will be sympathetic to the idea that all women and men are different. Although nurses may be overheard saying that so-and-so is a 'typical depressive', more often than not nurses are to be found scratching their heads at the apparent conflicts existing between 'patients' with similar diagnoses. Nurses discover early on that every person is to some extent:

- like all other people;
- like some other people;
- like no other person.

Medical diagnosis helps us to appreciate how people with quite different life-stories might experience similar (though hardly identical) life problems. This strength can be viewed also as its major weakness: by drawing out the similarities between people it can obscure their differences. This issue is critical for nursing. Increasingly, nurses have begun to realize that they are not concerned primarily with the diagnosis and treatment of illness. They are more concerned instead to identify the needs of individuals – who may or may not fit within a broad diagnostic category. Nurses deal with the person's human responses to illness, disability, handicap or dysfunction, rather than dealing with these phenomena directly. If psychiatrists look for signs and symptoms of schizophrenia, nurses look for the human problems that occur when a person experiences what is commonly called 'schizophrenia'.

Sadly, this attitude has often been seen as an 'antipsychiatry' outlook. It is quite the reverse. Nurses acknowledge that when people are beset by any kind of dysfunction, disorder or illness – whether this is schizophrenia or lung cancer – they will experience a range of human problems from disturbance of their emotions to disruption of their everyday living behaviours. These human responses to illness are 'the proper focus of nursing'. The nurse's first responsibility is to meet the needs of the unique person who is, temporarily, standing in a queue along with other people-in-care. Increasingly, people who experience even the most severe forms of mental distress challenge nurses and other mental health professionals to 'see the people and not their illness' [26]. Seeing 'patients' as 'people' may be the biggest challenge that faces us.

Behavioural assessment – is there any other?

It should be apparent from what I have said already that I favour 'learning from the person' – listening to the person's life story or personal narrative. Where this is not possible, or difficult, I favour the careful description and measurement of what the person does with himself and others and (if we can establish this) what he says to himself or others. I favour these forms of reporting rather than making wild judgements about the significance of what he appears to do or say. I shall expand upon the use of inference and extrapolation later. For the moment let me offer some kind of rationale for emphasizing the study of the person through his behaviour.

Recent years have seen significant developments in methods aimed at identifying and measuring discrete patterns of behaviour. These methods have largely replaced the use of projective methods, which sought to make comments upon concepts such as personality. These methods have reminded us, should we need such reminding, that we cannot make inferences about concepts like 'personality' without first making observations upon how the person behaves, even if this involves no more than 'verbal behaviour' – their answers to our questions.

In any situation where we observe people, we can later draw more general conclusions about the meaning of their behaviour in that situation, and what it says about the person overall. However, we cannot make either of these more general comments without first taking specific notes on how the person behaves. For example, if we observed a young man who is shown a photograph of a naked woman by his friend while both of them are standing in the street, what can we say about the young man's attitude [27]? Well, virtually nothing – at least not until we have made some notes on his behaviour. How does he react to the situation? Does he smile, blush, laugh, look away? What does he do next? Does he take the picture to study it more closely? Does he tear it up? Does he turn and walk away? Does he say anything to his friend which can be interpreted as positive or negative comment? From these simple observations we might make some guesses – or inferences – about his attitude towards female nudity, and perhaps towards women in general. Does his behaviour seem to suggest approval or disapproval? Of course, we could save ourselves much time and trouble by simply asking the person what he thought? If we stepped into the situation and questioned him – directly or indirectly – about the situation, what might he say? On the basis of what we observed and heard we might go on to make further inferences about (for example) his personality: does his performance under these very limited conditions suggest that he is shy or introverted, or gregarious and extroverted, a sexist or 'new male'?

All such 'observations' begin with information which records what we saw the young man doing and heard him saying. We cannot make any inference without first having access to observations. Such observations are worthless unless they also take account of the context within which the person exists – where and when the action observed took place.

These happenings make up the basic data from which other inferences are made. Although the kinds of observation we have talked about could hardly be called scientific, they may be fairly accurate in terms of building a picture of this young man in this situation. However, we would need to see him performing under different conditions to find out if his attitude towards female nudity is a constant one, or one that is influenced by circumstances. Would he, for example, show the same 'attitude' (or behaviour) if his parents were present; or if the picture was of a member of his family, or perhaps a woman friend? When we are talking about the person's behaviour we mean what we can see the person-in-care doing and can hear him saying. We also mean what he can tell us about what is happening 'within' him: his awareness of his 'internal life', especially his beliefs, various thought processes and emotional reactions.

Behaviour can also mean the 'hidden' aspects of human functioning that are involved in 'outward' shows of behaviour: the various functions of our autonomic or central nervous systems. Behaviour is often presumed to refer only to what is observable. It may be more appropriate, and helpful, to include the many forms of covert (hidden) behaviour – thinking, remembering, fantasizing and imagining – among the many cognitive functions; and the action of smooth muscles and the discharge of hormones among the various functions of the autonomic system. These hidden behaviours play an important part in assisting the performance of more open or overt patterns of behaviour. As we shall see in subsequent chapters, our assessment of the person-in-care often involves looking for evidence of the function of these hidden behaviours.

Some readers may disagree with my rather catholic definition of 'behaviour'. Let me suggest that – if nothing else – it might be a convenient definition. What do nurses do when they assess a person-in-care? They begin by studying the person's behaviour – what they can witness him doing, what he says he feels and what he says he thinks and believes.

Inferences

The act of observation involves the use of sensory apparatus to collect information about the person under observation. The observer uses her eyes to record what she has seen; her hearing to record what the person-in-care said; her tactile sensation to judge weight or power in a limb; and her sense of smell to note any particular odours. She might also use her sense of taste to determine (for example) how bitter or sweet some food is, before asking the person-in-care to judge it in a similar manner. All such information is called **data**: or rather, it is most often called information, but it becomes data when transformed into a numerical format. However, the correct definition of the term 'data' is 'the assumptions that form the basis for an inference or conclusion'. This definition is important. It reminds us that we collect information – or data – with a view to making some more general comment, or coming to a conclusion.

When we weigh someone we arrive at some assumptions about his 'weight'. We might suggest that this means something, for example that he is obese: this is an inference drawn from our study of the data. We might also say that this level of obesity is pathological: here we are making a more complex inference, suggesting the possibility of an unfortunate conclusion. You might be wondering what the relevance is of all this. I am trying to emphasize that, although we often talk as if we can make immediate judgements about people-in-care, we cannot come to any real conclusions without collecting some data. We use these data to make inferences about what we think is happening, and may then proceed to come to some conclusion about the situation. Inference is the process of reasoning by which we come to a conclusion. We cannot come to a conclusion without reasoning – without making some inferences. More importantly, we cannot make inferences without some basic data: some 'real information'.

I emphasize this point for another reason. Nurses, and indeed many other staff members, have a tendency to devote too much energy to 'making inferences' and not enough energy to collecting data. Figure 1.4 shows the levels of inference possible in making increasingly more general – and less specific – comments about a situation.

The nurse notices that a person is crying. She might conclude that this means that he is upset; this means that he feels threatened; this means that he is vulnerable; this means that he feels inadequate.

Let us take as an example the young man discussed earlier. Our 'basic data' involved notes about what he said and did in that situation. Based upon what we observed we could make a first-level inference: here we make a general comment about what we believe these observations tell us about him. Since this is only a first-level inference, the conclusion we draw will be fairly conservative. We might infer that his behaviour showed that he was embarrassed. We do not **know** that he was embarrassed; we merely infer this from what we saw.

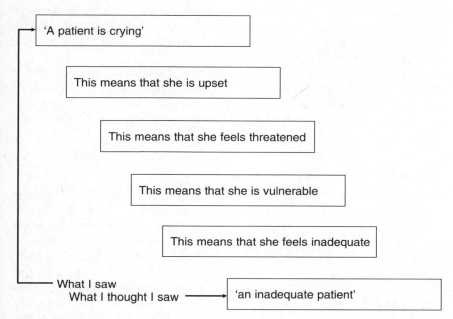

Figure 1.4 Levels of inference.

We could take the inference game a stage further by saying that he was embarrassed because he is uncertain about his attitudes towards women. It is clear that we cannot really know this: again it is an inference, but this time a more extravagant one.

We could become increasingly extravagant in our inference game, suggesting at the next level that he is embarrassed because he has a deep-seated fear of all women, a fear which is stimulated by seeing them adopting sexually provocative poses. And so we might go on, descending into the depths of inference, or climbing up into the clouds of 'unreason', as we move further and further away from the information that provided the starting-point.

I am not suggesting that we should not make inferences about behaviour. We cannot say anything of any great moment about a person without making some inference. I suggest only that we avoid making too many inferences. I am merely acknowledging the danger of losing sight of the original data by clouding it with fanciful inferences.

As I noted above, there is a tendency within psychiatry to 'jump to conclusions' about the person-in-care. Perhaps we do so because we spend insufficient time collecting basic data. A rather strict and moralistic father who observed his son looking at pictures of naked women in the street might infer that this meant that his son was immoral or, indeed, that he had gone to the devil. We might excuse the father on the grounds that he did not study the situation closely enough or that he had misinterpreted the facts. More importantly, we might suggest that he had failed to acknowledge the 'context' within which the action had taken place. We should take care that we – the professionals – remember always to study situations closely, and at least avoid making rash interpretations.

This assumes, however, that we do not need to make inferences. A major dilemma in psychiatric and mental health nursing is: to what extent should we accept the behavioural presentation of the person? This leads us to ask how far we should go in interpreting the wider significance of the person's behaviour.

Normal humans: where can they be found?

Psychiatry has always been interested in abnormal behaviour. It has been estimated that around 20 million people in the USA suffer from some distur- bance of thought or overt behaviour sufficient to merit psychiatric attention. The same sort of proportional estimate has been made in the UK. Some of these people will refer themselves for professional consultation, while many others will deny that they have any problem and a few may be treated forcibly by agents of the state. From even this casual observation it should be apparent that ideas about 'what is normal' can be held by the individual or by society.

On many occasions society and the individual may be in conflict. When, for instance, a person says that he can't cope, needs help or is otherwise distressed in some way, and we, the professionals, decide that he is not seriously disturbed in any psychological or psychiatric sense, then such a conflict is evident. In the mid-1990s British psychiatry was overtaken by the 'unscientific' principle that a distinction existed between the **worried well**, and people with **serious and/or enduring mental illness**. Given that the 'worried well' might include (among others) people with depression, personality or relationship problems, eating disorders and dementia, the assumption that the only 'serious' forms of mental distress involve psychoses is open to question.

On other occasions the roles may be reversed: we may try to encourage the person to think that he needs our care and treatment, and the person may reject the service we offer him. In either example the behaviour of the person- in-care is seen as 'abnormal': in the first case it deviates from the norm set by the person-in-care himself; in the second from our norms – social norms. Any pattern of behaviour – whether it involves action, thought or belief – is usually called deviant when it does not comply with some standard, most often the most common pattern of such behaviour (average) within a population.

We talk frequently about behaviour being within normal limits: this merely means the range shown by most of the population. People who are very tall or very short are un-average or atypical, as they fall outwith the range that covers most of the population. The same is true of people who are very intelligent or who are not very bright: they too fall outwith this 'normal range'.

Since such people deviate, or branch off, from the 'normal standard', we could call all such people deviants. However, where the term is used at all it is usually restricted to behavioural characteristics considered to be unwholesome or to be discouraged in some way: criminal or antisocial behaviours.

Just because a pattern of behaviour is 'deviant' does not mean that it is a cause for concern. Some people dress in an unorthodox manner. In terms of the strict usage of the term they are 'dress deviants'. We are more likely to refer to such people as 'eccentric', although increasingly little attention is paid to such 'deviations'. Other people may engage in even more unusual patterns of dressing, such as dressing up in the clothes of the opposite sex. Traditionally, such behaviour has been called a 'sexual deviation'. Such labelling reflects a cultural unease about such behaviour, assuming that it is in some way unhealthy or unwholesome. As attitudes change towards sexual behaviour in general, 'cross-dressing' has been seen less as a problem.

From a different perspective, people who do charity work in their spare time, men who give up their seats to women on buses and people who go to church regularly could also be regarded as deviants for the simple reason that such practices are not performed by anything like a majority of the population. However, we would not label such practices as deviant. Although we may not practise such behaviours ourselves, we assume that they are either noble or at least innocuous.

We have focused much attention on definitions of 'normal behaviour' since the 1960s, when many Western cultural conventions were called into question. However, the difficulty in determining a specific definition of 'normality' within psychiatric nursing has long been recognized. More than 30 years ago Altschul observed that: 'It is often said that we are all "a bit abnormal". Is this true or is it obvious nonsense? Is it any easier if the word "normal" is replaced by "healthy", or is it normal to be a little unhealthy?' [28]. This illustrates how the word 'normal' may be used in more than one sense. Altschul noted that it might be found that, by a certain age, most people have lost their teeth and are wearing dentures. She acknowledged, however, that we would hardly suggest that it was 'normal' to wear dentures by the age of 50.

When we come to consider mental health Altschul suggested that a person might be defined as healthy: 'if he manages to deal with the demands made upon him by society in a manner which is ideal both for society and himself. He is "ill" to the degree that he has failed in his adjustment, to the detriment either of society or himself' [29].

While I am sympathetic to this broad definition of 'normality' and 'health' it is not without complications. More extreme forms of human experience and behaviour can be accommodated easily within this definition: often presenting the person and society with similar challenges. However, throughout history patterns of behaviour that were once deemed to be antisocial and unhealthy have become better accepted. In present times this would include the more diverse range of sexual preferences and more generalized patterns of drug-taking. Such behaviours, once deemed illegal, immoral or symptomatic of some psychological disturbance, are now accepted as examples of personal choice or orientation. Derek Jarman once observed wittily that 'heterosexuality is not normal, only common'. We might consider the wisdom of this aphorism when we are tempted to judge the relative normality of any pattern of behaviour or reported experience.

Our interest in assessment lies mainly with the study of the person-in-care's behaviour: what he says, does, thinks, feels, etc. However, although it may be a relatively straightforward exercise to identify and measure such patterns of behaviour, it is more difficult to answer the question 'What does it all mean?' Once we have assessed a pattern of behaviour, how do we go about judging whether it is normal or abnormal? How do we determine whether or not any pattern of behaviour represents 'a problem'? Arriving at such a decision is rarely easy, since normal behaviour can vary from one person to the next, from one culture to another, and can be influenced by different laws even within the same country.

Our behaviour is, however, associated most with the culture within which we live. Most of our behaviour is learned: human beings appear to be poorly supplied with instincts, unlike our animal and insect relations. Even infants of only a few weeks old have already begun to learn how to respond to their environment: their behaviour is not preprogrammed before birth. We have no instincts or other biological endowments that help us to tie shoelaces, cook food, order a beer, comb our hair, catch a bus or open a window for fresh air. All these mundane behaviours are acquired through learning and are all part of the culture to which we belong. Were we to move to a different culture – like an underdeveloped country or a hospital ward – such behaviour might be redundant or might even be discouraged. Those features of our behaviour that are at present normal might become 'abnormal', deviant or at the very least unusual.

When we come to consider the behaviour of people in the psychiatric setting there is a common assumption that their behaviour is either normal or abnormal. It might make our task a lot easier were this 'absolute' situation in fact the case. The reality is not, however, quite so black and white. As I have said, normal behaviour appears to be defined by cultures. Even within a culture, discrete subcultures may determine different patterns of behaviour. Take, for example, the young man holding the picture of the 'pin-up girl' mentioned earlier. Within Western culture the study of 'pin-ups' is seen as 'normal' male behaviour, where expressions of sexual fantasy are deemed normal, if unfortunate. Within such cultures there are, however, subgroups of men who, for intellectual, religious or moral reasons, would refuse to display such 'characteristically normal male behaviour'. Such men might well be scorned by the majority for their soppy, effeminate, un-male stance.

I have no idea how one determines which of these attitudes is right. Each is 'right' given the subcultural context. I use this example as an illustration of the wide divergence of functioning that can exist within cultures, within subcultures, even within sexes.

There would appear to be few, if any, universal norms as far as behaviour is concerned. One might assume that murder, incest and child abuse would be viewed as unacceptable by all societies and cultures. Sociologists would argue that this is not the case. Many cultures, admittedly some of them 'uncivilized' by Western standards, will tolerate, even encourage, such practices under certain conditions. I take note of this simply to sharpen our focus when it comes to studying so-called abnormal behaviour within the field of psychiatry. We should not forget that even manifestly exceptional behaviour – such as the experience of hallucinations – is relatively common in some cultures. I noted above Romme's Dutch research into the hallucinatory experience. These findings are part of a longer history of enquiry that questions some of our established beliefs about the nature of 'madness', many of which are culture-bound by the Western tradition.

In a study in the early 1960s Lee noted that out of a random sample of Zulu women more than a third had reported visual and auditory hallucinations involving 'angels, babies and little short hairy men' [30]. In the same study he found that more than half of the women engaged in 'screaming behaviour', often yelping for hours, days, even weeks. Either of these reported behaviours would be viewed as grossly abnormal in the West. Yet few of these women showed any other signs of mental disorder. Within their own culture their hallucinations and screaming were legitimate. More recently, African psychiatrists have reported that persecutory delusions are more frequent in African, Jamaican and Caribbean subjects than in any other groups. They explain this finding by attributing the delusions to beliefs in witchcraft and voodoo, common to their cultures [31]. This has been reported for over 30 years by other researchers [32], who suggest that the beliefs (which we call delusions) held by West Indians diagnosed as psychotic are the same as those held by 'normal' West Indians, the only difference between the two groups being the abnormal reaction (or behaviour) of the so-called 'psychotics' to these beliefs.

We shall return to these issues in subsequent chapters and will discuss the 'problem' of normal behaviour in the penultimate chapter, where the ethical and moral dilemmas associated with the concept will be highlighted.

The search for an educated guess

In this chapter I have attempted to define my objectives for writing this book. I may have patronized some readers who were already aware of many of the issues: diagnosis versus assessment; normal versus abnormal behaviour, etc. I have expounded at some length on these issues since I am aware that all too often we think of assessment only in terms of specific instruments – the methodology of measurement. If we are to develop our knowledge about and our practice of assessment we must consider what assessment might mean in the broadest sense, as well as what procedures it might involve. I have tried to emphasize the ordinariness of assessment. It is different only in quality from assessing how much seed will be needed to cover the bare patches on the lawn, or how we might undertake a trip around the world. Anyone might make a wild guess as to what these exercises might involve. There is no substitute, however, for the 'educated guess' made by the keen gardener or the regular traveller. The calculations here are based upon knowledge and experience.

In the chapters that follow I shall try to discuss some of the facets of assessment and the interpersonal experiences with people-in-care that combine to produce an understanding of the term. It is an understanding for which we appear to be constantly reaching, but which always seems to elude our grasp.

NOTES

1. Barker, P. (1985) *Patient Assessment in Psychiatric Nursing*, Croom Helm, London.
2. Jones, G. H. (1974) Principles of psychological assessment, in *The Psychological Assessment of Mental and Physical Handicaps*, (ed. P. Mittler), Tavistock, in association with Methuen, London.
3. O'Toole, A. N. and Welt, S. R. (eds) (1994) *Hildegard E. Peplau: Selected Works – Interpersonal Theory in Nursing*, Macmillan, Basingstoke.
4. Ashworth, P., Castledine, G. and McFarlane, J. K. (1978) The process in practice. *Nursing Times (Suppl.)*, 30 November.
5. It is noteworthy, however, that an interest has been shown, again, in nurses' use of formal diagnosis, in the US (Caldwell, personal communication, 1993), UK (Baguely, 1995; Gournay, 1995) and Australia (McMinn, 1995). This ranges from the adoption of a 'common language' to nurses diagnosing forms of mental illness (*sic*). It is also noteworthy that in recent years in the USA and internationally there has been considerable debate over the validity and reliability of their diagnostic classification system (see Chapter 11). As a result the *Diagnostic and Statistical Manual* of the USA is now in a fourth version (DSM-IV) and the *International Classification of Diseases* is in its 10th version (ICD-10). (Baguely, I. (1995) Evaluation of the Tameside Nursing Development Unit for psychosocial interventions, in *Community Psychiatric Nursing: A Research Perspective*, vol. 3, (eds C. Brooker and E. White), Chapman & Hall, London; Gournay, K. (1995) What to do with nursing models. *Journal of Psychiatric and Mental Health Nursing*, **2**(5), 325–7; McMinn, B. (1995) Diagnostic classification systems and nursing diagnosis of collaborative problems. *Australian and New Zealand Journal of Mental Health Nursing*, **4**, 124–31.)
6. Hines, F. R. and Williams, R. B. (1975) Dimensional diagnosis and the medical student's grasp of psychiatry. *Archives of General Psychiatry*, **32**, 525–8.

7. Barker, P., Reynolds, W. and Ward, T. (1995) The proper focus of nursing: a critique of the 'caring' ideology. *International Journal of Nursing Studies*, **32**.
8. Robinson, L. (1983) *Psychiatric Nursing as a Human Experience*, W. B. Saunders, London.
9. American Nurses Association (1980) *Nursing: A Social Policy Statement*, American Nurses Association, Kansas City, MO.
   American Nurses Association (1982) *Standards of Psychiatric and Mental Health Nursing Practice*, American Nurses Association, Kansas City, MO.
10. O'Toole, A. and Loomis, M. (1990) Classifying human responses in psychiatric and mental health nursing, in *Psychiatric and Mental Health Nursing: Theory and Practice*, (eds W. Reynolds and D. Cormack), Chapman & Hall, London.
11. Ward, M. (1988) The nursing process, in *Applied Psychiatric Mental Health Nursing Standards in Clinical Practice*, (eds M. J. Schriger Krebs and K. H. Larson), John Wiley, New York.
12. *Ibid.*, p. 26.
13. Peplau, H. E. (1995) Another look at schizophrenia from a nursing standpoint, in *Psychiatric Nursing 1974–94: A Report on the State of the Art*, (ed. C. A. Anderson), Mosby/Year Book, St Louis, MO.
14. *Ibid.*
15. *Ibid.*
16. Parse, R. R. (1995) *Illuminations: The Human Becoming Theory in Research and Practice*, National League for Nursing, New York.
17. Peplau, H. E., personal communication.
18. MacIntyre, A. (1988) The story-telling animal, in *Twenty Questions: An Introduction to Philosophy*, (eds G. L. Bowie, M. W. Michaels and R. C. Solomon), Harcourt Brace Jovanovich, London.
19. *Ibid.*
20. The original Greek word *telos* meant 'end', which in this context emphasizes how we are always moving – or apparently not moving – towards endpoints or goals in our lives.
21. Barker, P., Reynolds, W. and Stevenson, C. (1996) The human science basis of psychiatric nursing theory and practice. *Journal of Advanced Nursing*, in press.
22. Kipling, R. (1902) *Just So Stories*, Macmillan, London.
23. The 'law of parsimony' is attributed to William of Occam, the 14th century English philosopher. This law suggests that a more complex explanation should never be offered where a simpler one would suffice. Hence we get the idea of Occam's Razor – trimming explanations down to their 'bare essentials'.
24. Sullivan, H. S. (1953) *The Interpersonal Theory of Psychiatry*, Norton, New York.
25. Romme, M. and Escher, S. (1993) The new approach: a Dutch experiment, in *Accepting Voices*, (eds M. Romme and S. Escher), MIND Publications, London.
26. Bayley, R. (1993) Hear our voices. *Nursing Times*, **89**(25), 32–3.
27. When I entered nursing in 1970 neo-Freudian theory still held sway and virtually everything in life was explained by reference to sexuality. This early induction may explain – in part – my choice of this illustration.
28. Altschul, A. (1963) *Aids to Psychiatric Nursing*, 2nd edn, Baillière, Tindall & Cox, London.
29. *Ibid.*
30. Lee, S. G. M. (1961) *Stress and Adaptation*, Leicester University Press, Leicester.

31. Ndetei, D. M. and Vadher, A. (1984) Frequency and clinical significance of delusions across cultures. *Acta Psychiatrica Scandinavica*, **70**, 73–6.
32. Kiev, A. (1963) Beliefs and delusions of West Indian immigrants to London. *British Journal of Psychiatry*, **109**, 356–63.

The interview: a character in search of an author | 2

One of the best rules in conversation is, never to say a thing which any of the company can reasonably wish had been left unsaid.

Jonathan Swift

When you don't quite know what to do, it is best to do nothing.

Napoleon

I cannot tell how the truth may be; I say the tale as it was told to me.

Sir Walter Scott

The pith of conversation does not consist in exhibiting your superior knowledge on matters of small importance, but in enlarging, improving, and correcting, the information you possess, by the authority of others.

Sir Walter Scott

INTERVIEW AS CONVERSATION

An old Chinese proverb suggests that: 'to listen well is as powerful a means of influence as to talk well'. More importantly, it goes on, 'listening is essential to all true conversation'. What better starting point for our discussion of the art of the interview? Any interview is a special kind of conversation.

In this chapter we shall explore exactly what kind of conversation can truly be called an interview. Not all conversations are interviews, and not all interviews have the hallmarks of what the Chinese philosopher saw as 'true conversation'. In a simple sense a conversation can be seen as people talking. However, traditionally, conversation has been seen as something of an art form: hence the modern complaint that – with the advent of television – the art of conversation has died. In good conversation ideas and emotions are communicated in a meaningful, creative and often entertaining manner. Where such ideas and emotions are passed from one person to another in a challenging or amusing fashion, an impact is made upon the listener. The listener may be stimulated, enlightened or otherwise impressed. Verbal information, the stuff of all conversations, can assume great power when handled in a lively or creative manner. However, as the Chinese philosopher observed the speaker is not the only influential figure. A 'good listener' has the power to draw more information from the speaker, or even to guide the content of his speech.

Most of us have witnessed the situation where someone appears not to be listening, or appears uninterested. Once we become aware of this, stilted or stifled conversation invariably results. Eventually, we stop talking. Although the ability to handle words and concepts is central to 'the art of conversation', we also need to be able to flip the 'conversation coin', adopting the role of a 'good listener' – supporting the speaker, giving his communication a good landing, thereby drawing deeper, more enlightening insights from the depths of his experience.

We need to begin our study of the art of the interview with the listening aspect. Most of our attention in this chapter will be upon talking: questioning the person-in-care and summarizing what he has said. Our efforts will, however, be wasted if we are unable to listen correctly, if we cannot encourage him, largely through our silence, to plumb his hidden depths.

This marriage of speaker and listener has intrigued some of the great minds of all civilizations. Most of them came to the same conclusions despite being separated by time and culture. Plutarch, the Greek essayist, was a great supporter of the strong silent type: 'Know how to listen, and you will profit even from those who talk badly.' More recently, William Hazlitt, the early 19th-century writer, commented that 'silence is one great art of conversation', the other, presumably, being the complementary art of the speaker. As I have noted already, no matter how hard you try to make conversation, on occasions the listening skills of your partner will fail to satisfy you. Another such 'conversation killer' is where your partner is an impatient listener. He is so eager to put forward his point of view that he has little time to listen properly. La Rochefoucauld, the 17th-century French moralist, thought that: 'the reason why so few people are agreeable in conversation is that each is thinking more of what he is intending to say, than of what the other is saying'.

This is another facet of the poor listener syndrome. Since there is no real passing and receiving of meaningful information communication will be frustrated. Laurence Sterne, the Irish writer, also commented upon this traffic in conversation. To have meaningful conversation we must have something to 'trade': we must be able to swap or exchange ideas, emotions or experiences with our partner. If we do not reciprocate in this way we should be able, at least, to show our appreciation or understanding of what he has said. As Sterne noted: 'conversation is a traffic – if you enter into it without some stock of knowledge to balance the account perpetually betwixt you and another, the trade drops at once'.

So what sort of conversational principles can we draw from these writers that might help us in our dealings with the person-in-care? It is apparent that we need to be able to listen. However, this is not just a passive act. We need to do more than sit back and let the other person do the talking.

- A good listener is a more positive force, helping the speaker to talk more, either in general or about specific areas of his experience.
- We need also to beware of impatience. We need to curb our desire to give opinions or summaries before they are needed.
- Finally, we need to be aware that interviewing is not an activity to be taken lightly.

All of us are experienced conversationalists: we can talk about the weather, our work, our families or just ourselves. Conversations with people-in-care most often are different from such everyday chatter. The interview is one such example: here we need special skills to help us interact with people who may either have difficulty in making relationships or be uncertain of the answers to the questions we might pose.

We also need to have some understanding of what is taking place to use as currency in this conversational traffic. It would be wholly inappropriate to approach an interview with a disturbed or distressed person in the same way as we might someone standing in a bus queue. Our first responsibility is to be aware of the potential importance of our interaction with the person.

CHARACTERISTICS OF THE INTERVIEW

An interview is the simplest way of obtaining information from the person-in-care. It can also be the most complex. An interview involves asking questions from which an evaluation of the individual or her circumstances can be made. Interviewing someone in a psychiatric context differs little from interviewing someone for a job. Both involve an imbalance of power, no matter how hard we try to dismiss it. Both may involve an 'open' as well as a 'hidden' agenda. Only the questions and perhaps the format will differ. The aim, common to both situations, is to build up a picture of the person through the medium of question and answer – through a conversation.

Interviews usually involve a face-to-face meeting between two people. Although interviews could be conducted over the telephone, this is reserved for special situations. The meeting is usually arranged for formal discussion of a specific issue: to find out something. The important feature of the interview is that it involves a pattern of interaction in which the roles of interviewer and respondent are highly specialized. We need no special qualification or training to be interviewed. People undergo interviews almost every day – when seeking employment, asking for advice from their boss or a friend, applying for unemployment benefit or a loan for a mortgage. The interviewer – by contrast – needs special training if she is to fulfil the requirements of this special position. The four main features of the interview are as follows.

- It usually involves a face-to-face meeting.
- The aims and objectives of the interview are known to the interviewer, although not always to the person being interviewed.
- It involves a restricted range of topics. These are controlled by the interviewer to obtain the maximum information in the shortest possible time.
- Specific roles are adopted by interviewer and respondent. Often this will influence the way the two speak, tone of voice, language and terminology, as well as the degree of formality, all being subjected to some control.

The interview is not, however, just another conversation. It may look like one but for those involved it has an atmosphere of purpose, direction and business not found in such everyday interactions. Nurses often confuse the two, concluding that an interview involves simply 'talking to the person-in-care about his problems'. This does not mean that a casual conversation cannot throw up useful information. However, it may not be the most efficient way of doing so.

The interview has three major goals or purposes. It may be descriptive, diagnostic or therapeutic.

- The **descriptive** interview involves collecting information about an individual from which a picture of this person may be developed. The nurse-interviewer is interested in John Smith the person – who may have been diagnosed as suffering from schizophrenia – rather than John Smith 'the schizophrenic'. The picture can only be developed from a broad factual base. The nurse might need information about the person's physical state, occupational history, family background, leisure interests, educational attainments, social activities, etc. Here we are not simply addressing the person's problems, we are attempting to consider 'John Smith' as a whole person.
- The **diagnostic** interview may involve nurses in describing the person with a view to assigning a psychiatric diagnosis. Although this is primarily a medical responsibility, I noted in Chapter 1 how some nurses are accepting this responsibility as an extension of the role of the nurse. Even if the assignment of a diagnosis is not the main aim, nurses may collect information that may help their medical colleagues confirm their diagnosis. Often, such information is accessible only to nurses.

However, there is a need also to make a **nursing diagnosis**, which will reflect 'the changing pattern of a client's problems and their effects upon the ability to function independently of others' [1]. Whereas the medical diagnosis might confirm the view that the person is suffering from 'anorexia nervosa', the nursing diagnosis might state that the person 'refuses to eat any food because she says she is fat and ugly'. This is not 'just an opinion, or even a wise judgement on the part of the nurse, but a statement or conclusion about an observed pattern of behaviour' [2]. The diagnostic interview provides nurses with an opportunity to explore the relationship between the person's thoughts, feelings, beliefs and behaviour. It also provides an opportunity to reach some agreement between the person and the nurse responsible for his care as to the exact nature of the problem at that moment.

- Finally, the **therapeutic** interview may be used to help the person-in-care. It can help clarify his problems and perhaps even arrive at some solutions. We can use our 'face-to-face' meetings with the person as a major force in the helping process: we can use our meetings for 'psychotherapeutic' ends.

The law of parsimony

Inadequate assessment is the biggest obstacle to the presentation of successful treatment. The person-in-care's problems must be seen in their totality: we should avoid assuming too much and should always try to see problems against the 'backdrop' of the person involved. However, a word of caution is needed here. We can never find out 'everything' about a person-in-care, or even about a specific problem. I should add that neither should we want to. In the past nursing assessment often tended to be overly simple or non-existent. We must take care not to fly to the other extreme. Certainly we should try to be thorough, but we must try to avoid examining areas of the person's experience that are either irrelevant or unnecessary for our needs.

Some critics of traditional 'psychiatric interviewing' have estimated that as much as three-quarters of the material covered could be left out without any appreciable loss. This view is taken on the grounds that this information plays little or no part in the plan of treatment [3]. Such 'over the top' interviewing is not only inefficient but also raises an ethical issue: what right have we to subject aspects of the person-in-care's life to needless enquiry? The answer is probably 'none'. For this reason it is important to plan the interview carefully. If we engage the person in idle chatter we may end up asking a lot of questions about things which are of little or no relevance to his eventual course of treatment. We may also omit many of the areas which are of crucial significance. Any interview should, therefore, be a controlled exercise. The golden rule is: 'Find out everything you need to know and no more'. This principle reflects the law of parsimony [4]: a law which can be useful in curbing what is often no more than our natural curiosity. Idle curiosity has no place in a professional interview.

The structured interview

Like a good story, a good interview should have a beginning, a middle and an end. To work through these stages the nurse needs a format or structure. The kind of interview I am discussing in this chapter is one that follows a particular course of enquiry. It takes a highly specific route to answer the two basic questions:

- What kind of help does this person need?
- How might nursing meet this need?

The structure of the interview is a metaphorical skeleton. The interviewer hangs questions on this framework, giving it bulk, substance or body. The design of this basic framework will influence the outcome of the interview as surely as any skeleton determines the outward shape of the person. However, this framework is flexible. It provides some guidance as to the kind of topics that might be covered. It does not dictate the kind of questions that need to be asked.

The sophisticated interviewer often looks as if she is engaging in a very casual conversation. She carries no notepad, no scribbled questions. She appears to be simply chatting to the person. The appearance may be highly misleading. The sophisticated interviewer has all her topics arranged clearly in her head. She also has a bank of questions, developed through experience, to draw upon.

For the novice interviewer, who is less confident, there is no shame – and a lot of sense – in working from a framework that has been committed to paper in advance. Perhaps all of us are novices in this sense. Failure to use such a framework may result in running off at tangents, getting muddled or getting lost altogether. A structured interview is likely to provoke less anxiety for both nurse and person-in-care. Structure provides security.

The aims of the interview

The interview can be an end in itself, but often is a preliminary for some other kind of assessment or a preamble to the offer of some kind of help. Before we begin to explore the structure and content of the interview in more detail, it may be worth reviewing the fundamental reasons for nurses undertaking an interview [5].

- **Relationship-building**: If the person-in-care is to be offered nursing – as a health-care intervention – then a relationship is necessary to serve as a medium for that intervention. The 'admission' or 'initial' interview provides the nurse with an opportunity to **establish a relationship with the person**.
- **Trust-building**: It is assumed that the person-in-care will not merely accept help from anyone. If this had been the case then family, friends, neighbours and colleagues might have met his needs already. It is assumed that the

person-in-care needs a special kind of relationship; one within which he can begin to trust someone who might assist in addressing his needs. The interview provides the nurse with an opportunity to **develop a basis for trust**.

- **Professional collaboration**: If the person-in-care is to begin to address his problems of living, this must begin with identifying and sharing his experience of these problems with someone who might help him further. The interview provides the nurse with an opportunity to **develop professional closeness and collaboration**.
- **Problem identification**: The person-in-care brings some kind of problem of living to the nursing situation. The identification of the nature and function of that problem – as it exists now – is the first stage of the therapeutic process. The interview provides the nurse with an opportunity to **begin to identify problematic patterns in the person's behaviour**.
- **Problem resolution**: The therapeutic goal of nursing is to help the person to resolve or reduce the distress associated with his human responses to problems of living. The interview offers the nurse an opportunity to **identify problems that are amenable to change and personal resources that might help resolve these**.

The nurse's educative function is to help bring these five interpersonal functions into the awareness of the person-in-care. By facilitating this awareness the nurse will help the person become more aware of what he needs to do, is doing and also what is left to be done. By furthering this 'self-awareness' he will also become aware of what exactly the nurse is doing in the name of nursing.

Direct *versus* indirect interviewing

Interviews, like assessments in general, may take two forms. We may examine the person-in-care directly: questioning him, discussing his life, his problems and possible solutions. Or we may be more indirect: examining similar concerns through others' experience of the person-in-care. When the nurse asks the person's family: 'What kind of man would you say Mr Johnson is?', or when she asks 'What do you think is troubling Janet?', she is engaging in an indirect examination of the person-in-care. Usually this course of action is taken because the problem cannot be studied at first hand, perhaps because the person-in-care is unable to discuss the matter. In other cases these 'second-hand' views may be sought to provide a back-up, or alternative perspective, to more direct interviewing. In either case, such indirect interviewing must be undertaken with care. The views of family – or indeed any 'significant other' – may be very different from that of the person-in-care. The nurse must be open to the possibility that the needs of 'others' – including professional carers – may conflict with the proper needs of the person-in-care.

THE RELATIONSHIP

Interviewer characteristics

The goals of the interview can be achieved only through a carefully thought out process. Before we discuss some of the mechanics of the interview let us consider how the nurse can use her 'self' to promote these aims. If the goal of interviewing is to 'shine a light upon the person-in-care and his problems' then clearly we want as much information as possible by the shortest possible route. How can the nurse ensure that she attains this objective? Let us talk first about what the interviewer needs to **avoid** doing.

It hardly needs stating that someone who is abrupt, rude or officious is unlikely to be popular. We might assume that no nurse would dream of adopting such attitudes. Similarly, it is clear that a nurse who is cold or indifferent is unlikely to generate the trust needed to allow talk about any delicate or highly personal material. Such attitudes are more likely to silence the interviewee. In many situations people will make statements that may appear shocking – admissions about suicidal intent, sexual practices, past misdeeds which have inspired guilt or material considered bizarre or delusional. Such topics may be disturbing, especially to the novice. Any expression of surprise, astonishment, reproach or even 'stunned silence' will stifle any further admissions or self-examination.

In view of the negative effect of all of these attitudes towards the person-in-care it is generally acknowledged that any interviewer should strive to appear warm, friendly and accepting. These attitudes seem especially important in the psychiatric field. Your intention should be to help the person-in-care feel 'Here is someone I can talk to'; 'Here is someone who understands me; and who is not sitting in judgement over me'. It has been argued that interviewer characteristics such as empathy, warmth and genuineness can help to promote self-disclosure and self-examination [6]. However, the evidence to support this view has been questioned. This has led some people to argue that the questions – rather than the way they are asked – are all-important. This reaction is unfortunate. Although such interviewer characteristics as warmth, openness, honesty, genuineness, etc. are difficult to measure in 'value' terms, this does not mean that they are unimportant.

It may be sensible and safe to assume that the questions and the way they are asked are of equal importance. The nurse interviewer should set a number of targets, aiming for accuracy, objectivity and organization – these will help her gain a recording of important information, reflecting a minimum of bias. At the same time she should display signs of warmth, empathy, genuineness and unconditional positive regard, to encourage the person or his family to provide this valuable information.

Reflecting on some of the points raised in the opening pages of this chapter I would suggest that the 'human characteristics' noted above are essential features of the good listener. These personal skills not only help us to achieve the aims of a single interview but help build a positive relationship with the person-in-care that can form the basis for therapy or help-giving. It is crucial that these 'conversations' get off on a good footing: if we make a bad start, it is often impossible to repair the damage. With this in mind, it is apparent that we cannot take the role of our 'personal relationship skills' at all lightly.

Prejudiced before you start?

No interview can be conducted in a vacuum. We need some kind of philosophy to guide our questioning. Traditionally, nurses have asked questions about the person-in-care's history, trying to establish how his condition originated and progressed. This was a reflection of 'medical history-taking' – assuming that all forms of mental disorder were some kind of 'disease'. Such a theoretical stance was a kind of bias. It led nurses to ask some questions and not others. Various kinds of bias, or preconception, can influence the line that an interview takes. For instance, an ardent socialist might view the person-in-care as a victim of circumstance. She might assume that he is depressed because of the effects of unemployment, bad housing, poor financial status, etc. This view would lead her to frame questions that would look for information to support this model of depression. Someone with alternative political views might assume that the person's problems are his responsibility and no one else's. This might lead her to frame questions that would highlight the personality weak-nesses of the person-in-care: his failure to make efforts to resolve these problems; his overall 'lack of personal responsibility'.

This issue of bias is another ethical problem for nurses. We all have biases and prejudices, some more strong than others. Often these biases are so much a part of us that we rarely give them a second thought. We may not even recognize them as biases. As I noted in the first chapter, psychiatry itself has a number of biases. There are few clear models of cause or treatment for any particular condition. Instead there is a range reflecting different viewpoints or biases. If we accept a theory that suggests that mental disorder arises out of interpersonal conflicts, we are likely to study the person-in-care's dealings with others as the basic material of our assessment. On the other hand, if we assume that his disorder is a function of some physical cause, our enquiries will reflect this viewpoint; we will look for physical signs and symptoms. There is little I can say to resolve this dilemma. Indeed, a critique of models of mental illness is not one of the aims of this book. However, this dilemma suggests other kinds of bias and prejudice to which we can be alerted and over which we can exert some control.

Let us assume, for the sake of illustration, that you hold strong religious views. These views may lead you to feel that certain patterns of behaviour, like suicide, homosexuality, drug abuse or even swearing are repugnant in some way. I have no way of knowing whether or not your 'attitudes' are right or wrong: like most other belief systems they represent opinions that are difficult to prove one way or another. However, I can predict with some confidence that unless these views are brought under some kind of control they will prejudice your relationship with the person-in-care. Your views will distort the 'picture of the person' which you see before you. Your beliefs, which in many aspects of your life are positive and life-enriching, may obstruct your efforts to help the person-in-care.

I use the example of religious views merely as an example. An alternative example might be someone who believes that organized religion is a disruptive social force. She believes that religion is the 'opium of the people'; that it takes away people's individual responsibility; that, in some cases, it can drive people to suicide. These are not academic examples. I have met many nurses who held such views. I highlight these extreme views simply to remind us of the need to keep our personal philosophies out of the care arena. Ideally, the nurse should act as a kind of advocate, attempting to act for the person-in-care, especially where he is not in a position to act for himself. We are not expected to act as his judge and jury, evaluating his behaviour, his life or his beliefs from the vantage point of our own personal philosophy. In this sense the profession of nursing involves sacrificing some of our personal selves. Often we need to suspend our 'personal' beliefs, at least temporarily, to act for the person-in-care. If we are fortunate, we shall already know what we think. What we want to know is: what does the person think, feel or believe?

Accuracy

It is not enough simply to obtain information about the person-in-care. That information should be accurate and should be reliably recorded for future reference. How do we set about ensuring this accuracy? Some nurses have tried to resolve this problem by writing down everything the person-in-care says in a verbatim transcript [7]. Although most of us would use such an approach with no more than a tiny fraction of those in our care, there are some important principles inherent in this practice. First of all, research has shown that inaccuracies can creep in even when interviews are written up as soon as they have taken place. This means that even if we set aside time to write down what has taken place, as soon as it has taken place, we are bound to get some of this 'reporting' wrong. This may have something to do with the sheer demand of having to record so much information in a short period of time. One way of getting round this problem is to summarize the interview. However, when we 'condense' the interview we may isolate and report upon certain items that are relatively unimportant; and we neglect to comment upon others that are crucial. Clearly, some kind of compromise is needed, as far as writing up the interview is concerned.

Some nurses tape-record interviews with people, using this recording as a memory aid when writing up their notes later on. However, this also may be too time-consuming. Perhaps the simplest procedure is to decide in advance upon the key areas of the interview: these can function as headings, to which we can append brief notes during the interview. These notes can then be extended into longhand as soon as possible after the interview. We must accept that we are likely to make mistakes in reporting our conversations with people-in-care. The reporting process that we finally adopt should attempt to reduce the risk of mistakes: it may be able to do no more.

The idea of a verbatim transcript is an interesting one. This means that we write down word for word what was said. We do not report what we thought the person-in-care meant, only what he said. In the early stages of any assessment I think that there is a great advantage in describing 'the events' of the interview, and leaving it at that. Often we are sorely tempted to interpret these events. Although there is a role for such interpretation, I do not think that it is in the early stages of assessment, or within the interview. Our aim in writing up a report on an interview is to have something to reflect upon, something to remind us of what took place so that we can give more thought to what was said. When we are in the heat of the interview – trying to listen attentively, making brief notes, thinking of the next question – it may be difficult to digest what has been said. For this reason we need a verbatim account of what the person actually **did** say. We can then study these notes, recollecting how certain comments were made, and come to some conclusion about what it all meant. The other advantage of this verbatim account is that we can discuss with other members of the care team 'what the person said'. Instead of saying: 'I interviewed John Wallace today and felt that he was very depressed; almost suicidal, I would say', we can tell our colleagues that 'I interviewed John today and these were the sort of comments he was making'.

It is all too easy to stray away from what the person-in-care actually said by adding layer upon layer of our 'professional' judgements. To maintain accurate reporting we should try to stick closely to the 'basic data': to what the person actually said or did.

So far three key points have been emphasized:

- To achieve the aims of 'good interviewing' we should strive to establish a positive, therapeutic relationship with the person-in-care. We try to gain his trust. We try to show our understanding. Most of all we try to show our willingness to listen.
- In preparing ourselves for the interview we should be aware of possible biases or prejudices that might influence our perception of the person or might lead us to judge him by our standards – standards that may not be wholly appropriate.
- Finally, we need to pay some attention to how we are going to record this important event. How are we going to retain what might be a vast amount of information? Short notes – detailing what the person-in-care said and did – may act as a memory aid for more detailed reporting, should this

prove necessary. In any case these notes will serve as a reminder of the responses made by the person.

I shall consider now in more detail the relationship that the interviewer has with the person-in-care, and in turn how the person-in-care relates to the interviewer.

Interviewer's attitude

In the interview you aim to find out 'Who is this person?' In a traditional diagnostic interview your interest would lie only in finding out 'What is wrong with this person?' I assume that most nurses want, and need, to know more than this. They want to look behind the 'patient' label; avoiding treating the person as the mere carrier of certain signs and symptoms. I assume also that people resent being viewed merely as a collection of symptoms, or typecast as some classic disorder. Maslow commented that many people dislike being pigeon-holed [8]. He suggested that they hated being treated like some kind of specimen, declaring that 'I'm me, not anybody else'.

Traditionally, we have tended to make a distinction between the person-in-care and his condition. Perhaps we have believed that the problems that we deal with inhabit a separate world from the person who is the person-in-care. Cohen has commented upon this situation within medicine by saying that: '[the] doctor is not so much interested in [the patient] as in his malady. He examines the patient's body as if, indeed, the patient were not there' [9]. Sadly, this dehumanizing experience is still a reality for many people when they submit to medical treatment. Some 30 years ago, Laing suggested that similar problems existed within psychiatry. He suggested that we have a choice between relating to the patient (*sic*) 'as a person or a thing' when he acknowledged that:

> no matter how circumscribed or diffuse the initial complaint may be, one knows that the patient is bringing into the treatment situation, whether intentionally or unintentionally, his existence, his whole being-in-his-world ... every aspect of his being is related in some way to every other aspect, although the manner in which these aspects are articulated may be by no means clear' [10].

The tone of Laing's argument is philosophical and perhaps may appear a little abstruse. The basis of his statement is, however, quite simple. All who are required to use mental health services were people before they became 'patients'. As psychiatric nurses the world over are pressured to participate more actively in the medical treatment of 'disorders' – such as schizophrenia – Peplau has reminded us all of the need to treat such 'patients as persons' [11]; especially those carrying a diagnosis of psychosis – since they may most easily be dispossessed further. They do not cease to be 'people' when they enter their 'career' as psychiatric patients – a career that is certainly not of their choosing. We might do well to remember this fact. That Peplau still needs to emphasize the need for a more manifest humanistic emphasis to care suggests that Laing's 30-year old message still retains some currency.

Interviewer beware!

I have made some observations already on the importance of the building of a positive relationship. Let us now consider some actions that might prejudice that relationship, or which might not be in the person-in-care's best interests.

Concern

It is important to appear interested and concerned about the person-in-care's plight. This rule applies even where 'the problem' may appear minor or trivial. The person may, in such cases, have a wholly different perception of his situation. In this context we should guard against suggesting that the person's problems are 'not real' or are in some way 'imaginary'. Most psychiatric problems involve the experience of some human difficulty. In this sense it may appear non-existent or insignificant to others but it is very real to the person-in-care. Take care to avoid embarrassing or alienating him further by suggesting that his problem is not really a problem. Instead, try always to appear interested and reasonably concerned for him.

Reaction

I have mentioned already the problem of 'shocking' or taboo material. During the course of the interview the person-in-care may say something that might shock or surprise the nurse. Such a reaction will depend, of course, on her background and experience. However, it is important to try to avoid showing surprise. Following what I have already discussed above, it is also important not to show too much concern: this may increase the person-in-care's natural concern. Instead, simply acknowledge what has been said, nodding, as an expression of acknowledgement and understanding, accompanying this with simple verbal encouragement: 'Yes, I see' or 'Uh-huh ... go on' or 'Tell me more about that'. This shows that the nurse has heard and understood. More importantly, it makes it clear that she is not judging the person. Any judgement the nurse might make is made privately and kept private.

Sympathy

Where the person is discussing highly distressing material – such as extreme anxiety or suicidal thoughts – the nurse should try to avoid becoming emotionally involved in this situation. However, there is a very thin line between 'overinvolvement' and 'lack of concern'. It is important to show some support for the person in such circumstances. This should not be extended to become grave concern or unnecessary reassurance. As I noted earlier, in such instances the nurse might disapprove of the person's actions or intentions. It is important here to avoid appearing unsympathetic. This does not mean that the nurse should be 'oozing' sympathy: this may only make the person embarrassed. Beware what might be a temptation to blame the person for his present difficulties. Resist what might appear to be a natural inclination towards being unsympathetic.

Interpretation

There are a number of rules related to the nurse's attitude towards the material that emerges from the interview. Remember that the main aim is to collect information. Consequently, an 'open' system is needed. Beware the temptation to interpret what is being said. This can be done later when all the information is available. Beware 'digging' into personal areas, concerning experiences or attitudes, which the person-in-care might wish to keep secret – at least for the time being.

VALUES AND BELIEFS

I have emphasized the need to be non-judgemental. I have also acknowledged that the person's 'life-philosophy', his values and his attitudes towards himself and others, may conflict with your own. It is important to avoid appearing narrow-minded, especially where the person-in-care is describing material that might be viewed as bizarre, irrational or unorthodox. It is also important to accept the person's value system, even where it conflicts with your own. You are not being asked to agree or disagree. You are not being asked to join his life, far less to live it. You are simply being asked to acknowledge what he 'is'.

   In this respect it is advisable to avoid discussing political or religious material. If he tries to engage you in such a debate, invite him to tell you in what way that might be helpful to him: 'In what way would that be useful to you?' If he offers what you consider to be a 'good reason', proceed. If not, you might suggest that this is not an appropriate line of enquiry, unless of course **you** have good reason to think that such a discussion is relevant. If he continues to press you directly for comment, admit that your opinions are not important right now: 'What I think is not important'. This is an 'honest' reply: you are not suggesting that you have no opinions.

   In this respect it is a good idea for nurses to keep their own 'selves' out of the relationship with the person. This raises, of course, the criticism that the so-called 'collaborative relationship' is somewhat one-sided. This seems entirely right and fitting, since the nurse is not – at least for the moment – defined as the person with a need for nursing. The nurse can act as an important model during psychotherapeutic treatment, where she might disclose feelings or thoughts of her own, to help the person identify with her. However, there is little room for such disclosure within the assessment stage. Discussion of the nurse's views, experiences or problems that have an affinity with those of the person-in-care may serve only as distractions. They may draw attention away from the real area of concern – the person-in-care's experiences and problems.

Patience

Very few interviews are without difficulties. Problems may arise where the person is viewed as uncooperative, uncommunicative or inarticulate. These three characteristics all combine to present one specific problem: a lengthy, and possibly frustrating, interview.

Some people-in-care are unwilling to talk about any aspect of their problem: they may have been over the same ground repeatedly with other members of the health care team. The person needs an explanation of why this interview is important. But most of all they need time – time to find out about you, the interviewer, and time to change their attitude towards the interview.

Other people-in-care may find it difficult to answer your questions, as the material they wish to communicate may be too distressing, or they may find it difficult to find the 'right words'. Again, patience is essential. In other cases the person-in-care may appear to be skirting around the subject, going off at tangents, taking a long time to answer your question or appearing to be avoiding answering at all. These responses may be an indication of difficulty. Again the person needs time, not criticism – whether overt or veiled – or further pressure. Avoid showing signs of impatience: beware of checking your watch, as you will invariably be spotted.

There is, of course, only a limited amount of time for the interview. Suggest that the person 'keep time'. Not only might this in some small way 'empower' the person, but it will allow you to give him your full attention throughout. By asking the person 'How much time do we have left?' or 'How are we doing for time?' you offer the person a degree of control over the course of the interview.

Conflict-resolution

No matter how open you are, there are likely to be some people in your care whom you do not like. They may be the same people who exasperate you, as noted above. Or they may be people whose past actions, personalities or attitudes and values you find repugnant. I see no real problem here providing that you do not show your intolerance. Ideally, all members of the 'caring professions' should be tolerant, accepting and non-judgemental. However, despite more than a century and a half of the myth, nurses are not ministering angels: it is clear that we all have feet of clay. While we pursue the ideals of caring, let me make a few practical suggestions. Take care not to:

- argue with the person-in-care;
- belittle the person;
- blame him for his failings.

In general, avoid being 'punitive' or making moralistic judgements. Many people-in-care have had more than their fair share of conflict already. What they have been, or what they are, is in conflict with what they would like to be. Avoid adding to that conflict.

Professionalism

During the course of your conversations the person-in-care is likely to disclose details of conversations he has had with other staff: nurses, doctors, social workers, etc. In such situations beware of being drawn into criticism of your colleagues. The person-in-care may say: 'This morning Sally said to me .... What do you think of that? That can't be right, can it?' The appropriate response, as noted earlier, is: 'What I think is not important. It's what you think that is important. If you don't think that is right, maybe you should ask Sally to discuss it again with you. For now, what does that mean to you?'

We may find it satisfying in some way when someone asks us for our 'professional' opinion: it reinforces our professional esteem. Such pleasures, however, may have painful consequences. Team morale and loyalty may be prejudiced by innocent yet indiscreet remarks. The person-in-care may also be confused by receiving conflicting messages from different team members.

In this context it is also important to emphasize the confidentiality of the interview. Somewhere at the beginning of your conversation you must reassure the person-in-care that everything he says will be treated in the strictest confidence. There can be complications resulting from this 'confidential relationship', as I shall discuss in Chapter 11. However, you are obliged to give this assurance. Without it your interview may not even get started.

The collaborative relationship

We have discussed the nurse's attitude towards the interview, and the person being interviewed. What about the person-in-care? What kind of problems will the interview pose for him?

As I have noted already, the interview is an unnatural form of conversation. This may be even more true for the person-in-care: at least staff have a chance to become more 'natural' through practice. The unusual nature of the interview may promote a lot of anxiety. The person may be unaware of 'why' he is being interviewed; or may simply feel uncomfortable when questioned closely about the private corners of his life. This is a natural anxiety. Most of us feel uneasy when under such 'direct fire'. The nurse should be sensitive to this, even when the anxiety is not obvious.

Many people can disguise their discomfort, displaying their uneasiness more indirectly through hesitant answers, short replies, or apparent 'striving to please' – always answering 'Yes', or agreeing with everything you say. Some of this anxiety can be reduced by the line of questioning. Always begin with non-threatening material; simple questions about who he is, where he lives, etc. These should be phrased to allow very short answers. Avoid asking for opinions or 'self-analysis' in the early stages, as it is too demanding. If the interview has progressed beyond this stage and the person again becomes anxious, postpone the questions that appear to upset him. If he becomes manifestly distressed it may even be appropriate to return to more mundane topics. This will give him a chance to regain his composure. The interview can return to the 'threatening' material gradually, allowing the person-in-care to regain his confidence through active participation.

In some cases it may be appropriate to ask the person when he is 'ready' to return to such a line of questioning: 'We spoke earlier about ... do you feel ready to return to that just now? If you don't want to discuss it just now, just say so.' Giving the person a chance to influence the direction of the interview is of crucial importance. This way he becomes a 'partner', instead of something manipulated by the interviewer. This partnership should begin early. The nurse's first responsibility is to tell the person-in-care what she would like to do; why she wishes to do this; and what will be the person-in-care's role in the whole proceeding.

Perhaps the simplest question is – paradoxically – the one that might get to the very nub of the issue by the shortest possible route. The nurse might ask the person: 'What have you brought along with you today?', or 'What brings you here?', or 'So ... how would you like to use this time?' Such questions hold no obvious 'hidden agenda'. They represent the simplest forms of enquiry. The last question is perhaps the most sensitive, and offers the person an opportunity to control the proceedings. This kind of question may well help build the kind of confiding relationship that the nurse most desires.

Another important question – and one to be asked at the very outset – is: 'Do you want to ask anything before we begin?' This may be the best guard against anxiety, since it removes much of the threat of the 'unknown'.

There is some likelihood that the person-in-care may not be enthusiastic about being interviewed. This is often true when people are first admitted into the 'care system'. The person may already have seen a long line of such interviewers and may be irritated by the prospect of another. The nurse should acknowledge that such irritation or annoyance is natural and appropriate. She should emphasize her awareness of how the person might be feeling. This acknowledgement shows that the nurse is trying to consider his feelings: he is not just another name on a list. However, this interview is slightly different, as it may be helpful in ensuring that he gets the right kind of care. Rather than suggesting that you might help him, it might be useful to suggest how you 'hope he will be able to help' you in this way.

I am talking here about what is commonly referred to as 'resistance'. However, instead of blaming the person-in-care for his 'poor cooperation' I am suggesting that there might be a value in trying to see the interview from his angle, so that we might prevent such 'resistance' developing.

Some people-in-care may be unhappy about being grilled or cross-examined. This seems to be quite a reasonable objection. We need to ask, however, why the interview should be so unpleasant. It must be something to do with the line of questioning or the way that questions are asked. It is important that we do not assume that person should want to answer our questions. The interview should be designed to encourage this 'participation'. Even where people are not resistant they may not be overly enthusiastic. Again this may be a reflection of the interview format. Are you simply rushing through a routine checklist, ticking off answers, looking as though you have done this a hundred times before? If this is the case the person-in-care may feel that this is not very important, and may be disinclined to 'work' at the interview. There is great value in trying to make each interview a stimulating prospect, for the person-in-care and interviewer alike. Even if this is the hundredth time this month, try to tailor the interview to suit the person: make it something personal to him. He may appreciate it.

I have written much more about the interviewer's attitude since I am able to draw upon my own experience, my own failings. I have said very little about the person-in-care's attitude since it is important to have as few assumptions about the person as possible. The one assumption I have made is that all people-in-care want to be treated as people. They want to be given a chance to be themselves – even when they feel at odds with themselves. They also resent being patronized, treated like children or treated as if everyone knows what is right for them, except them. It is a sad fact of psychiatric life that, even today, few people-in-care get full – or honest – explanations about what is being done to them. We accept that we should give everyone a chance to participate, even in a small way, in their care and treatment. Evidence from research suggests that such an approach to care provision makes life easier, for carers as well as the 'cared-for'. If we do not offer the person-in-care an opportunity to participate fully we should expect that he might become 'resistant' or at the very least unmotivated. In preparing to interview the person we should try to respect his true status as a full person. This will make the interview process more satisfying for him and for us.

AN OVERVIEW OF THE INTERVIEW

So far we have talked about some of the considerations which influence the interview. Let us now discuss some of the mechanics of interviewing – what we need to do and how we ought to do it.

Phrasing the question

Questions are the central feature of the interview. The first priority is to avoid confusing the person-in-care. He may be confused or otherwise 'at a loss' already.

Specificity

The first priority in phrasing a question is to avoid ambiguity. Avoid questions that may have more than one meaning. Focus your question so that it will draw information on one aspect of the person's functioning or experience. If you do not get the answer you expected, you may not have asked the question you meant to ask.

Length

Brevity is another key issue. Avoid asking long rambling questions. Avoid making general observations about the person or his situation, including a question somewhere within this statement.

Don't ask
'You were saying earlier that you feel pretty tense all the time ... that must be pretty awful. I can see that you are tense right now. You're sitting all sort of hunched up ... is that what you mean? Like you said a moment ago, I mean ... is that how you feel ... all tense, anxious, nervy, like you said. Is it?'

Do ask
'You said a moment ago that you often felt tense.' (Pause)
'Tell me more about that.' (Await reply)
'When you feel tense ... what does that mean for you?' (Await reply)
'So ... how do you feel right now?' (Await reply)
'You are sitting sort of hunched up. Is that how you usually are when you feel tense?' (Await reply).

The rambling question, rolled up in some observations, may be appropriate on a TV chat show. In a clinical interview it may simply lose the person. If the question is not direct, or specific enough, it is more difficult to answer and may increase the person's anxiety. The same is true of the string of questions. Ask one question at a time, unless you have very good reasons for acting otherwise.

Time

The question should also specify the time clearly, where appropriate. 'How do you feel now?' or 'How have you been feeling over the past two or three days?'

Where the time-scale is necessarily vague, you might ask: 'Can you tell me what sort of things you were able to do when you felt you were well?' or 'How did you feel when you were well?', following up the reply by asking 'And how long ago was that?' Be aware that many people who are highly distressed feel that they have 'always' been like this. Help them sharpen the time focus.

Open and closed questions

There are two main kinds of question: those that elicit a short reply, perhaps just 'yes' or 'no', and those that require fuller answers.

'Are you still feeling depressed?'
'Your husband left you. Do you think that made you depressed?'
'Do you hear voices a lot?'

All these **closed** questions can be answered 'yes', 'no' or 'don't know'.

'How are you feeling today?'
'How did you react to your husband leaving you?'
'You say that someone is talking to you, in your head. Tell me more about that.'
'Give me an idea of how you are feeling right now.'

All these **open** questions provide the person with an opportunity to talk at length, should he wish to do so.

Closed questions may be appropriate in the initial stages of the interview, as they put fewer demands on the person-in-care. In this sense they are also appropriate when the person is very distressed or withdrawn. Open questions will, however, provide more information about what it is like to be him – more information about his experience.

Reflection

When the person says something that appears interesting or significant, you may want to develop this theme, or gain more information. The simplest and least intrusive way to do this is to reflect – or bounce back – his reply. Hopefully he will pick this up, and amplify his meaning.

Person. I get so confused sometimes I just don't know whether I'm coming or going.
Nurse. Coming … or … going?
Person. That's right. I mean … I just don't seem to be able to cope with things. I feel so useless all the time.
Nurse. I see … you feel **useless**? Tell me more about that.'

Emphasis should be given to certain words to show that you are phrasing a question, and not simply repeating what the person has said. Reflection should also be used with discretion. If you repeatedly reflected the person's answers he might think that he was answering the questions badly, or that you were making fun of him.

Reflection can be taken a stage further by using the person's actual phrasing to frame another question: 'You say that you don't know whether you are coming or going. Can you tell me what you mean by that?'

The key feature of reflection is that you provide the minimum of guidance. You interrupt the person no more than is necessary. This allows for more efficient interviewing: you encourage the person to give as much information as possible, for the minimum of interviewing time. More importantly, it provides the person with an opportunity to talk as much as possible, without losing the necessary structure.

Perceived threat

Some questions will be disturbing or threatening to the person. Avoiding such questions is not a solution. Instead, questions about sensitive or distressing subjects should be carefully framed to reduce their impact. It is not possible to list all such perceived threats. These can vary from one person to another. However, even in today's liberated society detailed questioning about sex is often perceived as a threat. The same is true of domestic violence.

Don't ask
'How often do you and your partner have sex?'
'Do you ever hit the kids?'

Do ask
'You talked about you and your partner ... is there any aspect of your relationship with which you are not entirely happy?'
'What happens when you lose your temper?'

If the person-in-care feels threatened by direct questioning he may simply deny the existence of any problem. By taking a more oblique line of questioning the 'glare' of the searchlight is reduced. Such 'indirect' questioning may make it easier for the person to admit to problems of which he is ashamed.

Devising a framework

Any interview needs a structure. This can, however, be rigid or flexible – depending on the demands of the situation. The 'structure' most commonly refers to the kind of questions which you will ask. For example, a typical interview might begin with very 'open-ended' questions, such as 'Would you like to tell me what's bothering you at present?' Gradually, more specific queries can be introduced, such as 'How often has this happened?' Eventually, the person-in-care's perception of his 'problem' can be narrowed down to finer detail: 'How severe is this at present, on a scale of 1 to 10?'

These stages – beginning, middle and end – show how the interview begins with very broad concerns and gradually sharpens the focus on one or two problems. A first interview might be devoted entirely to drawing up a list of the person's problems. Subsequent interviews might take individual problems as 'topics', devoting the time to trying to understand each one better, through closer analysis.

A flexible framework, where the interviewer decides upon her line of questioning within the interview itself, is usually reserved for the 'expert'. Most of us need some preparation. We need some simple framework of questions to provide some security, so that we don't get lost for words. Our aim is to have a 'conversation' with the person-in-care. We want to talk to the person-in-care as normally as possible. If we have a general outline of the questions we want to ask – the areas we want to explore – then these guidelines may make us feel more comfortable. We may decide to use such a framework as a guide to notekeeping during the interview, or we may simply memorize the question areas. If we need a rule it is: 'select the approach that is most appropriate to you or the person-in-care'.

Some people-in-care like to think that their problems are being dealt with seriously: a more formal interview may be appropriate for them. Others will find this uncomfortable. Finally, we need also to consider the needs of the nurse. What sort of format would she be comfortable with?

Troubleshooting

Interviews rarely ever turn out the way we plan. It is important to prepare for problems: we need strategies 'up our sleeve' to avoid getting lost or grinding to a halt.

Failure to respond

The person-in-care may find it difficult to give the information you want, especially at the first interview. How far should you 'press' him? Should you press him at all? If the person fails to answer 'appropriately' (i.e. to your satisfaction) it may be that the question has been badly phrased. It may be impossible to answer in its present form. Try presenting the question from a different angle.

When there is conflict within the family, what kind of coping strategies do you employ under such conditions? (No answer – try again)
Well, let me put it this way ... when there's an 'atmosphere' at home, how do you deal with that?

The first example may look like a 'spoof' question but is actually drawn from a published transcript of an interview. The second example asks the same question, but uses some of the person's own language to aid communication.

Difficult to answer

The person may be able to answer, but may be unsatisfied with his reply. It is appropriate here to offer some words of encouragement, helping him to find the words he needs to express himself. Beware, however, of putting words into his mouth. Instead, try to shape up his answer through discreet feedback.

> **Nurse.** So how did you feel when that happened?
> **Person.** Oh, I don't know. Just lost ... sort of ... eh ... I – oh, I don't know.
> **Nurse.** Uh-huh, you felt 'lost': lost in what way?
> **Person.** Lost, yes. Didn't know what to do ... what to say.
> **Nurse.** Lost for words?
> **Person.** Yes ... lost for words. Didn't know what to say to her. Felt powerless. No, that's not right. Can't seem to think straight.
> **Nurse.** You were lost for words. You didn't know what to say to her – or you felt that you couldn't tell her how you felt?
> **Person.** Well, maybe that's true. I knew how I felt, but I just couldn't face her. Yeah, I guess I couldn't bring myself to tell her how I felt.

Refuses to answer

In some instances the person may not answer at all – which is an answer of sorts: 'I am not willing (or ready/able) to answer'. What should we do? Rephrase the question? Try to nudge him gently? Or simply respect his wishes, leaving this issue for another time, or another place?

My sympathies lie with the last solution, although there are bound to be occasions when it might be appropriate to try the others. If we choose to 'postpone' a question, however, we should let the person know why we have done so.

> You don't seem to be too happy with that question. (Pause) Maybe it was the way I put it. Perhaps you don't feel ready to discuss that with me just yet? (Pause) Maybe we could come back to it some other time, when you think you're ready. OK? (Pause) We were talking a moment ago about ... (Progress to next question).

Tangents

You cannot expect to find answers to all your questions in a single interview. Ideally, one question leads to another and so on, and may span several interviews. In practice, however, one question usually produces a number of answers, some aspects of which are relevant, others less so. The nurse must decide whether or not to follow up such 'tangents' or to stick to the core questions. If she decides to deal only with some of the person's replies she should make it clear that she is doing this. Let us take an example of someone who is being asked how she feels about going into town on a shopping trip.

> **Nurse.** You were talking yesterday about going shopping in town.
> **Person.** Oh, I don't know. I get terribly tense in the crowds. Then there's my Harriet, I should have rung her. She doesn't really manage well on her own. I worry about her ever so much … and I promised to take Johnny … he's just 11 … to the game on Saturday. I keep letting him down. He can hardly look at me. It's all so pointless.
> **Nurse.** Uh-huh. I see. Your family obviously mean a lot to you. You worry about them a great deal. Maybe we need to spend some time just talking about that. We should really give it the attention it deserves. Do you want to talk about that, or do you want to continue discussing the shopping trip you had planned? What do you think?

The nurse had a decision to make here: either to respond to the person's 'need' to discuss his worries about his family or to stick to the agenda of the interview. She chooses to turn the decision over to the person, thereby 'empowering' his decision-making. No agenda is ever 'fixed'. Providing that you review the change of direction that is mooted, the interview may follow any course that is deemed appropriate.

The setting

We should look upon the interview as a 'formal' conversation, since the outcome may be of crucial relevance to the person. Interviews need not, however, be structured in a formal manner. On occasions, it may be appropriate to interview the person in his bedroom on the ward, his sitting room at home, a consulting room off the ward, or an 'interview room' at a clinic. All are standard settings for conducting interviews. It may be just as practical, however, to interview the person in the hospital grounds or while walking his dog in the park. The important consideration in the selection of the venue or setting is: 'Will we have privacy, peace and quiet?' The person is unlikely to want to discuss personal problems within earshot of other people and may become distracted if there are repeated interruptions. In some cases 'walking in the park' may feel more private and distraction-free than a consulting room.

The setting is also important for 'putting the person at his ease'. A distressed person may feel more comfortable 'chatting' over a cup of coffee in the corner of the hospital cafeteria or when walking in the fresh air. The restrictions of a small interview room may enhance his anxiety and may make communication more difficult. However, in some cases it is appropriate to pick an awkward setting. If the person has identified a situation that appears to 'trigger' his problem it may be appropriate to conduct the interview there. We might take someone with social anxiety out into the street. If the person was suffering from a grief reaction, we might take him to a setting that evoked special memories of his loved one. In both examples the setting selected would serve as a trigger for certain emotions, thoughts and memories which might be less evident in a more formal interview setting.

Communicating with the person-in-care

Some people do not like being interviewed. Often this stems from bad experiences in other interview situations at the hands of the over-efficient, the cold or probing interviewer. I have emphasized already the need to be warm, non-judgemental and genuine. In addition to these classic features it is also important to talk to the person-in-care in language he understands. He may be baffled by the language of professionals, who often use jargon, vocabulary or grammatical structures that are beyond his capabilities. In addition to easing tensions, the use of a common language – especially where the person-in-care speaks in some dialect – may be helpful in establishing a positive relationship.

> **Nurse.** You're looking pretty down today, Geoff. Would you like to tell me what's troubling you?
> **Geoff.** Oh, I'm just proper ... scunnered, like. Been like this for weeks.
> **Nurse.** You feel **scunnered** (emphasis). What ... with everything?
> **Geoff.** Yeah, just sick of everything. But especially myself.
> **Nurse.** Tell me more about that.

By picking up on the person-in-care's use of the expression 'scunnered' – meaning sick or tired of – the nurse may strengthen her rapport with the person-in-care. She hopes the person-in-care will think, quite literally: 'this person is someone I can really talk to'.

Indeed, the nurse need not actually 'know' the exact meaning of the key words she picks up and reflects back. By using the person's language she establishes rapport; encouraging the person to amplify the point he is making. The more the person is encouraged to express himself, the more information the nurse will receive and the more she will be able to build up a picture of 'what it is like to be this person'.

Respect

In the same context it is worth picking up the use of more technical terms – like 'depressed', 'anxious', 'alienated', 'paranoid', 'hostile'. These words, which have very special meanings in our professional language, have become part of the vernacular. However, we should not assume that because such expressions are in everyday use their meaning remains the same. Where the person-in-care uses such 'technical expressions' as part of his description of self, ask him to clarify what he means.

In a related vein, it is important to avoid translating the person-in-care's words into our convenient shorthand:

Nurse. Tell me more about how you feel.
Person. Oh, blue.
Nurse. You mean that you're depressed.
Person. (Sighs) I guess so.

In this example the nurse missed an opportunity to engage with the person by using the words he has used to describe his experience. If he had intended to say he was depressed, he would have chosen that word. We might argue that this is mere semantics: it is not! Using the person-in-care's language – at least in the initial stages of the assessment – is respectful. We acknowledge that the person knows his experience better than anyone. Indeed, only he has access to that experience. The words he uses to communicate that experience are supremely important. The value we place upon them denotes the value we accord to the person.

In some situations it may be appropriate to encourage the person to talk about the problem without even naming it. Where the problem is a source of embarrassment, or the person does not feel prepared to trust the nurse, talking about the problem 'in the abstract' may represent a solution.

I get the feeling that you are not ready to talk about this situation yet. I understand … in fact … there is no need to tell me about this … whatever it is. Not until you are ready to. What about if we just called it X? Maybe you could tell me how X is a problem for you?

Alternatively, the nurse could ask 'How does X make you feel?' or 'How long has X been a problem for you?' or 'When did X first become a problem for you?' Indeed, providing that this arrangement is acceptable to the person-in-care, the nurse can explore the problem fully without ever asking for a definition of what it is.

It might be argued that this approach conveys maximum respect for the person and his experience. Where the person has identified a problem that presents the nurse with some difficulty, alternatives are available that maintain the respectfulness of the relationship. Peplau discusses the problem that might be posed by the discussion of hallucinatory phenomena [12]. She acknowledges that the experience of hearing voices (or seeing illusory figures) seems real; but from the nurse's theoretical standpoint these are illusions, autistically invented. Peplau suggests that:

This distinction between the patient's and nurse's perception should be clearly emphasized in what the nurse says to the patient. For example, when a nurse says 'tell me about the voices' she has, in effect, linguistically accepted the voices as real. It is possible to maintain the distinction when the nurse says 'tell me about these so-called voices of yours' or 'talk about the voices you say you hear', or 'when did you first notice these so-called voices of yours? [13]

Although, as Peplau has observed, these kinds of question are more cumbersome, they carry the advantage of: (1) attributing the hallucinatory experience solely to the person – the nurse neither confirms nor denies it; and (2) keeping the perceptions of the nurse and the person-in-care quite separate. In my view, this is another way to show respect for the experience of another.

PRESENTING THE INTERVIEW

Preparation

Whether the interview is to be formal or informal, taking place in a clinical setting or under a tree, the nurse should always be prepared. By preparation I mean knowing:

- the aim of the interview;
- how best to conduct it; and
- how much time is available.

As I noted earlier, the aims can vary enormously from one interview to another. This means that some preparation is necessary to ensure that you cover all the points you wish to cover. A general outline of what you intend to do is helpful for the following reasons.

- It acts as a guide to the line of questioning, guarding against getting sidetracked.
- It helps you follow a logical, sensitive line of questioning, in most cases beginning with non-threatening material, building up gradually to more sensitive material.
- It guards against duplication of lines of questioning followed by other members of the health-care team. In some cases such a 'follow-on' may be recommended. Doctors may ask nurses to pursue certain questions on their behalf to gain more information.
- It guards against taxing the person's concentration (e.g. by being unduly long), and guards against time-wasting (e.g. by spending too much time on general issues) before reaching the key questions.

Prepare to conclude the interview at least 10 minutes before you need to. This allows the person time to regain his composure or to ask any further general questions.

The plan

We have already discussed various ways of phrasing the questions. It is also helpful to distinguish between higher- and lower-order questions [14].

Lower-order questions

There are four main kinds of 'lower-order' question: in general, these are simpler forms of question. The first involves the **recall of information**. Here the person might be asked: 'Have you ever felt this bad before?' – to which he can answer 'Yes' or 'No'. Alternatively, he might be asked to recall more information: 'When did you last feel this bad?'

The second kind involves **rephrasing** or 'rewording' certain concepts or ideas: 'Can you tell me, in your own words, what you mean by "helpless"?'

In the third class the person-in-care is asked to **compare or contrast** situations or experiences: 'In which situations do you normally feel worst? Can you tell me, then, where you would feel OK?'

The last class of lower-order question invites the person-in-care to present **alternatives** to what they have done in the past: 'How could you handle that differently? Given what we have just discussed, how would you tackle that situation in the future?'

Higher-order questions

This class of questions involves more complex answering. These questions invite the person to **analyse** a situation: he is required to give some indication of why something happened. These motives or causes cannot, of course, be drawn simply from memory; the answer needs to be more 'creative' and is therefore more difficult. 'Why do you think your wife stopped talking to you?' or 'How do you think you came to be depressed?'

This class also contains questions that invite the person to make **predictions** or to discuss complex ideas: 'What would happen if you did that?' or 'What would be so bad about that?'

Ideally, the plan of the interview should begin with lower-order questions, which require the person-in-care to 'dip into' his memory or require simple problem-solving answers. As the interview progresses, or as the person-in-care becomes more comfortable, the more complex questions, relying on complex reasoning, may be introduced.

Seating

In the classic interview the interviewer sits behind a desk, with the interviewee facing him. This 'job interview' arrangement is wholly inappropriate in psychiatry given the messages about power, and its control, that are communicated.

Where two people face each other it may appear 'confrontational'. Where a desk is used it may appear to represent a shield (suggesting that the interviewer wishes to keep her distance) or barrier (placing the interviewee at a disadvantage).

The height and design of chairs are also important. If one person sits on a higher chair, this may appear to confer an advantage. If the person-in-care is given a stiff, high-backed chair, while the nurse sits in an easy chair, again there may appear to be an advantage; the person in the easy chair appearing more relaxed and comfortable. Ideally, both should sit on the same kind of chair, at roughly 60° to one another. This allows easy eye contact and orientation, such as is found in most normal social interactions [15]. Where 'odd' chairs are all that is available the nurse should offer the person 'first choice'. Where the nurse visits the person-in-care in his 'home territory', she should ask him where he would like her to sit.

The seats should be close together, registering the privacy and intimacy of the conversation. If they are far apart, this may be interpreted as a 'gulf' between the nurse and the person-in-care. However, as with other aspects of the interview, it is advisable to check with the person that such arrangements are acceptable before beginning.

Opening

The nurse should begin the interview by preparing the ground for what is to follow. She should tell the person what she intends to ask him. She will then proceed to conduct the interview, finishing by trying to summarize some of his answers. In her opening remarks the nurse should explain her 'aims', asking the person-in-care if he has any queries or objections.

Hello Mr Smith, I'm Jennifer Masters, Staff Nurse on the unit (Pause). I will be responsible for your care while you are here. I know that you are just settling in but I would like a little time with you later. I would like to get some more details about yourself. Just a few minutes, that's all I'll need. OK? (Pause) I'd like to ask a few questions about what led up to you coming in to hospital. (Pause) At the same time, if you have any questions for me – if there is anything you don't understand, or anything you need to know – just stop me. Is that OK with you?

Here the nurse is making it clear who she is and what she wants to do. She also tries to acknowledge that the person-in-care may feel inconvenienced and tries to encourage him to question her if he wishes. She also tries to make the whole affair as non-threatening as possible by giving him 'permission' to interrupt. She pauses briefly throughout her introduction, giving him time to speak, or to allow her words to register. This kind of honest opening may reduce the person's natural anxiety. The emphasis upon a kind of 'collaboration' may also raise the person-in-care's self-esteem.

The interview core

After this simple introduction the interview proper can begin. Here also it is important to emphasize the structure, marking clearly the beginning and end of each section and summarizing where appropriate.

1. 'To begin with, I'd like you to tell me a bit about yourself.' (This general question may be followed immediately by a series of specific queries: e.g. 'Do you live on your own? Who does your shopping for you? Where did you work before you retired?')

2. 'Good. That seems to cover everything there. Maybe we could talk for a moment about how you came into hospital? Now you said that you lived alone ...' (By recapping on some of the points covered in 1. above the nurse might move on to more open-ended questions: 'When did you first feel that you needed help? Who did you discuss these problems with? How did you feel about being on your own?')

3. 'That's fine. I have found that very helpful. Perhaps we might discuss some of the problems you have mentioned in more detail? Are you ready for that just now?' (If the person-in-care agrees, further questions of a 'who', 'where', 'when', 'what' and 'how' variety might be asked: 'Where did that first happen?' 'Were you on your own at the time?' 'What would be so bad about that?' 'In what way is that a problem for you?')

4. 'From what you have said a number of things appear to be a problem to you just now. First of all, you have some worries about your son ...?' (The information collected can now be summarized briefly. At the same time the nurse can check that her interpretation of the 'facts' is correct.

Promoting responses

As we noted earlier, the nurse must present a certain 'image' in order to encourage the kind of positive relationship essential to the success of any interview. So far we have discussed only the 'verbal' aspect of the relationship with the person-in-care. Let us now pass comment on some aspects of the 'non-verbal' interaction between the nurse and the person.

Many of the characteristics of the 'good' interviewer will be expressed through her non-verbal behaviour. Or rather, the person is likely to perceive the nurse positively or negatively on the basis of observation of these subtle characteristics. When we find people 'likeable' or 'unpleasant', rarely is this because of what they have said. More often it is the outcome of the way they said it, or some even less specific factor. Usually we say: 'It's something I can't put my finger on'. We should be aware that the 'impression' that the person-in-care forms will be based largely upon how we stand, sit, use our hands and look at him. It is not possible to cover all aspects of non-verbal behaviour here: the following represents just some aspects of 'body language', awareness of which may be helpful to the interviewer.

Spatial behaviour

I have already mentioned the need to sit close to the person, on an equal footing. This signifies the removal of status. If you wish to 'control' the other person, you try to look down at him or sit behind a desk. The side-by-side orientation recommended earlier will probably communicate your 'liking' for the person-in-care and may give reassurance.

Posture

The nurse should try to appear relaxed and comfortable during the interview. This should communicate 'confidence'. It may be appropriate to change posture during the conversation, leaning forward if the person is discussing confidential material or is distressed, or settling back in the chair if he appears able to talk at length. These posture changes may also communicate confidentiality or a willingness to listen. In general it is appropriate to sit turned slightly towards the person-in-care, leaning slightly in his direction.

Facial expression

Our faces provide a regular commentary on our speech, as we 'flash' our eyebrows, smile, frown, grimace, etc. The nurse should attempt to follow the person's conversation by displaying appropriate facial expression. However, this should always be controlled, otherwise it may look theatrical and insincere. If the person is discussing a harrowing incident it may be appropriate to acknowledge this by furrowing the brows slightly. Interest or mild surprise can be communicated by a slight raising of the eyebrows. If the person-in-care says something amusing, or laughs – even nervously – it is appropriate to smile, acknowledging his communication of humour. The nurse should partner the person, showing that she appreciates the meaning or significance of what is being said.

When meeting the person for the first time, even the first time each day, it is important to smile slightly. This should be enough to signal confidence or a positive attitude only. A beaming smile, of the 'have a nice day' variety, is not recommended. The person may interpret this as patronizing, or dismissive of the severity of his problems.

Eye contact

Usually, we look at other people in order to pick up the non-verbal cues just mentioned. However, gaze has another function: it adds emphasis to our speech and can be used to 'reply' to the other person. Although the amount of eye contact varies from one situation to another, rarely do we ever gaze constantly at the other person, except when we are madly in love or enraged with anger. 'Normal' gaze patterns involve looking and quickly looking away, result in about 75% of the time spent in eye contact. If we give more than this amount of eye contact we may appear 'confrontational' or aggressive; less, and we may look embarrassed, ashamed or 'shifty'. Many nurses think that they should 'study' the person all the time. If they try reversing roles for a few minutes, they will soon find out how uncomfortable this can be.

Gestures

We use our hands, like our eyes, to add expression to our speech. Gestures can play an important part in any interview, for example when we 'wave' to the person inviting further comment, or signal for him to stop for a moment. These gestures are direct signals from the nurse to the person. We can also 'signal' our attitude: for example, drumming our fingers on the chair or twiddling a pencil may signal impatience; resting our chin on our hands may signal 'thoughtfulness'. (I have a habit of stroking my moustache or pulling the end of my beard. This has been interpreted variously as 'a thoughtful look' to 'complete boredom'. It is interesting to note that some cultures interpret such 'stroking' as thoughtfulness **or** boredom, but never both. This suggests the need to monitor our gestures. I mention such 'autistic gestures' simply to remind you that you may be giving signals which you would rather omit.)

We also gesture by nodding or shaking our heads. The head nod is a valuable gesture, indicating agreement, acknowledgement, and also serving as an encouragement for the person to continue talking.

Physical contact

Contact between nurses and people in their care is often taboo. However, when carried out appropriately it can be a helpful adjunct to speech. It is important to recognize that the West is a 'non-contact' culture: most often, we only touch people anonymously – bumping into people in a crowd – or in highly ritualized situations such as the handshake. This convention extends to the psychiatric field and is broken only under certain conditions. If the person is distressed reassurance can be conveyed effectively by gripping him lightly on the forearm or resting your hand on his shoulder. I hesitate to suggest further in the case of adults, although in the case of some children much more contact may be considered appropriate. However, in the case of some children this may be highly undesirable. Some children with autism, for example, find close physical contact aversive; as might those who have suffered physical or sexual abuse.

It is apparent that some Western people have developed 'practised' forms of physical contact, which they use as an adjunct to their normal interpersonal style: hugging energetically, or stroking the upper arm of the other person in a 'supportive' manner. There is a danger that such contact may be interpreted as false, 'rehearsed' or otherwise 'non-genuine'.

Using non-verbal communication

Identifying these various facets of our 'non-verbal' communication is the easy part. How do we use such knowledge without appearing false; indeed, without giving out conflicting messages? Ideally, we should aim to communicate naturally – rather than in the rehearsed fashion noted above. Perhaps the only way to become aware of our 'non-verbals' and the hidden messages they display is to invite feedback, especially from our colleagues and supervisors. We need to accept, however, that the process of self-discovery probably involves lifelong vigilance. It is all too easy to become complacent.

Abuse of the interview

I have suggested in this chapter that the interview can be used to elicit all kinds of information from the person-in-care, from identifying who he is to asking him to comment on his role in life, if not his thoughts on an afterlife. Interviews are not restricted to the assessment phase and may figure in the caring phase itself, or even in the follow-up. At each end of the care spectrum questions are asked to elicit information about the person-in-care's history, his expectations of treatment, his attitude to treatment received, his relationships with family, friends or other people, his anxieties about the future or his plans for life after discharge. The uses to which the interview may be put are probably endless. However, in all these situations the interview is designed to achieve the following:

- to provide a situation where nurse and person-in-care can get to know one another, or can re-establish relationships of a positive nature – this is the rapport-building level;
- to gain basic information to help orientate the care staff towards the person, placing him in identity, time, place, etc. – this is the history-taking phase;
- to collect detailed information of a qualitative or quantitative nature, which will help us plan the kind of care he needs;
- to help the person assess or evaluate himself and his life situation by helping him to look at facets of his own functioning and relationship with his world;
- to help the person feel that he is a collaborator in his care and treatment; to make him feel that we are interested in him as a person, not as a ragbag of disparate psychiatric symptoms.

I summarize these aims to remind myself that many interviews fail to achieve these fundamental goals. These aims are not in any way idealistic: many more refinements and additions could be suggested. The main aim of this kind of interview is to provide a supportive, reassuring, non-judgemental environment in which the skills of the nurse and the assets of the person can combine to shine some light on the mystery of the patient.

It is quite easy to turn the interview from this positive, creative exercise into a third-degree inquisition. Although in some cases it may be necessary to look at aspects of the person's life he might rather leave alone, we should avoid making him feel worse. Providing that awkward or threatening material is handled sensibly and sensitively, the person may even feel that he has achieved something by confronting his problem. There is, however, a danger in taking such a 'confrontational' approach to extremes. Indeed, nurses often hold extreme views on the issue of upsetting people. Some believe that everyone should be confronted with their problems. I am not sure that such a generalized attitude is ever sensible. Other nurses might take the opposite view, believing that they should never upset anyone, in any way. Again, this extreme view seems illogical. I would suggest that we should only stimulate strong emotion in people if we have reason to believe that we can handle this, and that the person can emerge from the experience with some definable 'gain'.

In many interviews it is likely that the information you desire may not be forthcoming. It is important here to avoid becoming frustrated or exasperated. It is not necessary to remain forever tolerant and smiling. However, allowing your emotions to surface 'under their own steam' is to be discouraged. Instead, give the person some 'feedback': let him know that you do not seem to be getting the information you need. Does he not wish to answer these questions? If necessary, tell him that you are getting lost, finding it difficult to conduct the interview – even that you are becoming frustrated or annoyed. Better to tell the person 'intellectually' than to let him experience this 'emotionally'.

In some situations the information the person offers you could be interesting for reasons other than professional curiosity. Where he describes some behaviour, belief or emotion that appears to you strange, resist the temptation to question further simply to satisfy your own curiosity. This problem seems particularly prevalent where sexual behaviour and marital relationships are under discussion. In the same vein it is important not to stray to the other extreme. Some nurses are afraid to ask any sensitive questions about sex or relationships. The rule is: only ask about what appears to be relevant to the problem in hand. We might avoid such abuse of the interview if we were more knowledgeable about our own motivation before we began to study that of the person-in-care.

To achieve the basic aims of the interview, we must guard against these three examples of abuse. We must beware of using the interview as a means of dismantling or devaluing the person-in-care, as we should be concerned only with his development. We must beware of becoming emotionally entangled in the interview process, especially when it begins to fail us. Instead of using our status as 'interviewer' as an excuse to ventilate our feelings, we should try to construct solutions through more reasoned 'contracting' with the person-in-care. Finally, we must beware of idle curiosity. We should acknowledge the responsibility vested in us to probe and pry no more than is absolutely necessary.

CONCLUSION

In this chapter I have discussed the use of conversation to gain insights into the unique world of the person-in-care. I have emphasized the need to focus the interview on the person behind the patient label, studying his experience; what Laing called his 'being-in-his-world'. The basic interview format needs to be adapted to suit the individual. Factors such as age, sex, cultural background, values, beliefs and presentation will influence how we prepare or conduct the interview. These adaptations influence the structure of the interview, what we do and say, how long it lasts, where it takes place and how we record the outcome.

The interview has no single purpose apart from eliciting information. It may be used for a multiplicity of purposes, from finding out who the person is to evaluating how he thinks he has changed. Throughout this range of conversations some basic principles remain constant. The interview should be seen as a two-way process and the person should be given every encouragement to collaborate. He should also be kept informed of the progress of the interview, and wherever possible informed in advance of 'what is coming next'.

I illustrated how the person should be encouraged to participate in the control of the interview: in certain cases he might be asked to decide when he is ready to discuss certain aspects of his situation. Of supreme importance is the need for the interviewer to be unbiased, isolating any preconceptions or prejudices hidden in her view of the person. Instead, the person's value system should be accepted, although this need not mean that it is given active approval. The person's perception of his world and himself is used as the vantage point for the assessment. The interviewer tries to see the world through his eyes, at least for the time being. Later, in the treatment phase, it may be decided that his view of the world is his problem.

I have paid some attention to the mechanics of interviewing. Various ways of eliciting the person-in-care's thoughts, feelings and beliefs were described briefly. These responses are used to supplement the nurse's observation of the person's presentation. Emphasis was also given to the need to be as unobtrusive as possible. The person should be given every opportunity to speak. This rule is amended only where he is uncommunicative, where there is an expressed need for a talkative interviewer.

The interview can be a highly sophisticated interaction. In many ways it can also be therapeutic. If handled properly the person may discover aspects of his functioning of which he was unaware. Sometimes these revelations can be traumatic, the 'gains' often being seen as 'facing up to the problem'. In general, I have defined a 'good interview' as one that will ultimately benefit the person-in-care. Even a difficult or distressing interview yields an abundance of such fruits. I warned, however, against possible abuses. The status of the nurse should never be used to manipulate the person. The potential for damage to the person's esteem should be noted with care. Finally, we should take care not to allow our natural inquisitiveness to dominate our clinical judgement.

NOTES

1. Ward, M. (1988) The nursing process, in *Applied Psychiatric and Mental Health Nursing Standards in Clinical Practice*, (eds M. J. Schreiber and K. Larson), John Wiley, New York, p. 33.
2. *Ibid.*
3. Peterson, D. R. (1968) *The Clinical Study of Social Behaviour*, Appleton-Century-Crofts, New York.
4. This principle was noted briefly in Chapter 1. The principle, as stated by William of Occam, is correctly *Entia non multiplicanda sunt praeter necessitatem*: 'Entities ought not to be multiplied beyond necessity'. As an example of this principle Robert Bierstedt describes the experience of two 17th-century chemists, Stahl and Becher, who proposed a theory of combustion according to which something called phlogiston was present in the fire to make it burn. When Priestley discovered oxygen the phlogiston theory was no longer needed and was dropped as an explanation of combustion. Bierstedt noted that Occam's Razor is used, one might say, to shave the metaphysical stubble off the physiognomy of science. See Bierstedt, R. (1963) *The Social Order*, McGraw-Hill, New York, p. 21.
5. Simpson, H. (1991) *Peplau's Model in Action*, Macmillan, London.
6. For a detailed discussion see Truax, C. B. and Carkhuff, R. R. (1967) *Towards Effective Counselling and Psychotherapy: Training and Practice*, Aldine Press, Chicago, IL.
7. Altschul has described the 'practice on which much of American psychiatric nursing is based; that of one-to-one establishment of relationships, usually of a psychotherapeutic nature .... Some half-hour of a one-to-one session between patient and nurse requires verbatim record keeping, termed a "process recording". Each half-hour session requires about 2 hours work subsequently from the nurse and a further 1–2 hours from her supervisor.' She goes on to say, 'I believe that this practice is good for nurses, but I don't know if I still believe it is good for patients'. Altschul, A. (1984) Does good practice need good principles? II. *Nursing Times*, **18 July**.
8. Maslow, A. (1962) *Toward a Psychology of Being*, Van Nostrand, London.
9. Cohen, J. (1959) The relationship of psychology to medicine. *Imprensa Medica*, **23**, 113–15.
10. Laing, R. D. (1965) *The Divided Self*, Penguin Books, Harmondsworth, p. 25.
11. Peplau, H.E. (1995) Another look at schizophrenia from a nursing standpoint, in *Psychiatric Nursing 1974–94: a Report on the State of the Art*, (ed. C.A. Anderson), Mosby Year Book, St Louis, MO.
12. Peplau, H.E. (1990) The interpersonal model, in *Psychiatric Nursing: Theory and Practice*, (eds W. Reynolds and D. Cormack), Chapman & Hall, London.
13. *Ibid.*
14. This format is adapted from Hewit, F. S. (1981) Communication skills: questions and listening. *Nursing Times*, **25 June**, 21–4.
15. For a detailed review see Argyle, M. (1975) *Bodily Communication*, Methuen, London.

Taking the history: disentangling the web

3

History is neither more nor less than biography on a large scale.

Alphonse de Lamartine

Biography is the only true history.

Thomas Carlyle

Out of monuments, names, words, proverbs, traditions, private records and evidences, fragments of stories, passages of books, and the like, we do save and recover somewhat from the deluge of time.

Francis Bacon

Not to know what has been transacted in former times is to be always a child.

Cicero

INTRODUCTION

In this chapter I shall discuss the construction of some kind of history of the person-in-care's present and past life. As I shall discuss later, I have some reservations about the role of the 'history' in care planning in psychiatric and mental health nursing. Despite having spent a quarter of a century as a nurse I remain undecided, as yet, about how it should be done. However, given the traditional role of history-taking in all spheres of health care, I would be foolish to neglect what is, at least administratively, an important subject.

I am also aware that other members of the health-care team take 'histories'. The 'psychiatric interview', conducted by the doctor, is one kind of history. Social workers, psychologists and occupational therapists, among others, complete histories, usually as a reference point for more detailed examination at some later date. Nurses have also conducted truncated histories as part of traditional practice. Since the advent of the 'nursing process' we have all been urged to be more holistic. This usually starts with extensive life-histories. At the outset, we should acknowledge that it would be foolish of nurses to conduct their own life-history survey if it simply reproduced information already available either in a medical or some other format. However, in some settings nurses may be able to gain more information than other professionals about the person's lifestyle. As a result, they may be the best people to conduct the 'history'. I see no sign, however, that such a history will ever replace the medical-psychiatric interview.

Even if nurses do not complete histories as a matter of routine, it is important that they should be aware of its contents. The information contained in the history will be of crucial relevance to nursing care planning. Who took the history in the first place is irrelevant. In many settings nurses may be asked to follow up certain facets of the person's life-history, within the context of the multidisciplinary team, where each team member contributes some (different kind of) information to the final history.

The biography

Although I have admitted my reservations about the history, it is clear that we cannot assess the person further without knowing something of who he is. Such a history is a badly written biography, drawing together important milestones in the person's life, identifying his interests, his passions, his obsessions, his work, his family, etc. Since the field of psychiatry is concerned primarily with human weakness, the history may pay scant regard to the person's assets. This is an area of imbalance that nurses may address.

The history is an important starting point for subsequent assessment since it is here that we begin to understand the relationship between the person and his life. As Goethe, the great German poet, observed: 'Life is a quarry, out of which we are to mould and chisel a character'. Our intention in trying to unravel something of the person's past is to try to understand how he became what he is now. This experience may be of value in the future. The utility of observing the past to inform the future was noted by Shelley, when he wrote: 'and thence will essay to glean a warning for the future, so that man may profit by his errors, and derive experience from his follies'.

The history should never be a 'routine administrative chore': it should aim to search out something of the real person. As Bulwer-Lytton, the 19th-century novelist, observed: 'There are two lives to each of us, the life of our actions and the life of our minds and hearts. History reveals men's deeds and their outward characters but not themselves. There is a secret self that has its own life, unpenetrated and unguessed'. Lytton may well have not been talking about the kind of 'history' we have in mind here, but his words are wise none the less. Nurses have a responsibility to look beyond the 'life of our actions' in an effort to establish some kind of record of the life of the person's 'mind and heart'.

I shall present this chapter in three sections. First I shall discuss the broad content of the history, then I shall suggest where it might lead us, in terms of further assessment. Finally I shall discuss the concept of the nursing care plan, since the taking of a history or the execution of any subsequent assessment must be seen within the context of the overall care process.

THE ORGANIZATION OF THE HISTORY

The admission profile

In this section I shall review those aspects of the history which should be taken on admission. By 'admission' I mean any point of entry to the care system: this applies equally to entry to community and hospital care systems. Of necessity, this discussion relates only to the initial entry to the care system. The admission profile represents the basic history: details of the person's identity and status necessary for administrative purposes. Since there are regional and national variations on the recording of such information, this will not be described in any detail.

- **Whom to interview?** People may be admitted to a mental health service by a variety of means accompanied by relatives, professionals or alone. They may present variously as lucid, mildly anxious or manifestly distressed. Common sense dictates how the admission profile should be completed. The person will be interviewed if willing or able. Failing this, a member of his family – or whoever accompanied him: friend, neighbour or some professional – might contribute useful information. In some cases community nurses 'admit' people-in-care who are on their caselist. This nurse may provide important information and may be a key liaison agent should the person require care and treatment in hospital.
- **Where to conduct the interview?** Ideally, the information should be taken as soon as possible after admission. The interview should be undertaken in private, except where a chaperone is considered advisable. The person should be encouraged to see from the outset that he will be handled with dignity and confidence in an atmosphere of privacy and confidentiality. Background details may be available either from the admitting agent or from earlier records if he has previously been served by the service. Where such records are available, these should be checked to rule out any change of circumstances, or omissions.
- **Content.** The person's identity should be carefully recorded: his name, including any aliases and all first names, should be checked for spelling and pronunciation. If the person has an unusual name it may help to establish rapport if you ask him for his preferences regarding pronunciation. It may also be appropriate at this stage to ask him how he would prefer to be addressed: e.g. full first name, abbreviation, some nickname or a full title, such as Mr Smith.

- **Age, sex, marital state.** The person's date of birth should be carefully recorded, along with a note on gender identity: this is important for record purposes where the person's name may not indicate sex, e.g. Frances, Vivian. Many care settings enter also whether the person is married, divorced, separated, widowed or single. Aside from identifying possible next-of-kin, it is not clear what such recording achieves. More importantly, such requests suggest that the married state is somehow the 'norm', and may be offensive to some people. In this context it is appropriate to ask women (in particular) how they prefer to be addressed in writing, e.g. Miss, Mrs or Ms. A married woman may well wish to retain her identity as a single person. In general, of course, such respect should be extended to everyone.
- **Family.** Details on the person's family should be recorded briefly. Where appropriate, does he have any children? Do they live with him? Details of age and sex. Does he live with parents? Does he have any brothers or sisters? Is he a member of an active 'extended family'? Whom does this include?
- **Domestic.** Where does he live? Does he live alone or with some 'significant others'? If homeless, does he have access to a contact address?
- **Occupation.** Is he employed at present? Where does he work and what is the nature of his job? If unemployed, what occupation did he last follow?
- **Socialization.** Who are his close friends? Does he have other acquaintances or relationships? Is he a member of any clubs or associations? Does he attend a church or have membership of any similar group?
- **Financial status.** In entering hospital, does he have any money with him? What access does he have to other funds? Does he have any outstanding bills at present? Make a careful record of any money handed over for safe-keeping.
- **Personal belongings.** A record should be made of significant items of clothing, jewellery and other possessions, especially if these are handed over to residential care staff.
- **Medical cover.** Name and address of the person's physician (and social worker if appropriate). Is he currently taking any medication? Has he been receiving any other form of medical or psychological treatment?

The purpose of this initial interview is largely to establish the identity of the person-in-care. Gaining access to such information can represent a major intrusion for the person-in-care. For this reason **the nurse should ask no question that is not absolutely necessary**. The information collected should be necessary for legal or administrative purposes, as a means of understanding the person's situation or as the basis for planning the subsequent care programme. It should be acknowledged, however, that the person is under no obligation to provide any of the above information. The nurse would do well to remember that the person is helping her to complete a necessary administrative record. It might be appropriate to register her gratitude for such assistance.

Although this information may be obtained in a few minutes, in some cases this will not be possible and the nurse may have to await the arrival of relatives to furnish these details. Most of the details fulfil administrative requirements. Other details, such as occupation and home background, give a broad indication of class background. Identification of marital status, family situation and relationships are important for identifying people who may visit the person shortly. If the nurse can quickly become acquainted with the person's family and cultural background this may enhance her status. Advance knowledge of this nature also helps avoid making an unnecessary *faux pas*, e.g. asking 'Will your wife be coming to see you today?' where the couple are separated. This information helps build a simple sketch from what he likes to be called to who may need to be contacted regarding his care.

In taking these notes it is important to emphasize that all such information will be kept strictly confidential. Many people are suspicious of such documentation. Similarly, the person or his relatives should always be **invited** to offer information, especially about relationships and finance. At no time should they feel that they are under any obligation to supply such details, however inconvenient this may be to staff. The nurse should also make it clear why she wants this information, not just for records, but so that she can get to know the person-in-care better, so that she knows who to contact if he becomes ill or needs someone and so that she can learn to help him during his time in her care.

The presenting problem

The initial interview of the admission profile involved simple questions of a factual nature. The second part of the history involves looking at the person's problems. Of necessity this is a more complex affair. This interview may follow from the admission profile, or some time may be allowed to elapse to let the person settle down before further questioning.

The aim in this next stage is to identify the person's problems, and to find out how they relate to various aspects of his life.

The problem

Some idea is needed of why the person is in hospital, has been admitted to the care of a community team, or feels that he requires care or treatment. This might best be answered by asking: 'Can you tell me what has brought you here?' This direct question is perhaps appropriate only for those who are not overtly distressed. The nurse must judge in advance whether or not the person can handle such an open-ended question. If he appears to need some help or reassurance the following, more indirect, approach might be tried.

Nurse. OK, thanks for giving me all that background information: that was very helpful. Now, I'd like to ask you a bit more about yourself ... is that OK? (Person gives assent). Well, how are you feeling just now ...? (Following reply) All right, now, I am aware that you have been having some problems. Would you tell me a bit more about that ...? (Following reply) So from what you have said, you seem to be having difficulty with ....and ... (using direct quotes from the person). Would you say that these are your main problems?

The aim at this stage is merely to get the person to specify, in fairly broad terms, the nature of his problem, e.g. 'Couldn't cope any longer' or 'Couldn't stand the voices' or simply 'I just don't know what is happening to me'. The nurse might consider guiding the person to reveal more details of his problem, using the following factors as anchors.

- **Functioning.** Has he noticed any change in his bodily function – the use of his limbs, speech, memory, eyesight, etc.? If so, what is the nature of these changes? How does the person-in-care contrast what he is like now with what he used to be like?
- **Behaviour.** Have any noticeable changes in his behaviour occurred? Is he concerned about things he used to do, or even things which he has never been able to do? (e.g. he used to be a 'good mixer' but since he moved to a new neighbourhood he doesn't seem to 'fit in'.) Is he doing things now which are upsetting to himself or other people?
- **Affect.** Does he experience any specific feelings associated with these problems: anger, sadness, fear, tension, threat, confusion, excitement, etc.? Can he describe how he feels these sensations: do they involve his body or his mind, or both?
- **Cognition.** Does he have any specific thoughts about these problems? Does he spend time ruminating? If so, what does he think about? Does he have any recurring thoughts, which just 'pop into his head'? How do these thoughts present themselves: as words, images, memories or daydreams?
- **Beliefs.** What does he think these problems mean? What does he believe is happening to him, e.g. does this mean he is going mad? being punished? being rejected?
- **Physical.** Has he experienced any physical problems associated with these difficulties: pain, loss of appetite, loss of sleep, listlessness, decline in weight and loss of interest in sex?
- **Relationships.** Have his relationships with family and friends changed recently? In what way, if any, are these changes related to his 'problems'?
- **General orientation.** Have any changes occurred in his relationship with himself? Is he concerned about: his view of 'reality'?; losing sight of his former goals?; changes in his personality?; losing contact with friends, neighbours, etc.?
- **Expectations.** What does he think is going to happen to him now that he has entered the mental health service – hospital ward or community team?

Is he going to be cured? have his problems taken away? learn to come to terms with himself? with his fears? Or does he want to change the way he lives? Does he expect to be involved in his own care and treatment? Do his family and friends have any expectations of him, or of the mental health services?

The first review of the person's situation is unashamedly 'problem-oriented'. Later it will be necessary to build a more balanced view of the person. However, for now, it might be inappropriate to study his assets. The person might even think that the nurse was afraid to grapple with his problems.

Developing the history

The information detailed above might be collected in the early days following admission to the hospital, or as part of the initial assessment in the person's home or at a clinic. The next phase of the assessment involves the development of this thumbnail sketch. The nurse now tries to expand the material, beginning with a look at his past history, his present circumstances and the way his 'problem' interferes with these aspects of his life.

Depending on the setting and the resources, this interview might take place within the first week of admission or at the second appointment – at home or in the clinic. This interview will try to develop a more balanced view of the person, emphasizing his positive features as well as his difficulties. Again, I shall discuss the interview under topic headings. There is no need, however, to follow these in strict sequence. The sophisticated interviewer may well 'hop' back and forth across topics.

- **Education.** A brief description of his schooling at basic and advanced level, especially his attitude towards his education: was it an enjoyable experience? Does he still enjoy learning? Did school put him off the idea of education? Since some aspect of his care may involve learning, in one form or another, these questions are of vital importance. Knowledge about educational background is also important in terms of judging his capabilities, e.g. for filling in questionnaires, handling abstract concepts, etc.
- **Occupation.** Further details about his present job or his previous employment. In some cases 'work aspirations' may be a more appropriate topic. Did he select his present occupation? past occupations? Was he forced into it by family or financial circumstances? How does he feel about his present job? Is there something else he would rather do? Is he proud of his position or indifferent? Does his present problem interfere in any way with his capacity to work?
- **Social network.** Is he 'a social animal'? Does he enjoy going out: cinema, clubs, dining out, the local pub? Can he describe his friends and acquaintances in terms of a network, extending from very close ties through to casual acquaintances? What kind of social life would he prefer, if any? Part

of this line of questioning may refer to the person's sex life. What does he want to say about his sex life? (Note: we should not assume that, because the person has no sex life, he is unhappy.) What improvements would he like to see in any of these areas? Is there any way that his 'problem' interferes with any of his relationships with people?

- **Recreation.** How does he use his free time? Does he have any hobbies or preferred activities – from passive ones (watching TV, listening to records) to more active ones (working for a political party, visiting people)? Is he happy with his recreation? In what way would he like to see it change or develop? Does his present 'problem' interfere with this in any way?

- **General health.** How has the person's health been during his life? How is it at present. How does he view his health: does he take every complaint to his doctor or does he tend to 'put up with things'? Does he try to maintain his health: through diet, exercise, moderate drinking, etc.? Does he see his health as his responsibility, or merely 'the luck of the draw'?

- **Drugs.** Does the person take any drugs? Are they prescribed, self-selected or illicit? How does he feel about taking drugs? How would he describe his use: regular, habitual or a last resort? What other 'drugs' does he use: cigarettes, alcohol, coffee? Has he ever tried to stop taking these drugs? Has he ever experimented with illicit drugs? What was his reaction? Does his present 'problem' cause him to use any of these drugs more often? Does he think that his present problems of living are connected, in any way, to his use of drugs?

- **Past treatment.** Apart from drugs, has he had any other form of treatment for his 'problem'? What effect did this have? Did he think that this treatment was appropriate? What did he think he needed at that time? Is there any form of treatment that he wishes he had received?

- **Coping.** The person meets with 'problems' on an everyday basis. How does he cope with these upsets? Can he provide details of how he stops himself doing things, or how he prevents problems from preying on his mind? How does he think that he is coping with his present 'problem'? What has he done, in the past, to manage, or deal with, this kind of problem? How could he handle it better?

- **Outstanding problems.** Are there any aspects of his 'problem' that the person feels are beyond solution? Has he ever felt that he couldn't stand things any longer? How did he feel like reacting – showing his anger, killing someone, committing suicide?

- **Life role.** Who is in the person's family at present (recap on first interview)? Are there members of his family whom he rarely sees? If they are important to him – such as family in Australia – how does he feel about them? How does he get on with his family: how would he describe their relationships? Do they have arguments? Does he think that this is a good thing? Do they spend much time together? What are his thoughts on this? In what way has his problem prejudiced relationships with his family?

What about his original family: what are his memories of growing up in that family? Was his family similar to or different from the family he belongs to now – if indeed he has a family? Does he model himself on anyone from his original family? What was important about this person that he wishes to imitate or emulate?

How would he describe his role in relation to either or both of these families? Is he an important or an unimportant figure? Why does he think that? What do other members of the family think of him? If he is married, how does he relate to in-laws? If he is in a stable relationship how does he relate to his partner's 'biological' family? Does he make rules and regulations for his family or partner? Does he abide by these rules himself?

The admission profile and initial 'problem analysis' are akin to a skeleton. In the development interview we attempt to put some flesh on these bones. By trying to establish some details of how the person-in-care functions and what his attitudes to himself and his world are we grow to 'know' him a little better.

This biographical interview is in no way peculiar to psychiatry: some journalists, even television chat-show hosts, may do this very well, getting to the 'nub' of the character. In the space of a few minutes – providing the person-in-care is willing – we have located him in time, place, context, culture and role. We should not delude ourselves that this is anything other than a further character 'sketch': we have done little more than scratch the surface of his life. However, a good interview, like a 'good' portrait sketch, often catches something of the sitter that disperses some of the mist which enshrouds him. Such carefully rendered features provide something of an insight into his character.

So far, we have asked a few questions and made some notes about the answers. A well designed computer might well have kept up this pace. We can take the history a stage further by making some observations on what takes place within the interview.

THE NURSE'S OBSERVATIONS

In addition to the information supplied, the manner in which it is offered may also be important. The nurse needs to make detailed 'mental notes' during the conversation of how the person-in-care appears, judging how he behaves, feels and thinks.

Appearance

The nurse should make a note of the general presentation of the person: any outstanding features, specific deformities or disabilities? Does he appear healthy, wasted, undernourished, overweight? What is his approximate height and weight? (These may be checked later at a physical examination.) How is he dressed: not so much in terms of fashion, but in terms of appropriateness to the situation? Finally, some notes on his interaction during the interview need to be made. How did he relate to the nurse: avoiding eye contact? staring? appearing distracted? What about his general posture? Did he appear tense, relaxed, edgy? Was he willing to converse? If he appeared resistant, in what way did this show?

Behaviour

Notes on his behaviour during the session should also be made. Did he use many gestures? Were they appropriate or manneristic? In terms of his overall activity level, did he appear restless or relaxed? How did he walk – hurried? limping? with any peculiar gait pattern? What about his speech? Did he speak audibly? too loudly or too softly? Did he speak too fast or too slow? Did he display any interruptions: stuttering, stammering, long pauses?

Affect

More detailed judgement of the person's affect should be made during the interview. Here we are interested in his emotional state. Here I am discussing only the person's mood or feelings during the interview: this might differ markedly from his mood at other times. How appropriate is his mood to the situation? This must be related to the topics under review. Does he appear serious when discussing serious material; relaxed when discussing lighter material – perhaps even showing humour? Or is his mood incongruous: not in keeping with what he is saying? There is a wide range of mood states that we might judge under the affect heading. The nurse should avoid looking only for stereotyped emotions such as depression, anxiety, etc. Below I have noted just a few of the possible emotions that might be expressed:

- 'Sometimes I just feel like crying. Like right now.' (Sadness)
- 'I guess that I enjoy life.' (Satisfaction/contentment)
- 'I feel trembly all over. See, look at my hands.' (Anxiety)
- 'I'm worried about what is going to happen tomorrow.' (Apprehension)
- 'What do you mean? I just told you, **twice**.' (Irritation/anger)
- 'I'm scared right now.' (Fear)
- 'I just feel lost. Out of touch.' (Alienation)
- 'I just can't be bothered.' (Apathy)

Although I have noted verbal associates of these emotions, it is possible to detect emotional state by non-verbal means. Excitement is often shown by speed of speech and movement, rather than content; pain, by ways of holding parts of the body; hostility, or suspicion by subtle looks or sidelong glances. Finally, in addition to noting how appropriate or **congruent** is the person's emotional state, the nurse should note the main affective theme. What is the main emotion shown? What is the main emotion that is voiced?

Cognition

It is a truism to say that most of the interview is a reflection of how the person thinks, or indeed what he thinks. We are not dealing with factual material. Instead we are inviting the person to give a report on certain aspects of his life. Some kind of judgement must be made as to the relative accuracy of this information. Is it true or false? Might it be distorted by his interpretation of the facts? The person's thinking – or cognition – can be considered in two ways: the way he appears to think and what he appears to think about: **form** and **content**.

Form

The form of the person's thinking can be looked at from a number of angles. I do not wish to encourage nurses to repeat the psychiatric interview. The psychiatrist's interview is designed to ascertain the form and content of the person's thinking. However, the nurse's interview should also include some observation on his thought processes. This may reinforce or help to modify the other opinion, or provide information to help the nurse's evaluation of progress at a later date.

Among the general characteristics that might be judged are the following:

- How fast does the person appear to think? Does it appear excessively fast or slow? Is he easily distracted? Does he flit from one idea to another as he talks?
- To what extent does there appear to be continuity of thought? Is he able to link the various themes in his conversation?
- Does he appear alert: sensitive to the line of questioning? Or does he appear dulled in some way?
- Does he volunteer answers in a spontaneous manner? Or does he continually wrestle with himself, looking for 'the right word or expression'?
- Is his speech coherent or does it appear fragmented, with parts of words fused together?
- Does he show any perseveration – repeating statements or words over and over?
- Does he appear to get 'stuck' on a single theme, mulling it over 'in his head'?
- Does he suddenly break off in mid-sentence, showing 'blocking' in his thinking?
- Does he seem unable to draw out ideas or be specific?
- Is his speech disrupted by disruptions to the normal association of ideas?
- Is he unable to think – or discuss ideas – in abstract terms?
- Does he coin new or unusual words?

- Does he 'invent' material as a false recall for failed memory?
- Does he constantly introduce highly personalized themes that appear to reject reality?
- Does he find it difficult to concentrate upon the interview, or to recall information?

I need hardly remind the reader that, important though these 'observations' are, they may be wildly inaccurate. Some of the disorders of thinking that have been noted briefly are very subtle. It often takes a highly trained interviewer to detect their presence. The assessment rarely relies upon the observations and judgements of a single person. Indeed, the singular viewpoint carries many hazards. Ideally, we would expect that any conclusions reached concerning the person will have involved the contributions – and discussion – of a number of parties.

Rather than fearing that we 'miss' some characteristic of 'psychopathology', we should be concerned with the danger of 'finding' something through the simple act of looking for it. If we applied these notes to an analysis of a conversation over coffee or in a pub, someone, somewhere, could be called 'thought-disordered'. For this reason I urge caution in interpreting the person-in-care's thinking.

Content

The major consideration regarding content involves the person's major themes. What does he spend most time thinking about, or talking about? Are these both the same? How does he think about himself? Does he evaluate himself positively or negatively? To what extent does he believe that he has a problem? These considerations are especially important in the case of the person who is being treated against his wishes.

At this point I need to declare my unease over the use of the term 'insight'. Often we accuse the person of lacking insight because his assessment of the 'facts' does not match ours. However, providing that we use it in its proper sense – meaning the extent to which he is aware of what is happening to him, and can think about these events – then it may be appropriate. On a similar level we should consider the person's ability to judge the significance of what is happening to him, has happened in the past or might occur in the future. What thoughts does he have about these aspects of his life?

What are the person's major worries? These may not be the same as his presenting 'problems'. Does he worry about things that have happened in the past, are happening to him or might happen? To what extent might these worries be described as 'real' or imaginary fears? How would he (or you for that matter) make such a distinction? Perhaps the simplest and commonest fear we encounter is that the person is afraid of going mad.

To what extent does the person describe material of a 'delusional' nature?

It is important to be scrupulously objective here. Many people have beliefs or ideas that are 'strange' to me. Does that mean they are delusions? Obviously not. We are concerned here with beliefs that have no discernible basis in reality. Even this definition is problematic. Some readers will own religious beliefs, or will have beliefs that might best be defined as 'spiritual' in nature. Given that these beliefs are not verifiable, does this mean that they are delusions? Again, I am obliged to conclude – 'obviously not'. I hope that the reader will concur with me.

It is easy to spot such delusions when they are extreme, but less easy to judge subtler variations on the delusional theme. For instance, if the person believes that he 'can't cope with life' and the facts suggest that he manages tolerably well, is he deluded? Perhaps again, 'obviously not'. The person may also refer to 'hallucinatory material', hearing voices or sounds, seeing sights, of which other people are unaware [1]. Again, I hesitate to say that these are not real. In the case of delusions and hallucinations I think the solution is simply to report what the person says. Rather than 'labelling' the material, let what the person thinks or believes speak for itself.

The person may also have various vague fears that preoccupy him: fear of dying, of impending doom, or of nothing in particular – just 'everything in general'. He may be preoccupied with performing certain mental rituals to prevent disasters occurring. His thinking may also project ideas about himself that appear extreme, overinflated, grandiose or unnecessarily worthless.

In this context it is important to identify any sign of suicidal thinking, which may be explicit or veiled. Is he preoccupied with morbid thoughts? Does he think a lot about death or dying? Does he ruminate about the trappings of death – funerals, death notices, graveyards? Or is he preoccupied with extreme religiosity? It is worth asking him directly whether he has ever considered killing himself. Some professionals still believe the myth that questioning a person about suicidal ideas may 'put the idea into his head' or make it more acceptable. If he is already thinking about it, and he gains an opportunity to discuss these thoughts and beliefs, the reverse is likely to be the case. Encouraging the person to discuss such ideas often offers some degree of relief. (A further discussion on the assessment of suicide can be found in Chapter 6.)

In addition to asking whether he has ever considered harming himself, has he ever thought about harming anyone else? What is his reasoning for this?

Finally, the nurse should try to judge the person's contact with reality. Typically, this can be tested by reference to the year, day, date, etc. It may be more appropriate to try judging his orientation to events that have occurred in the distant and more recent past, such as dates of weddings, starting a new job, period of last illness. This may be less obtrusive than a formal 'reality orientation' test.

WORKING WITH THE HISTORY

The concept of personal norms

The information drawn from this limited 'developmental' interview should help the nurse to summarize the person-in-care's problems, using the life history as a backdrop. We have found out a little of the stages in his life and what it means to him to operate under the name of John Smith, or whatever. We may also have discovered how his perception of 'John Smith' has changed during the course of his life. We have found out something of his problems: how they relate to various facets of his life; whether they are new or repeats; how they developed. We may have some idea of the kind of person he was before these problems emerged, and how they have grown, diminished or remained static over time.

The use of the personal history is, in one sense, less useful than it is in general medicine. In another sense it is a crucial part of the assessment process. In physical medicine, if a professional footballer breaks his leg it is clear that rehabilitation of this injury must aim at restoration of something akin to his former athletic ability. Most medical treatment involves this restoration process: find out what the person could do before he became ill and aim to restore him to 'health'. In psychiatric care the problem may not be so simple. In many cases it is not advisable for the person to 'go back'. Indeed, the idea that anyone might ever 'go back' is an illusion, since one can only 'go forward'. It may be, however, that the person's life-style before his illness was a contributory factor. Indeed, such a return to a former state of health may be entirely illusory. Perhaps the solution is to help the person-in-care to 'move forward' rather than backward.

However, the value of the personal history is in helping us to understand 'personal norms'. The 'disorder' which the person presents with today may be an exaggeration of his normal behaviour. However, his normal functioning might be viewed as 'pathological' if it was shown by someone else. For instance, a person who has always been independent, free and easy, with a joking manner suddenly becomes indecisive. He starts to have problems at work, feels obliged to plan everything very carefully and becomes very sober in his manner. He 'looks' just the same as his colleague, with whom he shares an office: indeed both behave in exactly the same way. But even he is saying, along with the rest of the workforce: 'What's the matter with you?'

Many of the problems we meet in the psychiatric field are not pathological, in the sense that oedema or diplopia are pathological. These problems represent signs of an underlying disorder that would constitute problems for all people. Changes in a person's psychosocial functioning may constitute a problem for him because this is a sign of a disruption of his 'personal norms'. Such problems may be unremarkable when found in someone else.

I said at the outset that I had reservations about the 'history'. As I have noted above, the history is an invaluable part of the assessment process. My reservation is that some nurses – indeed some doctors for that matter – seem to think that they can base care or treatment on this single assessment strategy. I have even more reservations about some of the narrower 'life-histories' that abound in clinical practice. Although it is far from exhaustive, the history model I have outlined tries to be comprehensive. It avoids looking at the person as though he were 'one-dimensional'. The questions I have suggested have some bearing on the 'problem': they either reflect ways in which the 'problem' intrudes on the person's life or they highlight assets that might be conscripted to help solve the 'problem'. Of supreme importance is the recognition that the person is defined largely by the social order around him: how he relates to this social world and the demands it makes, and the restrictions it imposes upon him. Unless this reciprocal relationship – the 'person-in-his-world' – is described in some detail, the history will be largely useless. The person does not inhabit a vacuum. The history must illustrate something of the richness of his past and present experience.

The history can tell us a lot about the person and his world. What it does **not** tell us may be more significant. The main weaknesses of the history are that it 'quantifies' so little and that what it does quantify could be so much fantasy. The problem we face in using the history as the sole assessment vehicle is that we have little of a measurable nature. How do we judge the size or scale of the person's problems? How can we use what amounts to an extended 'conversation' as a means of evaluating progress?

The second problem involves the medium of the interview. The person may present an image of himself here which is in stark contrast to his other 'selves'. Either he may heighten the intensity of his problems or he may underplay them. Although nurses often make great play of being 'non-judgemental', this stance can be taken only so far. We do not pass judgement when the information is offered to us. But once in our possession it is our responsibility, often an awesome one, to judge its validity. If we fail to honour this responsibility, the person – or some significant other – may unwittingly prejudice the course of care and treatment.

Opening doors

The nursing history can be seen as a way of gaining an overview of the person's problems against the broader canvas of his life, his world. Given the crude nature of the interview method, this picture can hardly be anything but impressionistic. This is not to say that it is not important. We need this character sketch to help us judge what we euphemistically call his 'mental state'. Without this judgement we could hardly proceed. We need to proceed further with our 'picture'. So far we have a sketchy outline of the person-in-care's problems, seen against the perspective of the world he inhabits and interacts with. From this overview we can decide where to focus our attention. Which part of his life needs to be drawn into tighter focus? We cannot, indeed should not, study closely every facet of his being. We shall use the history as a springboard for further, more detailed, enquiries. The history will help us to plan the rest of the assessment. Using some of the functional problems discussed in the next part of the book I shall discuss briefly how the history can open doors into the person's life.

The person who is dependent

A key feature of severe mental disorder is the loss of independent functioning. This is most evident in the case of a person who has become heavily dependent on family, support services or the hospital routine. Such people may suffer more from 'dependence' than from their original disorder. His reliance on others to help perform tasks or to make decisions may emerge from this introductory profile. This should lead us to consider assessment of independent functioning as a key target. We need to know: to what extent can he perform everyday routines? To what extent is he capable of, or motivated to, make decisions affecting his life? Although people who are limited in this way are likely to have many other problems, loss of independence may be a key area for closer study.

The person who is anxious

The experience of anxiety is natural to all animals. Without it we could not survive. We only stop to consider it when it gets out of hand, when it becomes unnatural. Anxiety can be a problem for a wide range of people. It is not restricted to those with so-called 'anxiety neuroses'. The history may reveal situations in which the person-in-care is unable to cope with work, relationships, stress or the myriad other 'threat' factors found in our environment. This may suggest that we need to look more closely at this experience of 'threat': what are the situations in which he feels anxious? how does it manifest itself for this person? and how severe is this problem? We also want to know: what is the effect of anxiety upon the person? his dealings with others? his life in general?

The person who is depressed

The person who experiences a disturbance of mood – occasionally feeling low in spirits, or swinging to the other extreme of euphoria and excitability – is the partner to anxiety as one of the commonest emotional problems. Depression of mood is the commonest problem and can also be seen in a range of people-in-care, including those not identified specifically as suffering from depression. The history may reveal situations where the person becomes depressed in the event of some noticeable 'loss': bereavement, financial crisis, failed opportunities. Often no obvious cause is evident. The interview may reveal evidence of depression, shown perhaps more by presentation and lack of motivation than by any verbal signals. This may suggest a need to study this area of the person's emotional functioning more closely. How can we gauge the changes in his affective state? What relationship do such changes have to his observable behaviour? In what way is this 'depressed' state a function of events in his life? To what extent does it interfere with the everyday living of his life?

The person with relationship problems

Any of the people mentioned above might also have problems involving their interaction with other people: other people-in-care on the ward, family, spouse, friends, neighbours, individuals or groups. Since much of the history focuses upon the reciprocal relationship between the person and his 'significant others', any problem met in this area should emerge quite quickly. This might lead us to study at closer range the exact nature of such problems. Does the person feel anxious in company? Does he feel 'unprepared' to deal with certain social situations? Does he have difficulty making friends or sustaining conversation? The relationship problems may be specific 'disorders' of psychosocial functioning. They might also be part of a larger problem: people who are described as suffering from depression, anxiety or schizophrenia may also experience problems in relationships. Either way, there is some advantage to be gained from defining and measuring more specifically the nature and function of such problems.

The person who is out of touch with reality

This is a rather poor alternative to the title 'someone who is psychotic'. I use this euphemism to include others who may appear to have major perceptual disturbance, but who might not be diagnosed as psychotic. People who see things or hear voices that do not appear to be there, or who discuss ideas that seem bizarre in the light of our experience, might be included in this category. As my overview of the history suggested, such characteristics may be evident from our conversation with the person. Alternatively he may tell us about his experience of such 'unreal' phenomena at other times in his life. As with the other problems mentioned, it may be desirable to collect more specific data on this problem. What exactly does he see, hear or think? Are other people aware of his bizarre status? How can we begin to measure what appears to be a facet of our higher consciousness?

Problems of living

This by no means exhausts the possibilities of 'doors' that might be opened. The corridors of mental distress are long indeed, and many are the doors that open into this area of the human condition. There are people who engage in sexual deviations and those who cannot engage in sex at all. There are those who prejudice their health by eating too much and those who starve themselves to death. There are people who attack and maim others and those who enjoy the experience of being brutalized, as well as those who harm themselves but, manifestly, not for enjoyment. The list appears endless. The illustrations of 'problems' that I have selected for the second part of this book are significant in two ways. First, they can be viewed as 'problems of living' as opposed to specific disorders: I have suggested this already by pointing out the way such problems may occur across a range of so-called 'patient' populations. Second, these problems appear to establish links, one with another, in many people who end up in psychiatric care.

Case illustration – the case of Harry

Harry was a young man of 25 when he was made redundant from his job in a tyre factory. He had a wife and two young children to support, and little money to do it. Two years later he had run up a pile of debts through trying to own what he couldn't afford, and was finally evicted from his flat for non-payment of rent. His wife returned to her parents, taking the children. Harry moved into a friend's house, leaving after a few months to lodge at a men's hostel. The hostel was for sleeping only, so Harry tramped the streets by day, avoiding any old friends or acquaintances, manifestly distressed by his downfall. Gradually, he stopped visiting his children on Sundays. Visiting his in-laws only induced great anxiety beforehand; leaving his children afterwards induced a raging despair. As his relationships dwindled he began to lose confidence. Even 'signing on' at the labour exchange became an ordeal. He thought that the clerks were laughing at his shabby appearance, talking about him behind his back. When he was called before a benefits panel, he felt he was being victimized. It was an elaborate plot to bring him finally to his knees. He began to drink heavily to relieve the depression. He drank alone. He drank to forget. When the anger inside him couldn't be stifled any longer he slashed himself repeatedly with a broken bottle, to ease the tension. The punishment was almost at an end.

The problems that we pick up in the history may be circumscribed. More often than not they will be diffuse, or linked tenuously with other disorders. In Harry's case his 'career' had a predictable quality. The loss of something prized leads to the loss of self-esteem. The loss of self-esteem leads to the loss of motivation. Loss of motivation leads to loss of action. When we fail to act, events overtake us. When the world starts to run over our heads, we are under threat. When we are under threat we need to do something to resolve the distress that threat brings. Hiding, avoiding, abusing drugs and eventually opting out of life are fairly common strategies for coping with such distress. Why mention Harry here? Well, he was one person whom I would have liked to do a complete history on: but sooner.

The history in the process

Some years ago Annie Altschul commented that the nursing process was 'the current vogue in nursing circles' [2]. Almost 20 years on she remained sceptical about its validity as a mechanism for organizing nursing care [3]. In Professor Altschul's view the choice between 'well organized "good care" ' or ' "well organized "bad care" ' seems to depend more on the skills at the nurse's disposal than upon any 'process' she uses. This is an astute observation and one that we often miss. If we plan care carefully but employ the 'wrong' information or the 'wrong' goals, we may be more likely to harm the person than if we had **not** planned so carefully!

The development of the nursing process was, primarily, an American tale with some Canadian inflections [4,5]. Only relatively recently has it become an established part of the psychiatric and mental health nursing scene in the UK [6].The development emphasizes the planning of more individualized care and a move away from task-oriented nursing. This led to the formation of the concept of holistic care [7]. Nurses have always used a planning and implementation model, even for the execution of tasks. The history of nursing would suggest that little attention was paid to the orientation of this model to individual people with individual problems. The concept of the nursing process is heavily imbued with mystique. It is heavily laden with 'scientific' jargon and 'humanistic' concern. At its root, however, the concept is simplicity itself. It may be the walking personification of 'good old-fashioned common sense'.

The care menu

As Altschul has pointed out, we must use a 'process' even when planning an evening's entertainment for friends. We need to decide what they should eat and drink and which music to play. We try to present a 'programme' that will meet general needs – promoting conviviality and satisfaction – and will also meet individual needs, such as dietary prejudices, or the execution of deviant behaviours, such as smoking. The host(ess) who devises the evening's entertainment makes judgements about which 'needs' to satisfy and which to ignore. A no smoking rule may be imposed, or an ardent carnivore may be encouraged to 'sample' the pleasures of a vegetarian dish. Here the hostess is not blindly accepting that all the guests' needs should be met. Instead a 'value judgement' is made, which may turn out well or become a disaster. The smoker may feel insulted, or may be happy that someone is trying to help him kick the habit. The carnivore may enjoy the nut cutlets, or may find his appetite unsatisfied. Where 'needs' are not met directly, such an unpredictable outcome is likely. At the end of the evening the host(ess) will evaluate the outcome of the party. What evidence was there that people were happy? What steps could be taken to ensure that the next soiree will be better?

The planning of nursing care 'à la process' seems little different from the plan of this evening's entertainment. We assess the person-in-care in order to identify his 'needs': these form the basis of the care plan. We then decide whether or not we should try to meet these needs. In some cases, one person's needs may infringe on another's, as in the case of the smoker. In other cases there may be an ethical objection to meeting a particular need. Finally, there may be the consideration that the needs of the majority will prevail over those of the individual. Once we have decided which needs to meet, we plan how to do this and, having done it, we evaluate its success. Have the person's needs been met? Is he satisfied? Have we achieved our nursing goal?

A nursing process format

This book is not about the nursing process. However, assessment is part of 'the process', thus making a brief discussion relevant. One of the more elegant formats is the SOAPE model described by Desmond Cormack [8]. Based on an original model described in the USA [9], this model cites five stages. First, information is collected about the person's complaints: subjective information, supplied by the person-in-care (S), is paired with objective information, supplied by the nurse (O). From these two categories of information an assessment is made (A). Cormack calls this the 'nursing diagnosis'. Then a plan is prepared: what the nurse will do to meet the person-in-care's need (P). Finally, the plan is evaluated, by hypothesizing what should happen as a result of the intervention (E)

SOAPE is rational, systematic and straightforward. Consequently it should be easy to use, at least with simpler, specific problems. Where the problems are more diffuse – or 'interconnected' like Harry's mentioned earlier – difficulties might occur. I have serious doubts about deciding on a single action to meet such individual problems separately. Take, for example, someone who appears depressed. He may show a wide range of problems:

- 'affective': he complains of being unhappy;
- 'behavioural': he speaks very slowly, gives poor eye contact;
- 'motivation': he says, 'I can't be bothered trying any more';
- 'cognitive': he thinks, 'I'm all washed up';
- 'physical': he eats little and sleeps even less.

Most of these problems are interconnected. Instead of individual solutions, perhaps we need a 'build-up plan', one that begins by motivating the person to become more active, which may have a spin-off to his affective level and may help improve his physical problems. Becoming more active may also reduce his low self-esteem. The next stage might involve tackling his negative affect, improvements in this area improving his behaviour, and raising his self-esteem. Then we might move on to look specifically at the cognitive problems, which might lie at the core of his difficulties.

I should emphasize that this 'build-up' care plan here is not of a different order to SOAPE, but simply an alternative formulation. I simply have an anxiety about drawing up lists of problems where they occur in a complex form and proceeding to 'pick them off' like plaster ducks in a shooting gallery.

Altschul too had reservations about 'the process'. She was particularly concerned that the care delivered by nurses should continue to 'express' the inputs of other professions. She emphasized that the care offered by nurses could not be divorced from the inputs of other staff. Altschul was concerned, too, about tabulating long lists of problems which nurses 'picked off' without due consultation with other members of the care team. As I suggested with my 'depression' example, some problems will resolve themselves, at least partially, as a function of gains in some other area. Where the person-in-care presents with highly complex problems, the basic nursing process model requires major revision. Perhaps, however, the major problem lies in the nurse's working relationships with other professionals. Can she promote a 'nursing' process that is not wholly congruent with the 'medical, psychological, social work, physiotherapy, etc.' process?

The concept of need

Most nursing theorists base their models of practice on the concept of fulfilling needs. One of the goals in the history, which figures centrally in the 'process', is the identification of the person's needs. Where I have talked about 'the problem' we could easily substitute the term 'need'. Before we close this chapter, perhaps we should consider the concept of need.

It is apparent that people have basic physiological needs for food, drink and warmth. Without these the biological self suffers and may die. We also have basic needs for comfort, shelter from the elements and security from danger. These are also concerned with preservation and maintain the basic quality of life. Much of 'basic nursing care' is concerned with meeting these needs. We assume that a person 'needs' a drink when he says he is thirsty or appears dehydrated. Usually we plan to meet these needs in advance, preventing desperate needs arising. Similarly, we arrange certain kinds of seating, or help non-ambulant people to move around, to avoid pressure sores, thus meeting the twin needs for comfort and physical exercise to stimulate circulation. In any 'basic care' situation we meet basic needs for food, drink, warmth, ventilation, comfort, avoidance of pain, injury, etc.

However, the concept of need can at times be a difficult concept. To begin with, it is largely hypothetical once we go beyond the stage of basic needs. What other kinds of needs might people have?

- a need for sex;
- a need for success;
- a need for recognition;
- a need for friendship;
- a need for control over situations;
- a need for happiness;

- a need for freedom from worry;
- a need for freedom itself.

The list is potentially endless. These needs are much more vague and subjective. I could offer you a list of 'my needs': what I think I must have satisfied to lead a full, satisfying life. Does this mean that all my needs must be satisfied, simply because I have said so?

Consider for a moment a person who experiences severe anxiety whenever he goes out. This anxiety makes him avoid leaving his house. He says that he feels insecure whenever he is far from home. He stays at home because it makes him feel secure: it satisfies his 'security need'. If a community nurse asked him how she could help, he might say, 'Arrange for my shopping to be done, and for my friends to call round, so that I needn't go out.' If we did this we would meet his 'need for security'. It may be that we would not have helped him. Would the situation be any different if the person described above was also diagnosed as suffering from schizophrenia?

A similar problem might occur with the person in hospital who is depressed. Each time he thinks about a distressing situation he feels the 'need to cry'. When asked how we might help him he says, 'Just leave me alone, I need to be on my own. I need to cry'. Again question-marks hang over whether or not we should meet these needs for privacy and emotional expression. Our great need in such situations is to be aware of the possible outcomes of providing the 'help' for which the person asks. Such awareness will help us to judge which needs to satisfy and which to ignore.

When we start identifying the person's 'problems' in the history we start to make judgements about what he needs. Someone needs to learn how to pay a compliment without feeling embarrassed. Someone else needs to learn how to cope with anxiety; to control anger; to ease the distress felt when thinking about unhappy events. In each case we are talking about the necessity for some change in the person-in-care's functioning. This is our judgement. The person may not see these needs at all. We might say that our housebound person needs to be able to go out without experiencing crippling anxiety. He sees his need for staying indoors, his need for security. The depressed person we see as someone who needs to be able to look at his life problems in a more objective manner. The person sees only the need for privacy and emotional expression.

I raise these points as a way of rounding off our discussion of the history. In the history we identify the person's problems. We see these problems against the backdrop of his life. I am suggesting that it may be incorrect to assume that the problems we identify represent needs in the person's eyes. In many cases what we see as 'needing' to be done may be the reverse of the person-in-care's need-goals. When our assessment is translated into the 'process of nursing', the needs that we identify in the person exist solely in our professional, clinical judgement. Our view should be influenced by the available body of knowledge about the identification and resolution of psychiatric distress. The needs of the person, and the needs we attribute to him, may well be in conflict. There is no obvious solution to this conflict. This is just one nettle of the assessment process that we must grasp without too much trepidation.

TAKING A 'HORSTORY'

An apocryphal tale is told about the famous American psychiatrist and psychotherapist, Milton Erickson. One day, he and a friend were in a field near his home when a horse trotted in through the gate, wearing a bridle but no saddle. Erickson waited until the horse had cantered to a stop, then he grabbed the bridle. 'I better take her back where she came from,' Erickson called to his friend. 'But you have no idea where she came from,' his friend called out as Erickson trotted off into the road.

The horse trotted along the road, Erickson gently holding the reins. Each time, the horse turned in the direction of a field, Erickson gently reined her back, and he continued on along the road. Eventually, they came to a turning and the horse took the left turning. After a couple more miles, and a few more turnings, the horse cantered into a farmyard, where the farmer grabbed his 'lost mare'. 'Hey, thanks for bringing her back .... I thought she was gone for good,' the farmer said, as Erickson dismounted. 'But where was she and how did you know where she had come from?' the farmer enquired. 'Oh about 5 miles due East', Erickson answered, 'and I didn't, but she did'.

Whether or not this story is true hardly matters. It illustrates the humanistic basis of Erickson's approach to therapy and the process of change. He assumed that the people in his care intuitively knew what was the nature of their problems and what needed to be done about them. Like the horse, people know where they have come from and – in a similar sense – where they need to go. The story is a metaphorical illustration of how 'gentle therapy' might work: when people are (metaphorically) lost, the gentlest kind of intervention involves guiding the person back to their life path and supporting them as they take their own route either back to where they came from, or onward to someplace else.

I have told my version of this story to many people over the years since I first heard it. Some have been captivated by the possibilities of such an 'empowering' approach to individual problem-solving, and personal growth. Others have told me that such metaphors are useless when dealing with real problems in mental health.

In my view the 'horstory' is the alternative to the 'history' that we have addressed so far. Whereas the history provides us with the story of the person's life so far, it offers us no indication of where the person might go in future. The reader may well comment that we have no idea where the person might be heading. Indeed, they would be right. However, given that nursing is primarily concerned with the person's human development, we need to consider how we might begin to establish where he might be heading.

Creating the future

One of the characteristics of human nature – indeed of human experience – is the ease with which we reflect on the past. Given that we have been there – the past – we can look back on it and may even learn from the experience of reflection.

Looking forward can be more complicated, since we have no real idea of what may lie ahead of us. If we are to develop a truly 'whole' picture of the person in our care, that story should include some consideration of his hopes and dreams for the future; as well as a summary of the life that has already passed.

The assessment of the person's future involves addressing his wishes, his dreams, his desires, his hopes, his expectations. These may appear – on first hearing – to be realistic or fanciful. This distinction is not as important as establishing what are the meanings – for the person – of these particular dreams, hopes, etc. In the 'horstory' we want to establish where – exactly – it might be meaningful for the person to move in the immediate or distant future. Such an assessment can be achieved – as with the history – by the use of fairly simple questions:

- 'Where do you see yourself going from here?'
- 'What do you need to do next?'
- 'What are your hopes for the future?'
- 'If you had three wishes, what would they be?'
- 'What have you always wanted to do with your life?'
- 'If you could wave a magic wand over your life, what would you change?'
- 'If, when you were asleep tonight, a miracle happened, what will you notice when you wake up that will tell you a miracle has happened?' [10]

The reader may have concerns that the person might fantasize or talk in manifestly delusional terms. At the risk of oversimplifying the process, I would suggest that even 'delusional' talk can help us develop our picture of the person.

Nurse. So, what would you like to do with your life?
Person-in-care. I don't know ... maybe ... start a rock band, play some gigs for all my fans.
Nurse. Uh-huh ... tell me more about that.
Person. Well ... like I said ... make some records ... play some concerts ... be famous.
Nurse. So what is it about that – being a rock star, having fans, being famous – what is it that is important to you?
Person. Being famous ... being **somebody**. Having people look up to you ... respected.
Nurse. And how important is that ... being respected? How important is that for you, right now?

Person. Really important. Of course it is.

I am assuming in this illustration that people always say what they mean even when they do not, necessarily, mean what they say. I assume that all people who express a need or desire to do something are, at the same time, saying something meaningful about themselves and their lives. The form in which that desire is expressed may not be as important as the underlying meaning. All of us have dreams. Many of us have 'pipe-dreams'. Rather than paying too close attention to the surface detail of such dreams, ambitions and desires, we might ask the person to tell us more about what those dreams mean for them 'as people'.

One of the therapeutic advantages of such 'futurology' or daydreaming is that it offers the person-in-care an opportunity to visualize himself as an effective, functional, fully-operating human being. Adopting this alternative view (or construction) of himself may be highly uplifting. It might also serve as a rehearsal for active steps he might take as part of his life-plan.

CONCLUSION

In this chapter I have discussed the role of the life-history in assessment. Some attention has been given to the general structure of history-taking, suggesting that three stages are evident: the administrative 'admission profile', the problem-oriented interview and the developmental interview – where more comprehensive coverage is attempted. I have compared the development of this history to the construction of a skeleton, followed by a gradual shaping of the human figure, who is the person-in-care.

This kind of assessment is based entirely on the conversational elements discussed in the last chapter. Information is supplied in response to questions, the nurse making objective judgements all along the route. From this combination of 'subjective' and 'objective' information emerges the picture of the person-in-care: necessarily crude, but a representation none the less. This picture can help us to open doors which, we hope, will lead to closer examination of important facets of the person-in-care's problems.

Finally, the profile, and all subsequent assessment information, needs to be compiled in some kind of format which will allow such information to be used as an aid to care planning and care evaluation.

NOTES

1. In the rare condition of **synaesthesia** the usual barriers between our different senses are dissolved. The 'sufferer' may be able to 'see' sounds or 'taste' textures. Such experiences are more than mere metaphors and have been reported, especially, by poets. There is a danger that such reports might be assumed to be an indication

of some hallucinatory process when, for the individual, such experiences are quite natural.

2. Altschul, A. (1977) Use of the nursing process in psychiatric care. *Nursing Times*, **8 September**, 1412–13.

3. Altschul, A. (1984) Does good practice need good principles?. *Nursing Times*, **18 July**, 49–51; Barker, P. (1995) *An Interview with Annie T. Altschul* (audio-tape), University of Newcastle-upon-Tyne, Newcastle-upon-Tyne.

4. Henderson, V. (1960) *Basic Principles of Nursing*, ICN, Geneva.

5. Little, D. G. and Carnevali, D. H. (1976) *Patient Care Planning*, J. B. Lippincott, Philadelphia, PA.

6. Ward, M. (1993) *The Nursing Process in Psychiatric Nursing*, 2nd edn, Churchill Livingstone, Edinburgh.

7. Beck, C. M., Rawlins, R. P. and Williams, S. R. (1983) *Mental Health Nursing: A Holistic Life-cycle Approach*, C. V. Mosby, St Louis, MO.

8. Cormack, D. F. S. (1980) The nursing process: an application of the SOAPE model. *Nursing Times*, Occasional Papers, **30 April**, 37–40.

9. Weed, L. (1971) *Preparing and Maintaining the Problem Oriented Record: The PROMIS Method*, Press of Case Western Reserve University, Cleveland, OH.

10. The 'miracle' question derives from the work of Steve de Shazer. See de Shazer, S. (1988) *Clues: Investigating Solutions in Brief Therapy*, Norton, New York.

Assessment methodology: an overview

Method ... makes the task easy, hinders confusion, saves abundance of time, and instructs (in) what to do and what to hope.

William Penn

Methods are the masters of masters.

Charles Maurice de Talleyrand

Every great man exhibits the talent of organization or construction, whether it be a poem, a philosophical system, a policy or a strategy. And without method there is no organization or construction.

Edward Bulwer-Lytton

INTRODUCTION

It has often been said that 'method' is like placing things in a box: a 'good' packer will get in half as much again as a 'bad' one. In this chapter I shall discuss some aspects of the methodology of assessment: ways of gaining information about the person for the minimum of effort. I want to consider some ways of obtaining a 'good' assessment: one which will be of use to nurses in the care-planning process; and to the person-in-care, in the therapeutic process. I do not intend, however, to discuss any of these methods in any great detail. Some of these methods will be discussed a little further in subsequent chapters. (An annotated bibliography is provided in Appendix B.) Neither do I intend to cover all the possible mechanisms of assessment. Instead I shall discuss here briefly some of the differences between the different methodologies, emphasizing their advantages and disadvantages.

I have discussed ways of describing the person and his life from the perspective of his personal history. This relies upon the collection of information through interviewing: the person, or a member of his family, is asked to report what he believes to be 'the truth'. This picture may be broadened by including observations made by the nurse: what she perceives to be the truth. Despite the importance of the history, I need hardly comment upon its inherent weakness, if relied upon as the sole method of assessment. Not only may the final picture of the person be of doubtful accuracy, but it may also lack the fine detail necessary for planning care or evaluating progress. As we approach the millennium, health-care systems around the world are being reformed. In the USA these reforms were driven primarily by demands made by health insurance companies. Although differences prevail across the USA, UK, Europe and Australasia, all are giving greater emphasis to the evaluation of care as a function of policy planning and funding. These changes present compelling reasons for introducing standardized psychosocial assessment methods into nursing practice. If used as part of the care planning and evaluation process, such methods help to gauge the person's response to care and treatment; and may also help us appreciate which care circumstances benefit which kind of people-in-care [1]. In this chapter I shall consider some of the methods which can add more precise and accurate detail to our assessment and evaluation of the person-in-care.

Careful study

The need for a 'system' of studying any situation is taken for granted in scientific or technological circles. In the past, many nurses have been unhappy with the concept of 'scientific method'. Often it has been seen as in conflict with the 'art of nursing', an activity that operated outwith the narrow confines of science. Nursing was often thought to be too flexible and pragmatic – not to say creative – to be defined in any systematic or scientific way. Without science, however, our view of the world would be uninformed or idiosyncratic [2].

We take for granted our use of scientific principles and knowledge in our everyday life. My labelling and interpretation of certain atmospheric events at the beginning of Chapter 1 may be simple, but are scientific none the less. The influence of science on our perception of the world is noted by Bronowski and Mazlish [3]. Commenting upon the way in which our view of the world changes in the light of scientific discovery, they argued that science influences our 'concept' of the world.

> A medieval traveller was not unobservant when he described what is obviously an elephant as an animal with five feet, one of which the animal uses like a hand. To us, the traveller's tale is ridiculous, because to us the elephant fits into the order of mammals and the unfolding of evolution ... but to the medieval man, the world had a different set of inner connections; it was organized differently.

Our conception of the world – how we **think** about it – is influenced by what we know from the world of science. In considering how we conceive that part of our world – inhabited by the people in our care – we must ask, 'What can the methodology of science offer by way of a positive influence?' In many instances, our view of our persons is often 'medieval' in character, so removed is it from the influences of contemporary scientific thought.

However, the need for some system, or systematic way of working, is not peculiar to the scientist. Even writers like Samuel Taylor Coleridge commented that 'the first idea of method is a progressive transition from one step to another on any course'. Joseph Addison, the 18th-century essayist, remarked wisely that 'irregularity and want of method are only supportable in men of great learning or genius, who are often too full to be exact, and therefore choose to throw down their pearls in heaps before the reader, rather than be at the pains of stringing them together'.

It is clear from the advice of these two eminent minds that method is an essential part of writing. It should also be clear that it must also be an essential part of the assessment of people in psychiatric care. We must give assessment the status it deserves. It is also clear from Addison's comments that the vast majority of us simply cannot afford not to be methodical. Assessment involves collecting information to construct and communicate some image of the person to others. We must be at pains to describe exactly what is there, within the parameters of as rational and 'scientific' a view of the world as possible; so that others may appreciate what we have witnessed.

METHODOLOGY: AN OUTLINE

Assessment involves collecting information and making some judgement about that information. How we go about collecting that information is the **method**. When we aim to approach the assessment of the person-in-care from a 'scientific' perspective, we often talk about the **methodology** that informs the actual mechanism of assessment. This means no more than the system of rules and methods applied within the scientific approach. When nurses try to establish a format of assessment that is reliable, irrespective of who undertakes the assessment, and provides a valid information about the person and his problems of living, the methodology they will use will – in one way or another – be scientific.

Information can be collected in two ways. We can ask the person to report on his situation, which might involve simply answering questions, or completing a record. In either of these cases we need to be confident that the person is willing and able to provide such subjective reports. We also need to be assured that he has no reason for wishing to mislead us. If we do not possess such confidence or have such an assurance, then this self-report method may be worthless.

The alternative is to invite other people to make observations on the person. It may be appropriate to ask members of his family to use their 'proximity' to the person to study him at close quarters. Where the person is in care, we may use the observations of the various members of the health care team to provide such reports.

Selecting the channel

Any of the methods discussed in this chapter could be used as subjective or objective reports. Wherever possible, information should be obtained direct from the person, either by 'self-reports' or direct observation – by studying him closely. The 'second-hand' observations often obtained from family and friends come a very poor second in this respect. We should be aware, however, that the person may mislead us – intentionally or unwittingly. In some cases the person may be unwilling or unable to provide the information needed, requiring you to fall back on the reports of others.

The comments and observations of other people can, however, serve an important function, providing information that may be known only to them, or as corroboration or contradiction of the story offered by the person. For instance, junior nurses on a ward may have much more contact with the person than the senior staff. The person may also behave differently with staff they assume to be of 'lower status'. Indeed, he may well divulge more information to more junior staff on the grounds that he feels closer to them than to senior staff or other therapists. Consequently these people can offer particular insights into the person's behaviour, known perhaps only to them.

Where the person describes a specific problem it is often helpful to ask 'significant others', such as family, or friends who know him well, to comment upon this. Their report may reinforce his description or may present a different perspective on his story. Even where the person's report is not substantiated this may also be significant: it may confirm that this is the way the person perceives the situation.

Collecting information from the person or his 'significant others' usually involves some 'informal' method of assessment. Information taken from staff is more likely to be 'formal', involving the use of some standardized method of observation or recording. The aim of the assessment will determine which information channel is selected.

- If you want to know how the person thinks or feels, or if you wish to identify his values or beliefs, ask the person.
- If you want to know what other people think or feel or believe about the person, ask those other people.
- If you want to know how the person behaves under certain conditions, either ask him to observe or reflect on his own behaviour or ask someone

else who is available to study him in these settings. (These two options may provide completely different reports.)

PSYCHOSOCIAL ASSESSMENT

Given the complexity of the human being who is the person, nurses may be expected to be involved in assessing the person across a wide range of dimensions. The various selves of the human being were discussed briefly in Chapter 1. The focus of assessment in this book is, however, wholly psychosocial in character.

Nurses might be expected, for example, to: participate in the collection of body fluids and their analysis; undertake routine physical assessments; or support physicians undertaking more complex diagnostic assessments such as CAT or PET scans. These biomedical assessment activities are often a critical part of the diagnostic process for some people, and may represent a valuable contribution to determining appropriate medical intervention. Although these assessment functions are important to physicians, however, they do not represent the 'proper focus' of nursing which was alluded to briefly in Chapter 1 [4]. The major assumption of this book is that nurses focus upon, address and subsequently become involved in the person's interaction with his environment. Given this focus the assessment methods discussed here and summarized in the bibliography emphasize this psychosocial world.

It is important here to acknowledge that the term 'psychosocial' is a very broad one, and includes consideration of the assessment of **individual factors**, such as:

- psychological and biological phenomena;
- functional (behavioural) performance;
- self-efficacy,

as well as ecological factors, which would include:

- relationships within the family;
- relationships with the wider social environment;
- interpersonal communication;
- social resources.

Judging psychosocial functioning

The psychosocial framework that has been adopted to guide the selection of measures for illustration in this and subsequent chapters, as well as the annotated bibliography, is Kurt Lewin's person–environment theory [5]. This assumes that the person's behaviour is primarily a function of his interaction with the environment. This theory recognizes that people do not function within a vacuum, but interact – creatively – with the world in which they live. The assessment methods and specific instruments summarized in subsequent chapters focus on individual 'vulnerabilities' and 'competencies'. In the same sense that people do not 'stand alone', it is assumed that these assessment methods do not function independently. Instead, it is assumed that nurses will interpret the levels of functioning revealed by any assessment, within the context of support currently available from the person's family, interpersonal or social environment.

As noted in Chapter 1, collecting information can be fairly straightforward. Making a judgement as to the significance of this information is a more complex affair. The crux of the assessment process involves a consideration of the interdependent relationship between the person-in-care and the diverse ecological factors necessary to ensure his physical, psychological and social survival. The concept of **holism**, which nurses have grasped readily as the fundamental basis of nursing practice, involves balancing these diverse and often conflicting ecological functions. Increasingly, this attempt to balance the competing influences on a person's behaviour – within the health-care arena – has been addressed by the **biopsychosocial model** [6].

THE MAJOR METHODS OF ASSESSMENT

Interviewing

Although interviewing was covered in Chapter 2, let us refresh our memory about its nature and function before we contrast it with other methods.

In an interview the nurse questions the person about his feelings, his thoughts, his behaviour or his beliefs. These questions may relate to his life in general or may be specific to things like his current course of treatment. At one extreme, an interview can simply mean 'sitting down and chatting with the person'. At the other, the person is simply asked to answer 'Yes' or 'No' to a series of questions on a checklist. These represent the extremes of highly unstructured and highly structured formats. Somewhere between the two lies the **semi-structured interview**.

In the semi-structured interview the person is asked a range of exploratory questions on various topics. His answers may generate some additional questions which need to be answered before moving on to the next topic. By contrast, the unstructured 'chat' may be seen as too rambling to lead anywhere conclusive. The rambling nature of the inquiry might even make the person uneasy, since he may feel that the conversation isn't going anywhere. At the other extreme the highly structured 'quizzing' of the person may appear impersonal and officious. Where the nurse is using a fixed interview schedule – where all the interactions are determined by the questions on the paper – the person may feel that he is being processed: that he has no part to play in this other than to supply these highly specific replies.

The semi-structured format is a common preference in virtually all situations. The conversation is orderly, without being regimented. There is room to break off at a tangent where appropriate, without losing one's place. This allows the conversation to 'flow', giving both nurse and person some security.

It needs to be acknowledged that the success or failure of the interview is tied up inextricably with the nurse's behaviour. Sources of error in the use of interviews – whether structured or semi-structured – are most often associated with the nurse, or her interaction with the person, and less often with the person himself. If the interview has been carefully constructed then any possible errors are bound to involve such 'human factors'.

The relationship

The success of the interview depends largely on the nature of the relationship which is established between the nurse and the person-in-care. This was discussed fully in Chapter 2. The interview should always be undertaken in a relatively quiet and relaxed setting. Initially, the nurse should open with general questions, aiming to achieve rapport and put the person at ease. The purpose of the interview should be given at the outset, in language that is appropriate to the intellectual and affective status of the person.

Motivation

Some people-in-care will feel threatened by the prospect of the interview. They may also feel inclined to deny, minimize or exaggerate the problems of living that they experience. For these reasons it is important to try to motivate the person to complete the interview fully and accurately. This can often best be achieved by relating the interview to the care planning process that will probably result.

The nurse's attitudes

The nurse also needs to consider, carefully, her attitudes towards the person-in-care and his problems of living before undertaking the interview. It is well accepted that if the interviewer feels uncomfortable, or feels negatively predisposed towards the person, this may prejudice his responses to her questions.

Following the method

It should hardly need stating that the nurse should follow the structure of the interview as laid down in the schedule. Some nurses choose to adapt interview schedules or take questions in a haphazard fashion, basing this on 'clinical judgement'. Such an approach will of course influence the outcome. Where an effort is being made to compare the person's experience with others, any adaptation of the interview schedule will render such comparisons invalid.

Recording

Most interviews require that the nurse makes some record of the person's responses. Ideally, this should be done during the interview, and should only be postponed until afterwards if absolutely necessary. Any postponement may, of course, lead to errors. Recording responses as they occur reduces the risk of a **halo effect** – where the nurse's judgement is information not directly related to the item addressed in the question. When the nurse postpones her recording until later, her scoring, or coding of a response to a question, may be influenced by other information only indirectly related to the question topic.

The person-in-care

It is generally accepted that the interview can have an effect on the information supplied by the person and his feelings during the interview [7]. The time of day can be crucial, especially where the person is affected by time-related variations in mood. On completion of the interview, the person should always be offered an opportunity to discuss the interview – in whole or in part.

Advantages of the interview

The popularity of the interview can be attributed largely to its simplicity. Many nurses can 'converse' with the person with little or no training. Suffice it to say that they might converse a lot better if they were properly trained. The interview may be most appropriate where the person is unable to use any kind of self-assessment. This is especially the case where the person is illiterate, or can speak the common language but has difficulty in interpreting it in writing. This may be the case where the person belongs to an ethnic minority population.

The interview also allows the nurse to check the person's understanding of a particular question. If he appears hesitant or puzzled she can rephrase it or amplify it in some way, to help him answer. This is not possible where the person is left to fill in a questionnaire or rating scale.

The interview also allows the person to give as much detail as he thinks is necessary. The semi-structured format noted above allows the person to develop a theme that may not be possible by any other means. Of course such a development is only possible if the nurse has the ability to recognize 'something significant' and can encourage the person to amplify his response.

Finally, the interview usually allows the nurse to design the rest of the assessment. Interviews are often the first 'port of call' in the assessment process. We may have no idea of what we should be studying until we have conducted a preliminary interview. This may give us the clues we need to introduce either other interviews, or other methods of assessment.

Disadvantages

Interviewing can be very time-consuming. In a difficult (or badly handled) interview, a lot of time may be spent for little reward. A successful interview may be equally costly: a lot of time is spent preparing the ground, asking general questions, probing the details and recording the person's replies. This does not take account of time lost following up 'red herrings'.

Secondly, the interview can be very demanding in terms of expertise. I noted above that many nurses are obliged to assess persons in this way with minimal training. Where the person is very confused or otherwise distressed we must challenge the wisdom of this policy, not to mention the ethics. Where the person is not distressed, but is anxious to resolve his problems, this may also tax the expertise of the nurse. Highly intelligent and articulate people can be as demanding as those who are less intellectually gifted or educationally enabled. In either case the nurse may need considerable skill to cope with difficulties or high expectations. One way to resolve this problem is to allow junior staff to develop their interviewing skills gradually, beginning with the highly structured 'quiz' which usually greets the person on admission to the service, working gradually towards a more semi-structured format.

A third problem already noted briefly is that the nurse may have a 'negative' effect upon the person. Some people become anxious during interviews, especially when they are uncertain about the aims of the interview or find it difficult to supply the answers. They may also be anxious about how their replies may be interpreted. It is clear that similar anxieties may be present when a person is asked to fill in a form. However, interview anxiety seems to stem from being looked at, when the person may feel that he is being 'scrutinized'. Although I suggested ways of offsetting this anxiety in Chapter 2, it is clear that the interpersonal nature of the interview may cause problems for some people.

Logs, diaries and records

A more formal way of collecting information from the person involves asking him to reflect on his own experience of himself. This may be undertaken by recording details of his behaviour, feelings or thoughts as they occur, during the course of everyday activity. A log or a diary will provide details of the person's actions and experience more or less as they occur. The diary may be completed once a day, such as the evening. Or the person may fill it in at 'rest points' in the day: lunchtime, at the end of the afternoon, before retiring to bed.

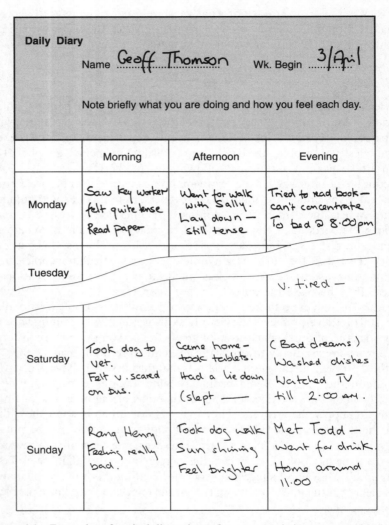

Daily Diary

Name Geoff Thomson   Wk. Begin 3/April

Note briefly what you are doing and how you feel each day.

	Morning	Afternoon	Evening
Monday	Saw key worker felt quite tense Read paper	Went for walk with Sally. Lay down — still tense	Tried to read book — can't concentrate To bed @ 8·00 pm
Tuesday			v. tired —
Saturday	Took dog to vet. Felt v. scared on bus.	Came home — took tablets. Had a lie down (slept ——	(Bad dreams) Washed dishes Watched TV till 2·00 am.
Sunday	Rang Henry Feeling really bad.	Took dog walk Sun shining Feel brighter	Met Todd — went for drink. Home around 11·00

Figure 4.1 Examples of typical diary sheets for a person being supported at home by a community nurse.

Figure 4.1 illustrates a typical diary sheet kept by a person who was being supported at home by a community nurse.

The person was asked to record what he did during the day, and any significant emotions or thoughts that accompanied these actions. In a sense this diary is no different from the traditional diary format.

This 'self-study' format can be formalized by breaking the diary down into sections, allocating space for action, feeling and thought (Figure 4.2).

This format might make it easier for the person to know 'what to record'.

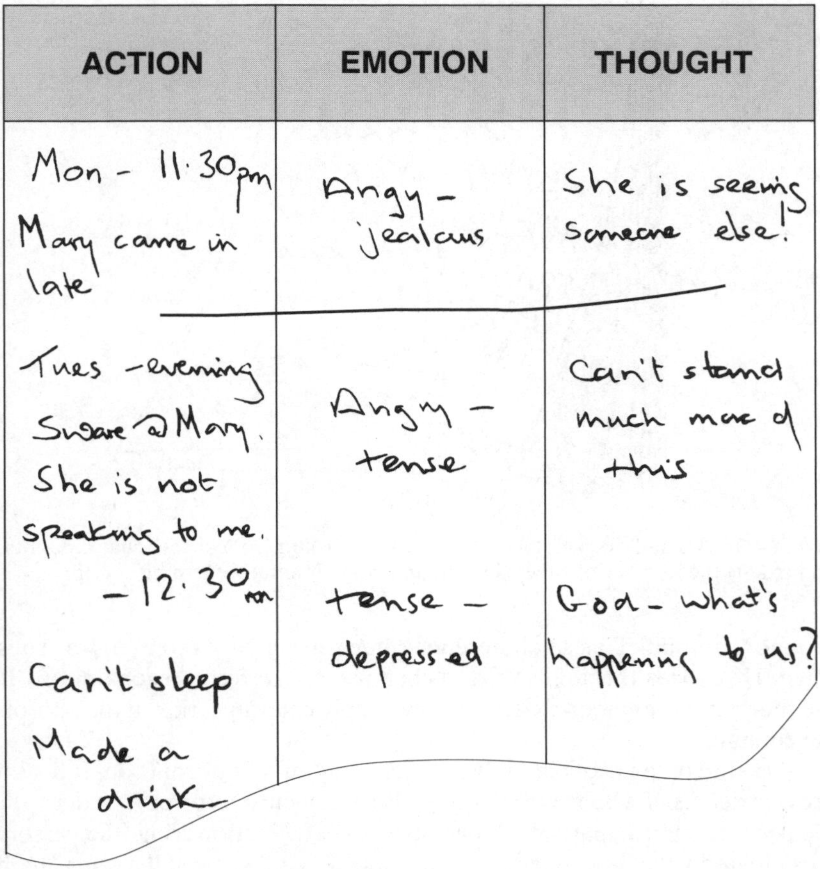

ACTION	EMOTION	THOUGHT
Mon - 11.30pm Mary came in late	Angy - jealous	She is seeing someone else!
Tues - evening Swore @ Mary. She is not speaking to me.	Angry - tense	Can't stand much more of this
- 12.30am Can't sleep Made a drink	tense - depressed	God - what's happening to us?

Figure 4.2 A diary sheet broken down into sections.

For example, if a person described a feeling of anxiety that came and went throughout the day, it might be helpful to monitor this. If the anxiety appeared to prevent him from doing things, the nurse might ask him to record any activity that was disrupted, when the anxiety began and ended, and how severe he felt it was. Such information not only provides more details about the presenting problem, but can be used to evaluate progress at a later date.

The 'daily log' format may be even simpler in structure, and can be used to record specific problems. Figure 4.3 illustrates a small notebook used to record specific 'obsessional' thoughts, and the number of times the person avoided doing things.

The person had tried unsuccessfully to use the diary format described above, but felt that the A4 size sheet was too bulky and obtrusive to carry

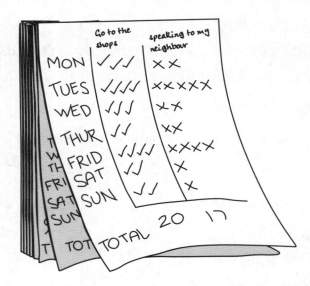

Figure 4.3 A small diary notebook used for recording (left) obsessional thoughts and (right) the number of times the person avoided doing something specific.

around with him. This small notebook, measuring 70 × 100 mm, was substituted. He carried this in his shirt pocket, using it to record each time he 'had the thought' or 'avoided an activity' by simply entering a tick in the appropriate column.

This kind of log provides only a limited amount of information. It does not provide details of where, when or how these incidents occurred, but does allow the person to participate in his own assessment. 'Empowering' the person to participate in the assessment process may be vital, especially where he has encountered failure previously with another format.

Where the person's problems tend to occur in a variety of places, at all times of the day, this method – which emphasizes the scale of the problem – may be the most appropriate.

Advantages

The main advantage of these diary formats is their simplicity. They can also be seen as 'cost-effective', since they can reveal a wealth of information for minimal staff time. This information can be 'qualitative', as the diary examples show, or 'quantitative', as in the case of the simple log. Where the person is already a diary keeper, these notes may be seen as a simple extension of routine 'self-study'. Where the person is less confident about committing his experiences to paper, it may be necessary to tailor the format to suit him. (An example is given in Figure 4.4.)

DAY	WHERE WAS I ?	WHAT WAS I DOING ? WHAT WAS HAPPENING ?	HOW DID I FEEL ?	WHAT WAS I THINKING ?
Mon	At work	J. laughed at me		Wan to run + hide
			Quaking inside Awful	
	Bus queue	Asked woman for change		
	on bus	sitting	embarassed ++	she thinks I'm stupid !

Figure 4.4   A structured diary format.

In some cases the person may make suggestions of his own as to how he might study his life experience. A young man who had been studying for an engineering degree used his home computer to design an elaborate daily diary, which included schedules for completing various activities, ratings of performance and satisfactions, as well as a section for 'failures'. This format was interesting since it was a more 'positive' record: it laid out what he wanted or needed to do – as a result there was less emphasis given to the things he failed to do.

On a final positive note it should be apparent that, if used correctly, these self-study methods may have an inbuilt therapeutic effect: they may reduce problems before treatment even begins. The student above began to focus more on his 'successes' in life as part of the assessment process. This produced a major 're-framing' of his overall view of himself.

Disadvantages

Although these diary formats require little investment of nursing time to complete, they can be costly in terms of analysis. This is the case where the person commits a lot of information to paper, some of which may be of little relevance. If the nurse asks the person to study only one area of his life experience, this advice may influence the person's observations – commonly called 'observer effect'. If the person is advised to make a note in his record each time he feels anxious, he may record more instances of anxiety than he was previously aware of. 'Looking for' anxiety may increase the person's awareness of his feelings, thereby increasing the severity of the problem. Alternatively, if the person is asked to record the number of times he avoided a situation or lost his temper, he may record less of these than we might expect. Since he is aware that these actions are 'undesirable', this awareness reduces his performance of such behaviour.

A further disadvantage with these methods is that, because they are so simple – even commonplace – the person may forget to complete them. If this is the only information that is being collected then the assessment of the person can be delayed considerably. In this context it may be helpful to design diary systems to suit individual people. If the format is seen as a special diary (like the engineering student) this may encourage the person to be more fastidious. Although this may generate more work for the nurse, the advantages of the 'personal' over the 'standard' form of record are many and varied.

Questionnaires and rating scales

This third class of methods also involves written information. However, these differ from the simple methods described above in the way they have been developed: they belong to the formal area of assessment methodology noted at the beginning of the chapter.

Questionnaires and rating scales are designed to gain specific measures of a problem area. (As we shall see later, this general rule can be broken.) These methods are usually developed from research projects, or are designed to augment scientific research. Various 'drafts' of the measuring device are tried out on a sample population, revisions or modifications being made depending on its success. When the research is complete, the questionnaire or rating scale should provide a reliable measure of a specific problem for the minimum of effort. A vast assortment of such methods have been developed to assess 'depression, dependency, disorientation or social competence'. (Examples of such scales are noted in Part Two and the annotated bibliography.) Each problem is a construct rather than a reality. Each problem comprises various behavioural, emotional or cognitive 'problems'. The questionnaire or rating scale provides only a global, or general, estimate of its severity.

Questionnaires

If the nurse wants to collect information on one aspect of the person's functioning, a questionnaire might help her do this for little effort. In Figure 4.5 an 'assertiveness' questionnaire is illustrated.

The person is required only to answer 'Yes' or 'No' to the questions. This will provide a 'total score' for assertiveness (the construct) and may be compared with the scores of persons with similar problems, or 'normal' subjects. The questionnaire can be completed by the person alone, or as the basis for a structured interview.

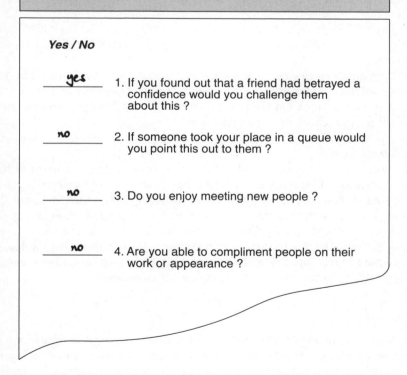

Please answer **yes** or **no** to the following questions :

If you have not experienced a situation personally, consider how you *might react* to such a situation.

Yes / No

_____*yes*_____ 1. If you found out that a friend had betrayed a confidence would you challenge them about this ?

_____*no*_____ 2. If someone took your place in a queue would you point this out to them ?

_____*no*_____ 3. Do you enjoy meeting new people ?

_____*no*_____ 4. Are you able to compliment people on their work or appearance ?

Figure 4.5 An example of an assertiveness questionnaire.

A questionnaire can also be used by the nurse to assess the person's 'orientation to reality'. The nurse asks the person to answer each of the questions, indicating whether his replies are 'true' or 'false'.

This is the simplest form of questionnaire. However, it should be apparent that the information produced by the responses will be equally simple.

Rating scales

The rating scale may also specify a problem area. However, instead of answering 'Yes' or 'No' the person is asked to rate the severity of a problem; or to rate his performance; or to indicate the extent to which he agrees or disagrees with certain statements. In principle, the rating scale may assess any area of human functioning. This might range from measures of behaviour – 'How often to brush your teeth': 'Never' (1) through to 'More than twice a day' (5); to measures of belief: 'Success in life depends on luck' – 'I agree strongly (1) through to 'I disagree strongly' (5).

Figure 4.6 illustrates a rating scale that assesses how the person might perform under certain conditions. This scale asks a range of questions about social functioning: the person indicates how he thinks he might respond, using the scale provided.

Figure 4.7 shows a scale that assesses the person's beliefs about his illness. The person is asked to record the extent to which he 'agrees' or disagrees' with the various statements.

Although there can be some variation from the standard procedure described, all such scales result in a numerical score. This score will reflect the extent to which some emotion is felt, some behaviour is performed, some thought is experienced or some belief is held.

The Likert scale

Many rating scales are described as 'Likert' scales after the originator of this scaling method. Likert found that the best results were achieved by five categories of response [8]. Rating scales invariably, therefore, measure the degree to which some behaviour is performed, emotion felt, thought experienced or belief held: usually from 0 = 'Not present' or 'Not at all' or 'Never' to 5 = 'Extreme' or 'All the time' or 'Maximum'. In principle, the Likert scale can be used to measure any phenomenon, and might also be used to measure 'change': 0 = 'No change' to 5 = 'Significant improvement'.

Advantages

The major advantage of standardized formats such as the questionnaire and rating scale is that a quantifiable measure of a problem area will be achieved for the minimum investment of time. We could spend 20 minutes interviewing a person about 'how they feel'. The use of a rating scale may require only a

How would you react to the following *everyday* situations ?

Please use the scale below :

> 1 = never
> 2 = rarely
> 3 = sometime
> 4 = often
> 5 = always

If a situation has never happened to you,
rate how you *think you would* deal with it.

Rating

___3___ 1. If you found out that a friend had betrayed a confidence would you challenge them about this ?

___1___ 2. If someone took your place in a queue would you point this out to them ?

___2___ 3. Do you enjoy meeting new people ?

Figure 4.6 A questionnaire to assess potential social functioning.

few minutes' explanation and a further few minutes' completion, and might generate a more manageable body of information for subsequent care planning and evaluation.

Secondly, since the same facets of the problem are assessed in each person, some comparison can be made between one person and another. Most published questionnaires and rating scales include 'norms', reflecting the range of scores obtained from the study of different populations – e.g. hospitalized persons or 'normal subjects'. It is possible, therefore, to compare the score one person gains on the measure with the available norms. It is possible, then, to say that 'this person is **very** dependent, depressed, lonely, anxious', etc. This judgement is not an opinion; it is made in the light of available knowledge regarding how people (in general) function.

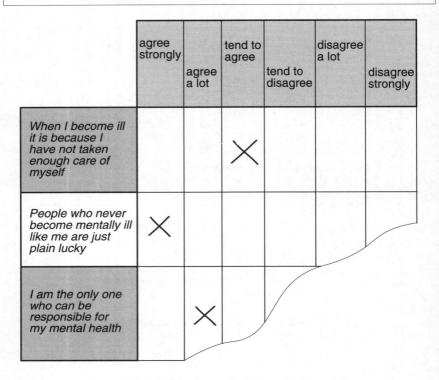

Figure 4.7 A questionnaire designed to assess beliefs about illness.

A third advantage is that these standardized methods often break a 'problem' into various component parts. This 'deconstruction' may help both us, and the person-in-care to appreciate what the problem involves. A scale measuring 'depression' might cover aspects of the person's motivation, mood, libido, appetite, etc. An anxiety scale might measure a range of anxiety-related factors: feeling tense, panic attacks, sweating, urge to pass urine, etc. These analyses are not simply whimsical exercises. The various items on the scale or questionnaire have been arrived at through careful study and experimentation. They refer to the phenomena experienced or exhibited by most people described as suffering from anxiety, depression, etc. As I noted in the opening chapter, these methods are the psychosocial equivalent of the measuring tape, the thermometer and the sphygmomanometer.

Disadvantages

The main disadvantage is that both of these methods are rigid and disallow the flexibility found in direct interviewing. The person may gain the impression that he is being 'processed'. We may appear interested only in certain facets of his problem and we may appear to spare no time in establishing what is the human significance of these facets.

A further disadvantage is that many people find it difficult to express themselves using a structured format. Where the questionnaire demands a 'Yes/No' response, the person may want to answer 'Sometimes' or 'Just in the morning'. The scale, however, may make no concession to these varieties of experience. Where ratings are involved the person, again, may feel 'stuck' if obliged to choose between 'agree' or 'disagree' categories: he may protest that 'sometimes' he does agree, but 'at other times' he disagrees. This may frustrate – or even infuriate – the nurse, who might be forgiven for thinking that the person is simply being difficult. Such a 'difficulty' may only illustrate the uncertainty of his experience.

Finally, it is apparent that some people-in-care are unhappy with the written format, even when this is completed by the nurse. The demands of the exercise may throw them completely, adding to their distress. For this reason it may be necessary to be selective where questionnaires or rating scales are involved.

Direct observation

This last category involves the most rigorous and methodical of the methods described here. Perhaps by virtue of the rigour required, it is the least practised of all the methods illustrated. That direct observation is difficult should not, however, discourage us from considering its potential value as a method of nursing assessment.

Direct observation may be carried out by the person himself ('self-monitoring'), by members of the staff team, or, less frequently, by members of the person's family. Although the principles behind the two approaches are the same, I shall discuss them separately to aid clarity.

Self-monitoring

This approach is an extension of the diary/log format. However, here the self-assessment is made more formal. The person is helped to identify specific 'targets', which are defined clearly and unambiguously, so that some kind of measure can be taken across time. The person may self-monitor any aspect of his experience, but in practice specific behaviours, discrete thoughts and clearly defined feelings may be appropriate targets.

Following the initial assessment the nurse discusses the person's problems with him, selecting the targets for self-monitoring. A decision must be made regarding the kind of measure to be taken. This usually involves an estimate of frequency – how often the person engages in the behaviour, or has the experience – or time – how long the behaviour or experience lasts.

In the **frequency count** the person records each occurrence of the target. I noted earlier how a person recorded each time he experienced an 'obsessional thought' and each time he avoided doing something. These recordings can be tallied up each day to give a daily score for each target. Alternatively, the person might be asked to record each time he:

- had a panic attack;
- drank alcohol;
- felt angry;
- spoke to a stranger;
- completed a task.

The only requirement for this technique is that each incident should be similar in size or severity to the others. Before beginning the exercise it may be appropriate to ensure that the person can distinguish 'anger' from 'jealousy' or even 'annoyance'. The easiest way to ensure this is to define what the person might do or say when he is angry, jealous, annoyed, etc.

If the intention of the assessment is to help the person clarify the nature of his problems, it might be appropriate to distinguish (for example) between 'feeling angry' and 'losing his temper'. In some examples the definition can be quite specific:

- 'drinking alcohol' can be defined in terms of units of alcohol consumed, rather than glasses of beer or gin and tonic;
- 'speaking to a stranger' might be defined in terms of the sort of interaction that could be included, which might be many and varied and might need to be listed to exclude any inappropriate behaviours, e.g. 'saying "Hello" to a neighbour'.

The best targets for a frequency count are those actions that have a clear beginning and end. The person might be asked to record every time he:

- drinks one unit of alcohol;
- introduces himself to a stranger;
- swears at his wife;
- slaps his son;
- smokes a cigarette;
- thinks 'I'm a failure';
- eats a sweet biscuit;
- refuses to do someone a favour;
- thinks he heard the voice of his dead mother.

All these 'actions' have fairly clear-cut beginnings and endings. Some may be more independent than others. However, it will be possible for the person to distinguish each occurrence of these actions, thereby ending up with a measure of at least one facet of his 'drinking', 'bad temper', 'greed', 'unassertiveness' or 'hallucinatory experience'.

In the case of other behaviour patterns it may be more helpful to measure how long the person spends engaged in the action. This is indicated where on some occasions the action may be short-lived (shouting for a few seconds) but on others it may last much longer (e.g. a violent argument lasting 20 minutes). Instead of counting the number of times the person loses his temper, washes his hands, checks the doors and windows or has a conversation with a workmate, he is asked to note roughly how long he spent engaged in the activity. These are usually called **duration measures**.

In a few cases a slightly different kind of time measure may be appropriate. Where the person is particularly slow at doing something, such as 'summoning up the courage to say "Hello" to someone' or making decisions, it may be appropriate to measure how long he takes to complete these actions from the time he started the action. This is often called a **latency measure**. In any situation where the person appears to take a long time to do something, this kind of measure is appropriate. He might be asked to record how long he takes to:

- get up in the morning;
- get dressed;
- answer a question;
- select a particular brand of peaches;
- sit down to dinner;
- answer the telephone.

These examples were all problems for one person, who described these problems-of-living variously as:

- 'I can't be bothered getting up';
- 'I can't decide what to wear';
- 'I can't think of anything to say';
- 'I can't make up my mind';
- 'I'm too busy, I'll be with you in a minute';
- 'I'm frightened who might be on the line'.

If we were to adopt a traditional psychiatric approach, these problems might be described variously as:

- apathy;
- indecisiveness;
- insecurity;
- obsessionality;
- anxiety.

If the nurse is interested in how the person lives from one day to the next, the problems all boil down to the same common denominator: the person took a long time to do any of these actions.

Self-monitoring is rarely easy. The person is required to 'watch' himself virtually all day long. If he has too many things to monitor, the activity may simply overwhelm him. If the exercise requires him to make detailed notes, it may interfere with his work or his social life and he may give up. Appropriate assessment targets and a simple observational method are of crucial importance. The person may be given a tally counter to carry in his pocket. He can clock up every 'worrying thought' or each time he 'thought people were laughing at me', without anyone noticing. Other ideas for frequency measures might be placing ticks on:

- the inside back page of a diary;
- the top of a newspaper;
- the back of his hand with a felt-tipped pen;
- the corner of a desk blotter.

These 'ticks' may be tallied up at the end of the day or week, whichever is appropriate. Alternatively the person might carry a plastic container of tiny cachous. Each time he felt 'gripped by panic' he might suck one of the cachous. If he counted the number of sweets in the box each morning and night, by subtraction, he would be able to record his frequency of panic attacks per day.

Time measures are more complex. However, with the advent of the microchip almost everyone is now sporting a stop watch within their wristwatch. Providing that one remembers to set and stop it, highly accurate timings are possible. These may be transferred to the top of the newspaper, back of the hand, etc. Such self-monitoring is unlikely to be noticed, since many people fiddle continuously with 'chronographs' anyway. Just because a simple measurement system is selected, however, it offers no guarantee that the person will continue with the self-monitoring. Unless he already is an avid 'self-watcher', such as a diarist, he is likely to tire of the chore. Consequently it is necessary to provide regular boosts of encouragement or offers of alternative ways of collecting the information. Otherwise the exercise may simply become another problem on top of many.

Too technical – too difficult?

Some nurses take the view that their 'patients' would not be capable of such apparently complex forms of self-observation. Although the methods outlined above may appear complicated, in practice, depending on the context, they may be simplicity itself. The issue here is not so much the method as the degree of collaboration with the person-in-care.

To a great extent people are 'empowered' or delimited by the nurses who care for them. All the examples offered in this book are drawn from my own clinical practice. More than a decade ago a colleague and I published a book that included examples of 'self monitoring', many of which appear – from an academic viewpoint – to be examples of 'sophisticated' assessment [9]. In reality, they were highly practical methods of collecting information in, often, less than ideal clinical settings. Their success attests only to the 'sophistication' of the nurses involved, who judged – carefully – the capabilities and motivation of the people-in-care involved. When I published an earlier version of this text [10] a psychiatrist colleague took the view that many of the methods described were appropriate only for a 'research context'. On reflection I am obliged to disagree. It has always seemed to me ironic that we use 'sophisticated' methods of enquiry in research, but whenever we are confronted with 'clinical' problems we think that it is acceptable to fall back on 'less sophisticated' methods of inquiry. The examples I have cited are examples of 'appropriate' self-assessment undertaken by people with serious forms of mental disorder in very average clinical settings. These examples should serve as an encouragement to all nurses to develop the methodology of self-assessment in everyday clinical practice.

Staff monitoring

The three simple methods described above can also be used by staff where self-monitoring is impossible or inappropriate. Take for example the case of Jeffrey, resident in an intensive-treatment facility.

It is 9.00 am. Jeffrey leaves the breakfast table and goes to his room. Here he remains for the next hour, pacing back and forth. Every so often he stops and rushes over to the window which he opens and closes repeatedly for several minutes. His pacing is accompanied by rhythmic waving of his arms, which he raises aloft. He talks aloud to himself, occasionally making a strange 'barking' sound over and over again. At less frequent intervals he stops, puts his hands over his ears, and sways backwards and forwards on the same spot.

What can we make of this behaviour? Is this some kind of psychotic manifestation? Is he engaged in some strange obsessional ritual? As I noted in Chapter 1, our task in assessment is, first of all, to collect some information about what is happening. Only when we are in possession of such detailed information should we begin playing the 'inference game' – drawing conclusions about what the information means.

Earlier in this chapter I suggested that we might help the person to study how problems come and go during the day, by noting when they began and ended and what was happening at those times. This simple analysis would be our first 'port of call' in the assessment of Jeffrey. We would be interested to know what he does, and the things that are happening around him, as he performs these various actions.

In Figure 4.8 I have illustrated how a nurse made some notes while sitting with Jeffrey in his room: similar observations were repeated at random intervals over a period of a week.

The nurse was aiming to find out whether Jeffrey's behaviour varied greatly from one day to the next. Her aim was to draw up a list of behaviours that

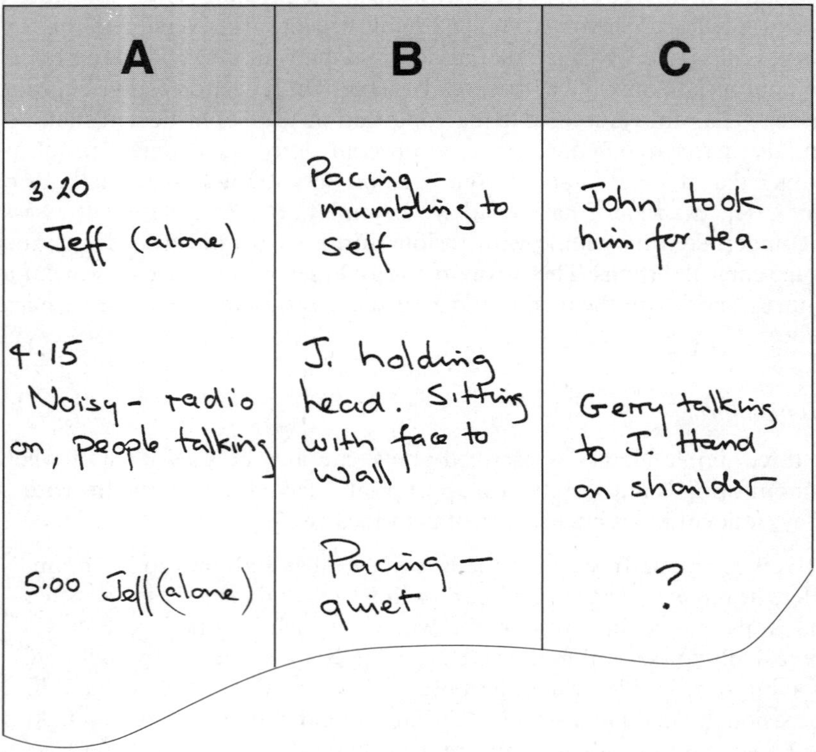

A	B	C
3.20 Jeff (alone)	Pacing — mumbling to self	John took him for tea.
4.15 Noisy - radio on, people talking	J. holding head. Sitting with face to wall	Gerry talking to J. Hand on shoulder
5.00 Jeff (alone)	Pacing — quiet	?

Figure 4.8 Notes made during staff monitoring of a person-in-care.

might be studied in detail later, in an effort to establish whether any events preceded or followed any particular behaviour. In effect, she was trying to establish whether or not there was any **pattern** to Jeffrey's behaviour. As the figure shows, the nurse recorded **what was happening around Jeffrey** — the antecedents of his behaviour (the A category). She also noted **what Jeffrey was doing** — his behaviour (the B category) during these conditions. Finally, when he stopped doing something she noted **any events that followed Jeffrey's behaviour** (the C category).

This simple **ABC** analysis aims to 'make sense' of Jeffrey's behaviour by trying to detect any 'cues' within the environment that might play a part in signalling the beginning of a behaviour, and any events that might lead to the termination or maintenance of the action.

What do these notes tell us about Jeffrey's behaviour? We might assume that he goes to the toilet area for 'a bit of peace and quiet'. Certainly, every time someone comes in he either begins swaying and covering his ears, or heads for the window. However, I do not wish to discuss possible inferences or interpretations here. I only note that through such structured observations a picture of Jeffrey's behaviour may be built up. This might prove helpful in trying to establish 'why' he does this or that. However, even where such an explanation proves elusive, these few observations will help us decide which aspects of his behaviour we might study more closely.

Sampling observations

The simple frequency, duration and latency measures could be used to quantify Jeffrey's behaviour. However, this would require a nurse to 'shadow' him constantly, noting each time he opened a window or how long he spent pacing the floor. In most situations such a detailed picture, although desirable, is an impossibility. One alternative is to take 'samples' of the person's behaviour. This is analogous to taking very thin slices at regular intervals out of a fruit cake. These slices give us an indication of what the whole cake is like, although only a tiny proportion of the whole cake is sampled.

Such a sample is reasonably accurate. However, depending upon where the slice was taken, a juicy currant or glace cherry might be missed. The same is true of the time sample. This involves taking very quick observations of the person at regular intervals. The nurse acts like a camera, taking a mental snapshot of what the person is doing at the very instant that she looked at him. These observations give us a flavour of the person's overall behaviour. If, however, the observations are too widely spaced, important pieces of behaviour – like the cake's glace cherries – may be missed.

Disadvantages

So what are the disadvantages with this method? Like the slices of the fruit cake, sampling measures only the behaviour shown where the sample is taken. Important behaviours may occur between the samples.

Another disadvantage involves the need to design new formats to suit each person. All time sample methods are similar. However, the list of behaviours to be studied and the time between samples must be worked out for each individual. Since each person is likely to show different patterns of behaviour, at different intervals, a standardized format is not possible. It is clear, however, that with a little effort a simple observational format can be worked out that will collect a lot of information for little cost in terms of nursing time.

The frequency and duration measures mentioned earlier are best used for single behaviours: counting the number of times a person loses his temper, refuses to do something asked of him, answers a question in an interview; or timing the length of conversations, hours spent working, or how long he can stand beside some feared object.

In certain instances it may also be interesting to time how long a person takes to answer a question, get dressed, remember his name, etc. These measures appear so simple that nurses are often blase about their use. Although they require little effort in their application, some planning and preparation is necessary to ensure that each nurse observes the person in the same way and records the information reliably. Many nursing reports describe the person as 'very disturbed this morning', 'hallucinated' or 'aggressive'. These observations may be accurate but, because they fail to quantify behaviour in any way they serve little purpose in evaluating change in the person. Indeed they are not observations but, rather, interpretations of something the nurse observed but has not written down.

Frequency, duration and latency measures help the nursing team to discuss exactly what the person did this morning. The report might then read: 'Jeffrey was observed to shout and scream three times this morning. He also paced back and forth, gesticulating and muttering to himself for half an hour before sitting down'.

Nurses have observed and recorded various patterns of behaviour of the people in their care for generations. With the advent of formalized nursing assessment and care planning has come the need for more rigorous forms of assessment. Today, as the effectiveness of more and more services is monitored through 'clinical audit', the simple recording methods noted here are gaining in popularity [11].

VALID AND RELIABLE?

So far in this chapter I have described four methods that illustrate the major differences between the main classes of assessment, beginning with the most open-ended observation, the interview, and ending with some measures of discrete behaviours. Two questions are worth considering, which may prevent you from wasting time using a method that is unsuited to the problem in hand or does not give you reliable results.

Validity – will the method I have selected assess what I want to assess?

It is always good policy to play your own devil's advocate. By being sceptical about what you are doing, you may see weaknesses that otherwise you might miss.

Let us assume that you have decided to interview the person, to find out how he feels. You have selected this approach because the person is articulate, intelligent, appears 'insightful' and does not appear to feel threatened when being questioned. But will this approach tell you what you want to know? Will this approach tell you how the person feels when he is under pressure at work, or alone at night? The person may be able to recall how he felt at these times. But is his memory of the event the same as his experience?

In the same vein, it is clear that what people say they have done, or are about to do, may not match their behaviour in real life. Helpful though the interview may be, it may only assess 'interview behaviour'. Any approach will only measure what it is able to measure.

Let's take another example. Let us assume that we want to assess a person's social skills. We decide to observe his interactions with other people in the clinical setting. We rate the content of his speech and his non-verbal skills, and we note the number of times he initiates conversation. This is a complex piece of observation. But are we measuring his social skills? Or are we simply noting how he functions under very specific circumstances? Will this tell us anything about how he interacts with family, friends, neighbours, workmates, authority figures, etc.?

Scepticism on this level is useful. It helps us judge the true merits of the assessment method we have chosen. Both approaches illustrated above have points in their favour. But both could benefit from some extension, either the addition of another technique or broadening of the format to cover more situations.

The question raised concerns validity. How valid is the information we are collecting? To what extent does the method measure what we set out to measure? What does the method we have selected really tell us about the person's feelings, social skills, etc.?

One problem in psychiatric assessment is our reliance on the use of what Robert Mager called 'fuzzies' [12]. These are the vague concepts that professionals often use carelessly. They are called 'fuzzies' because they are ill-defined, unquantified and – by ill-definition – unobservable. Mager popularized the use of the 'Hey Dad' test. Children tend to ask their parents to explain things to them, from their background of experience and greater knowledge. In the 'Hey Dad' test Mager illustrated how any 'fuzzy' could be distinguished from a 'performance': the performance being a description of something that is discrete, observable and quantifiable.

In Table 4.1 I have listed a number of 'fuzzies' in common use in psychiatric nursing. Beside each 'fuzzy' I have tried to restate the concept in performance terms. The novice nurse might – looking up respectfully to her patriarchal tutor – say, 'Hey Dad, show me how I can ....'

Fuzzies are a convenient shorthand. If pressed, most of us could tighten up a vague concept. We could translate it into performance terms. Often, fuzzies represent a consensus view of reality in highly simplified terms. Sometimes, however, fuzzies are grossly oversimplified versions of 'consensual reality': they are based on the assumption that we all are observing the same phenomena. It hardly needs stating that such an assumption can be hazardous to the welfare of the person-in-care.

If we do not take the time to clarify what, exactly, we mean by 'personal growth' or 'staff morale', an invalid assessment may result.

At a case review a nurse discusses a person with her colleagues.

Table 4.1 The relationship between 'fuzzies' and evaluable performances

Fuzzies	Performances
Assess this person's personality	Observe what he says and does under a range of circumstances
Study staff morale	Record attendance at work patterns and requests for transfers
Establish meaningful relationships	Listen to the person without interrupting or appearing bored
Help this person to get better	Set goals which can be monitored and evaluated
Help this person understand his illness	Identify his thoughts, feelings and illness behaviour, and how they relate to various aspects of his everyday world
Help promote my personal growth	Graph the number of times I use a performance description instead of a fuzzy and monitor if the trend is upward

Beryl has become more dependent over the last few weeks (murmurs of agreement). She is also acting out quite a bit. Sometimes she doesn't say anything but clearly is hostile (nods of approval). I think we need to assess her carefully and report back to the next team meeting – good! Pamela, would you help me progress this?

Similar conversations might be overheard in the medical, occupational therapy, clinical psychology or multidisciplinary team meetings. In each of them, although there is agreement that a problem exists, the truly independent observer might be uncertain as to exactly what the problem is. Alternatively, the independent observer might be forgiven for asking if everyone is murmuring or nodding their agreement in response to the same mental picture.

Unless a case conference ends with a clear and unambiguous statement of the goals of the assessment – in clear performance terms – the nurse's subsequent reports might be at considerable variance with the perceptions of other team members. Irrespective of how the assessment is conducted – by interview, rating scale, questionnaire, direct observation or all four – the first step must be to define, unambiguously, the target for the assessment.

Reliability – will the method give me the same information each time I use it?

This question is about reliability. By reliable I mean consistent. If any measure is 'reliable' we expect it to give the same results each time it is used. If it does not, then we might be forgiven for classifying it as unreliable.

A reliable assessment instrument or method is like a good friend: it can be trusted. If it doesn't, it is unreliable. Let us take an everyday example to explore this idea.

- A clock is a measuring device. It measures time.

- To be a valid timepiece it should always show the correct time – day or night.
- Therefore, to be valid, it must always be reliable.
- If, however, it sometimes goes slow or fast, it is unreliable. You can't trust it to tell the right time. Therefore, it is not a valid timepiece, because it is unreliable.
- However, it is possible for a measuring device – such as a clock – to be reliable, yet still invalid. The clock that always runs 3 minutes slow is reliable. You can trust it to be three minutes out – every time you check it.
- However it is not a valid timepiece. It is not valid, because it does not measure the correct time each time you check it.

Let us consider here, briefly, some examples of the assessment of people-in-care. If we give a person a questionnaire to complete, we can judge its reliability by asking him to repeat it the next day, checking whether the answers are the same. If the person repeatedly gives the same answers we might assume that the questionnaire is reliable. If we transfer our example to the physical world, this is akin to saying that if we measure our height, or weigh ourselves one day, we should expect the height and weight measures to be approximately the same the next day. If we discovered marked differences in our height and weight measures across two days we might conclude that our measuring devices were not reliable.

However, when we are measuring human phenomena – such as the behaviour, feelings, thoughts and beliefs of people-in-care – we cannot simply assume that these phenomena will remain constant and will not change from one day to the next. If, however, a measure of 'attitude' or 'generalized anxiety' varied across a short period of time, we might assume that the method of measurement was unreliable.

The issue of reliability in nursing assessment gained prominence a few years ago when a study found that thermometers in daily use gave a wide range of readings. In effect they did not measure temperature correctly. Some of the thermometers were highly consistent: they always recorded temperatures that were too high or too low. By definition, these thermometers were not unreliable: they were simply invalid. It is of little comfort to know that a measuring device is consistent. We also need to know if it is accurate: does it measure what it says it will measure?

Most standardized methods referred to in Part Two and summarized in Appendix B derive from research studies that include reports of the validity and reliability of the method or instrument. Careful scrutiny of such research reports is, however, variable in psychiatric nursing. Before we decide to use an assessment method we need to find out whether it will do the job we want in a consistent, reliable manner. Appendix A describes the process for the development of an assessment instrument which will be both valid and reliable.

ASSESSMENT GOALS

Assessment can be a many-headed monster, or it can be a bag of tools that can serve us well in unravelling the mysteries of the person. Assessment does not involve only one function. We can assess people to find out who they are – as in the life profile. We can also assess them to describe and measure their problems – the problem-oriented interview; or their assets – the global assessment.

We can also try to assess the scale of these problems or assets; here assessment becomes an evaluative tool, judging whether problems (or assets) appear to be diminishing, increasing or remaining at the same level.

Common to all these areas is the hope that through assessment we might grow to understand the meaning of the person's problems. Historically, in many areas of psychiatry there has been an assumption that the person's behaviour is merely a signal of some greater distress. I do not wish to debate this issue here. I believe that it is possible to follow this line of thinking only if we assume that the person's problems are encompassed by an idea. This idea may be held by the person himself, by ourselves – the professionals, or by society at large. However, it is not a reality of itself. The fact that many people believe in the idea of 'latent hostility' or 'repressed anger' does not make this idea any more real, only popular. Many of the problems that we are required to deal with in psychiatry involve such 'consensual realities': 'manic-depressive psychosis'; 'inadequate personality'; 'agoraphobia'; 'sociopathic disorder'. These ideas exist fundamentally in our thinking and reasoning. In a sense such ideas have a vicarious existence: they exist only through the behaviour of people whom we call 'manic depressives', etc. It is for this reason that I have emphasized the assessment of behaviour.

It is for this reason also that I have emphasized the psychosocial focus of nursing assessment.

Since the behaviour of the person is the stimulus for the generation of ideas about 'illness', 'disorder', etc., the behaviour of the person, and the real world that it inhabits, should be our primary target in the assessment process.

Stages of assessment

We have discussed a number of ways of describing the person. Through interviewing we build a picture of how he functions on various levels of experience and how he and others perceive that functioning. This is the least specific form of assessment. An unstructured interview will elicit a vast range of information about the person, his interactions with others, his past and hopes for the future. Most of this information will be non-specific: a catalogue of 'fuzzies'.

A structured interview begins the process of defining the person and his situation more clearly. Interest in the person's stream-of-consciousness begins to wane as we start to narrow our focus – looking for more specific kinds of reply. We begin to structure the situation so that his replies become more pointed, more specific and perhaps even more considered. Naturally, the person's 'freedom' to talk begins to be curtailed.

By the end of the structured interview we should have identified the areas of the person and his life that interest us. We may now wish to describe these significant aspects in more quantifiable terms, perhaps beginning by asking the person to summarize aspects of his life, his behaviour or his beliefs (his thoughts) through rating scales or questionnaires. These may produce a quantifiable measure of a certain idea, e.g. anxiety, social interaction, independence, depression. These will reflect either how the person sees himself or how he is perceived by others. These are only indirect measures. They are based upon the person's perception of himself. At a stage slightly beyond this lies the perception of the person held by others, e.g. staff, family or friends.

At the next stage in the assessment we can tighten the focus further by assessing the discrete patterns of behaviour that have been highlighted by indirect methods. By studying what he does, where, when and with whom, we can begin to quantify in greater detail the 'personality' before us. Staff or members of the person's family might record how often, or for how long, he engages in certain patterns of behaviour, under different circumstances. This would bring us closer to the target: the person's experience of these events. This is finally achieved when the person learns how to study himself closely under a range of conditions. Using logs, diaries, self-ratings and any one of a number of simple self-monitoring techniques, he can begin to describe himself in terms of his functioning in different settings.

Crude though these methods may be, they represent a form of 'personal science' wherein the person might study himself in much the same way as a naturalist might study a butterfly or bird. Of course the person-in-care has an advantage over the naturalist, as he can assess his thoughts and feelings as well as his behaviour.

CONCLUSION

In this chapter I have provided an outline of the kinds of method that may be used to look at different aspects of the person's life. Through these methods the process of assessment can range from the broadest description of many aspects of the person's functioning, obtained through interviewing, to a close-up study of one specific problem by the person himself. In selecting these methods an effort is made to pick the approach that will do most justice to the problem in hand. Examples of the use of these methods with a range of problem areas will be given in the latter part of the book.

When nurses talk about assessment one gains the impression that they assume that it is just one thing: a singular noun. Ideally, assessment should be seen as a plural noun meaning 'a range of methods used to describe and measure the problems and assets of the person'. Many nurses appear to be involved in some kind of search for their Holy Grail: the single method (preferably encompassed by no more than two pages of paper) which will tell them everything they want to know about the person. I exaggerate, of course. Yet, like most exaggerations, this contains an element of truth. When nurses are under pressure the ides of completing more assessments can be a daunting prospect. Yet that is what assessment should mean: a range of methods, each with a different purpose and each producing a slightly different picture of the person. The person's best interests will be served by exposure to a variety of assessment methods, presented by a variety of people, from the interview taken on admission to the service to the assortment of assessments organized and delivered through the therapeutic team.

When we talk about assessment, we should try to think of a battery of methods, each highlighting different facets of the person. If our intention is to reveal something of the mystery that is the individual person, we need to acknowledge that this is unlikely to be a simple affair. If we are willing to accept that the person might occupy a range of dimensions – emotional, cognitive, behavioural, interpersonal, social and spiritual – then we should also accept that a range of methods might be necessary to do justice to the assessment of such human complexity. In this sense the development of an appropriate 'assessment battery' should become our Holy Grail.

NOTES

1. Increasingly nurses are participating in the documentation of change using standardized psychosocial instruments that were once the preserve of psychiatric medicine. See Acorn, S. (1993) Use of the brief psychiatric rating scale by nurses. *Journal of Psychosocial Nursing and Mental Health Services*, **31**(5), 9–12; O'Connor, F. W. (1991) Symptom monitoring for relapse prevention in schizophrenia. *Archives of Psychiatric Nursing*, **5**, 193–201.
2. It should be noted that considerable confusion still exists over the definition of what is or is not science. The paradigmatic view – that many different views of 'reality' and the 'world' are possible – emerged formally in the 1960s with the publication of Thomas Kuhn's landmark text: Kuhn, T. (1962) *The Structure of Scientific Revolutions*, University of Chicago Press, London. The debate that Kuhn stimulated was developed further in the 1970s: Suppe, F. (ed.) (1977) *The Structure of Scientific Theories*, 2nd edn, University of Illinois Press, London, and has continued up to the present day: Casti, J. L. (1992) *Paradigms Lost: Images of Man in the Mirror of Science*, Abacus Books, London.
3. Bronowski, J. and Mazlish, B. (1963) *The Western Intellectual Tradition*, Penguin Books, Harmondsworth, p. 134.
4. Barker, P., Reynolds, W. and Ward, T. (1995) The proper focus of nursing: a critique of the caring ideology. *International Journal of Nursing Studies*, **32**(4), 386–97.

5. Lewin, K. (1951) *Field Theory in Social Science*, Harper, New York.
6. Banchik, D. (1993) Psychiatric assessment and case formulation, in *Handbook of Psychiatric Mental Health Nursing*, (eds C. G. Adams and A. Macione), John Wiley, New York, and Evans, M. E. (1992) Using a model to structure psychosocial nursing research. *Journal of Psychosocial Nursing and Mental Health Services*, **30**(8), 27–32.
7. Brown, G. and Harris, T. (1978) *Social Origins of Depression*, Basic Books, New York.
8. For the original reference see Likert, R. A. (1932) A technique for measurement of attitudes. *Archives of Psychology*, **140**, 140–55.
A more recent classic theoretical text is Ghiselli, E.E., Campbell, J. P. and Redek S. (1981) *Measurement Theory for the Behavioural Sciences*, W. H. Freeman, San Francisco, CA.
9. Barker, P. and Fraser, D. (eds) (1985) *The Nurse as Therapist: A Behavioural Model*, Croom Helm, London.
10. Barker, P. (1985) *Patient Assessment in Psychiatric Nursing*, Croom Helm, London.
11. O'Connor, F. W. and Eggert, L. L. (1994) Psychosocial assessment for treatment planning and evaluation. *Journal of Psychosocial Nursing and Mental Health Services*, **32**(5), 31–42.
12. Mager, R. F. (1972) *Goal Analysis*, Fearon, Belmont, CA.

PART TWO

Some specific applications

The field of psychiatric and mental health nursing embraces a vast canvas. Once life was simple – so we thought – and involved nurses caring only for those who were manifestly ill. Now we have included in our focus the concept of promoting 'mental health' as well as addressing mental illness.

In Part Two we continue our search for what ails the person. Perhaps, by dint of our attention to this goal, we may also come to appreciate – if not understand – what exactly we mean by the concept of 'promoting mental health'.

Our focus in Part Two is upon the classic ailments associated with mental ill-health: anxiety, mood disturbance, relationships with 'reality' and relationships with others. These chapters involve, by necessity, a consideration of the person's relationship with himself and his 'world'. As a conclusion to this section a short consideration of the assessment of the environment is included, especially the world shared by the nurse and the person-in-care.

Method will teach you to win time.

Goethe

The assessment of anxiety: the rust of life | 5

Present fears are less than horrible imaginings.

Shakespeare

All fear is painful, and when it conduces not to safety, is painful without use.

Samuel Johnson

Better be despised for too anxious apprehensions, than ruined by too confident security.

Edmund Burke

INTRODUCTION

We tend to view anxiety as a circumscribed problem, sometimes even as a disease or illness. Anxiety is, however, a natural and relatively common experience. We cannot afford to live without some degree of anxiety for long: we would either be flattened by the convenient passing of a truck, or consumed by the first tiger seen in our suburb for years.

Clearly, many different kinds of anxiety exist. Also, there are different degrees of the experience. One constant is that anxiety always occurs when we are under threat – when we are too close to a speeding lorry or a creeping tiger – or when we interpret threat, an interpretation that may be a distortion of reality. Threat is the key. The greater the threat – perceived or actual – the greater the anxiety. We need to feel threatened to become anxious.

Despite the impression that anxiety is a modern phenomenon, born of our hi-tech age, it is clear that it has troubled women and men down the ages. Apart from stimulating essential fight-or-flight mechanisms, anxiety has also served as the fuel for many a literary and artistic mind. The expression of anxiety through art is common to most 'primitive' cultures, e.g. talismans, voodoo masks and dolls, highly formalized demons and spirits. Such 'abstracted images', which draw out anxiety-evoking stimuli from common objects or images, have been found in Western culture only since the beginning of the 20th century. Abstract art – whether primitive or modern – is thought, however, to reflect the deeper anxieties at large in a society.

The growth of abstract art in modern times coincided with growing preoccupations with themes of death and decay and the anxiety of living and dying in general [1]. In the world of literature such anxieties are well illustrated in the works of writers like Samuel Beckett and Harold Pinter, both from the world of the so-called 'theatre of the absurd'. It is now commonly assumed that the work of such writers reflects man's experience in a world shorn of all certainty; a world that generates a conflict between our hopes and our fears [2]. What such writers and artists are telling us is hardly new. When people lose – or believe they have lost – the ability to control or cope with their world, they become anxious. In art such loss of control may be symbolic – similar to traditional superstitions. Such fears may have a more practical base. Our 20th-century 'cultural anxiety' has been highly Eurocentric. It began with the aftermath of the ritual slaughter of the First World War; was calmed by the 'good fight' required by the Allies in the Second World War; rose sharply with the 'Cold War' scenarios of the 1950s; peaked with the insanity of the nuclear arms race in the 1960s to 1980s; and, following a short lull, is peaking again as Eastern Europe seems set to collapse within its own borders.

As we approach the millennium the West has lost its well-established 'bogeyman' in Communism and appears increasingly threatened by various examples of fundamentalism and nationalism. *Plus ça change* ...!

We might well argue, however, that such 'cultural anxiety' is justified – given the sociopolitical context. On the other hand, much of the anxiety addressed in this chapter will involve an **unreasonable** or dysfunctional fear of the unknown, or even the non-existent. Such fears appear to have plagued us through the centuries. Thomas Jefferson, the American president, complained once: 'How much have cost us the evils that never happened.' Another American statesman, Benjamin Franklin, advised us 'not to anticipate trouble or worry about what may never happen. Keep in the sunlight.' The problem seems to be, however, that it is difficult to follow Franklin's logical code. Nearer home, the Irishman Edmund Burke recognized the difficulty of quelling the threat that arises from within: 'No passion so effectually robs the mind of all its powers of acting and reasoning as fear'.

The 'fear' that our powers of logic and action are so vulnerable may have led Franklin Roosevelt to ask for a world that was founded upon four freedoms, one of which was freedom from fear. One way to be 'free' of fear is to rise above it – through the exercise of logic – or otherwise to sidestep it. The man or woman who can place his fear or threat in a logical context is likely to experience a reduction of anxiety. The trick is of course to be able to manipulate those scarce commodities reason and logic.

Anxiety as a construct

A construct is a statement about some aspect of a person's internal state. In simple terms it is the way we describe the private events that we assume have an influence, or bearing, on the public aspects of a person's behaviour. The construct 'anxiety' appears to derive from the translation of Freud's use of the term *Angst*. Originally derived from the Latin *anxietas* ('anxiety, trouble of the mind'), or the stem of *angere* ('choke' or 'oppress') [3] the term is used to denote the experience of negative affect and physiological arousal that is 'similar to the sensation of having food stuck in one's throat' [4]. Although Freud never defined specifically the important features of anxiety, it became the key component in his theory of behaviour disorders. Through time the term has grown in stature, almost achieving a status as a 'thing' in its own right. We often talk about anxiety as though it had a separate existence from the person's experience of it: something we **suffer from**. As we move – or return – to a holistic perspective of human functioning, we might reconsider 'anxiety' as something that defines who we **are** at some moment in time.

It has been noted that anxiety can be viewed from a number of angles, almost like a multiple personality [5]. Sometimes we look upon it as simple behaviour, when we talk about a person 'appearing anxious'; or as a personality type, when we say that someone is an 'anxious individual'; and even as an explanation of the way someone behaves – she drinks 'because she is anxious', or he behaves like that as a 'defence against his anxiety'.

Peplau [6] provided a highly detailed description of the characteristics of anxiety that are universal – including common elements, regularities occurring across ethnic and cultural contexts. Anxiety, in Peplau's view:

- is a subjective affective experience, felt as unpleasant uneasiness, apprehension, dread or uncanny sensation;
- is an energy that cannot be observed directly – what is noticed are its effects;
- is triggered cognitively by an input of real or imagined, internal or external, personal or situational material, perceived as threat;
- is an immediate physiological reaction, evidenced by increased heart rate, sweating, trembling, irritability, vertigo, etc.;
- is an awareness of apprehension, felt discomfort and physiological reactions, often in the absence of awareness of the precise nature of 'cause';
- is adaptive, in the sense that it warns of impending threat to survival – particularly the survival of the self-system;
- occurs in different degrees;
- may reflect a predisposition within families.

This description – besides providing a rich and concise overview of the construct – warns us against taking anxiety too lightly. As pressure on mental health services mounts, unscientific distinctions between 'serious mental illness' and 'the worried well' have arisen. People who experience anxiety are all too easily dismissed as 'the worried well'. However as Peplau has shown, anxiety embraces a dual threat:

- a threat to biological integrity, disturbing the homeostasis of temperature control, vasomotor stability, etc.;
- a threat to the self-system, disturbing the maintenance of established views of self and the values and patterns of behaviour used to resist changes in self-views [7].

Peplau noted that when our world view is destabilized – as when the firm earth beneath our feet suddenly collapses when an earthquake occurs – we become awash with anxiety, if not terror. She offers two clinical examples of how challenges to the self-system (a personal world-view) can stimulate anxiety and terror, which might appear 'inexplicable'.

Case illustrations

A woman with a very beautiful face tells the nurses, loudly and often, that she is ugly. The nurses (kindly) rebut the patient's self-view, telling her 'No, you are so beautiful', or 'I wish I had your lovely face'. The woman – using a razor blade – slashes her face: this confirms her self view (**now** she is 'ugly') and relieves the anxiety evoked by the unmet expectation.

During therapy, a woman tells how her father 'hated' her, her mother 'couldn't stand' her, her sister was always 'disgusted' with her – all her life 'nobody loved' her. The therapist tells her, 'Well, I love you', and the woman runs screaming through the unit, wrecking furniture, and finally is restrained and secluded [8].

When the world does not turn out the way we expect it to – unmet expectations – crippling anxiety may result.

If one thing is clear from the vast body of research conducted over the past 60 years, it is that anxiety is not any one thing. It is neither an emotional state nor a personality type, nor an underlying cause of behaviour. Perhaps the most succinct description was offered by Paul, who described anxiety as a shorthand term for a very complex pattern of behaviour, saying that anxiety 'is characterized by subjective feelings of apprehension and tension accompanied by, or associated with, physiological activity' [9]. These feelings – for clearly it is not one single feeling – can occur in response to things that happen to us (external events) or the way we think about what is happening, or has happened, or is about to happen (internal events). To some extent this may help us to appreciate how some anxiety can be seen as natural or 'normal' – for instance when we meet genuinely threatening events like a tiger in the High Street. The stereotype of 'abnormal anxiety' is perhaps the situation where people become anxious in the absence of any such obvious threat. Here, we conclude – rightly or wrongly – that the problem is all inside their heads.

Freud argued that anxiety occurred in greater or lesser degrees in almost every form of mental disorder. How anxiety manifests itself is the nub of the issue, and clearly suggests what might be 'going on' in the person's life. The 'agoraphobic' avoids certain places that generate anxiety. In doing so he does not feel anxious. If he did not engage in such avoidance he would feel helpless in the face of whatever demands being in public might make on him. The person with a 'separation anxiety' feels the absence of support or reassurance – perhaps from a parent, partner or some 'significant other'. The restoration of the 'support or reassurance' eliminates the anxiety.

Existentialist theory suggests that anxiety equates with our dread of being alone, or of being nothing. Without the reassurance given through a relationship the sense of self is threatened.

Channels of anxiety

The anxiety construct can be seen to operate through three main channels (Figure 5.1).

First of all the person shows certain patterns of **motor behaviour**. He may tremble, shake, stutter, back away from a situation or try to escape or avoid the situation completely. This channel represents aspects of anxiety that are visible to the onlooker: we can pick up 'signals' of what we assume to be anxiety. This is especially the case where the person appears uncomfortable, or is manifestly 'running for his life'.

The second channel involves certain **cognitive processes**: what the person says to himself about the situation and how he interprets his reactions to the situation overall. In this channel the person may attribute certain threatening characteristics to objects or situations that others do not interpret as threatening, or he may simply tell himself that he cannot face or cope with the situation. He may also 'report back' to himself privately, telling himself that his motor behaviour is further proof – if needed – of his inability to handle or cope with the situation. This is, of course, a very private channel. Access is

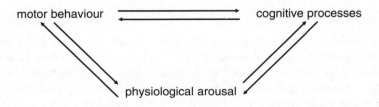

Figure 5.1 The anxiety triad.

only possible if the person agrees to report to the nurse what he is 'reporting back' to himself.

The third channel involves **physiological arousal**: the function of the sympathetic branch of the autonomic nervous system. Typically, the person reacts as though he were under serious life-threatening conditions. He may show changes in heart rate, blood pressure, respiration, muscle tension, sweating, etc. These are the classic features of autonomic arousal. Other less commonly reported phenomena may be evident that can lead to people assuming that they are going to collapse, or even die, since the display of arousal is concomitant with a state of severe illness.

All three channels of anxiety are commonly reported. All anxious people need not, however, report all of them to the same degree. Some people may experience severe arousal and 'report back' negative thoughts about the situation and their performance, but may appear calm and composed on the surface. Because they manage to control their motor behaviour they manage to disguise their anxiety. A person who is frightened of cats but who does not wish to make a fool of himself, might conceal his anxiety by failing to report it to others. This does not mean that he does not feel it autonomically, or register it cognitively: 'I felt as though I was going to collapse …. I just couldn't stop thinking about it looking at me … but I couldn't make a fool of myself by running away from it'.

In other situations someone might experience arousal and some avoidance behaviour – for instance, when speaking in public for the first time. However, he might attribute this to excitement, or 'a normal state of affairs': 'Oh, I felt terrible … couldn't stop shaking. I couldn't even look at the audience. But I guess everyone feels like that the first time'.

Finally, in the classic fear situation – the dentist's chair – people experience anxiety but make no attempt to avoid the situation. Presumably, the pain of any treatment is less than the discomfort of toothache. Although all three persons in these examples managed to cope with their anxiety, this does not mean that we should not assess it. These examples illustrate the need to establish what anxiety means for the person involved. What does the person do that denotes anxiety? What does he think about what is happening to him? And how does his body react to the situation in terms of autonomic arousal?

An unnecessary title?

Some authorities have argued that the term 'anxiety' is a redundant construct. There has been a strong drive, especially within behaviourism, to drop the term, even as a piece of descriptive shorthand. Instead, attention has been paid to the situations that give rise to anxiety, either within the environment or within the person's own information-processing and physiological functioning. I have some sympathy for this idea. As I noted earlier, there is a danger that we might attribute 'disease' status to something that is no more than one person's way of reacting to a set of circumstances. The advantages of using the three-channel model of anxiety can be summarized as follows:

- It provides us with a framework for collecting information about the manifestation of anxiety, or what is actually happening in the case of this person.
- This framework allows us to collect details of how the three channels operate across different situations, across time or across treatment.
- This information helps us to model our treatment or care plans. Careful examination should reveal the kind of behaviour, thought patterns and physiological arousal that should be the focus of any intervention.

Even if we accept the general construct of anxiety, and the implication that this is symptomatic of a personality type, we must question what we have gained by deploying such a label. To meet the needs of the person we must identify the function of his anxiety. Then we must ask, 'What does the label anxiety tell us about the person that is not contained in the three-channel description of his problem?'

THE ASSESSMENT OF ANXIETY – THE ANXIETY ANALYSIS INTERVIEW

The anxious person is rarely ever in any doubt about the nature of his complaint. He may be unaware of its origins, causes or other explanations. He is never ignorant of its presence. With this in mind I shall attempt to describe how the interview would try to unravel some of the mysteries of his anxiety state. Using the three-channel model described I shall illustrate a range of possible questions.

The nurse–person relationship

Before discussing the mechanics of the interview let us acknowledge that assessment of the anxious person is rarely easy. The temptation to 'spare no blushes' and 'get straight to the point' is a tactic that may, ultimately, be to the nurse's disadvantage. Many people may choose to discuss some trivial fear or phobia, perhaps as a cover for a more severe problem they find difficult to disclose, especially to a relative stranger. I am not suggesting that problems which are identified quickly should be disregarded in search of some deeper anxiety. Rather, I am warning against the danger of taking the person at 'face value', especially where insufficient time has been given to establishing a positive relationship within which the person may feel comfortable. He already feels under threat: if we want him to disclose details about his problem and his reactions to it, we must avoid threatening him further.

It is important to spend some time simply talking to the person about how he feels, in fairly general terms. Give him a chance to warm up for the interview proper. Many anxious people may feel inhibited about talking about deeply entrenched fears or worries to a complete stranger. Within this rapport-building session, ask the person how he feels about being questioned.

- How does he feel about being interviewed repeatedly by doctors, different nurses or social workers?
- Does he feel that this is an intrusion?
- How does he feel about you?

Give him a chance to articulate these worries, if they exist – anxiety about the process of the interview. This casual conversation will help the person find out something important about the nurse: that she is honest, open and sincere. She is not afraid of resistance or rejection. She is also interested in the person, rather than just his 'illness'. The nurse is trying to encourage the person to trust her: trust her with his deepest fears, his irrational-sounding worries, the concerns that at times he thinks are no more than foolish ravings and that cause him some embarrassment.

If the person expresses any disquiet about the interview, time can be set aside to resolve these anxieties before it begins. By offering the person 'the first shot' – a chance to make himself heard before the probing begins – the nurse may reduce his anxiety about the whole assessment significantly. The spirit of collaboration begins here, and forms the platform for the rest of the assessment. Once this rapport has been established, the nurse can begin to look with the person at the nature and context of his anxiety.

Exploratory questions

The opening question should be broad, allowing the person a clear field to say anything he wants about how he feels, thinks or acts when he is anxious. The nurse's task is to pick up statements, asking him to elaborate to gain more detail:

> 'You told me earlier that you get very anxious. Can you tell me what that means to you?'
> 'You feel awful? How exactly do you feel? Where do you feel it?' (Looking for physical sensations, such as giddy, sweating, palpitations, tense, etc.)
> 'You say that you just panic? What do you do when you panic? ... and what sort of thoughts are running through your mind when you feel like this?'
> 'How bad would you say this feeling is? I mean, is it always the same? Or does it vary? How long does it last? ... I see ... and what is "a long time"?'

In these open-ended questions the nurse tries to shape up a more detailed picture of anxiety, in the person's own words. This might cover:

- Motor behaviour: what he does. Does he fidget, get up, walk around, leave the situation, turn away, chain-smoke, talk a lot, get stuck for words?

- Thought processes: what does he think? What does he imagine or visualize? 'I can't stand it. I'm going to collapse. It's getting closer. They're looking at me. I must look a fool. My heart's going to burst.'

The nurse's intention is to help the person express himself, taking care not to put words into his mouth. Don't ask questions like 'Do you ever feel really tense?' unless the person is finding it difficult to express himself. During the interview reinforce the joint nature of the exercise by summarizing:

OK. Let's have a look at this. You said first of all that you .... Is that right? Do you want to change that in any way? I'm just trying to see it as closely as I can from your angle. So that I can understand how you feel.

If the nurse intends to make notes this should be discussed with the person at the outset, making explicit the aim of note-keeping – to act as a guide to greater understanding of the problem for nurse and person.

'When do you usually feel like this?'

This second question tries to identify the situations (or conditions) under which anxiety shows itself. Again the question is open-ended. Follow-up questions will try to nudge the person gently towards identifying objects, people, places, events, activities, etc. which relate directly or indirectly to his experience. His anxiety may be focused clearly: fear of dogs, heights, insects, injections, disease or confined spaces are examples of a range of 100 or more specific phobias. In some cases the person may feel anxious only when in the presence of this focal object, animal or situation. It is important to clarify that other situations have not been neglected, especially where one specific situation stimulates high anxiety.

The focus of anxiety

It is impossible to deal clearly with anxiety without relating it to the situation that 'triggers' or stimulates it. Within this question it may also be appropriate to ask further clarification questions: '... and what is it about spiders that you don't like?' or 'You feel anxious in shops? What is it about shopping – the store, the people, crowds, talking, the queues, traffic in town? Can you tell me exactly?'

The person may have more generalized problems, where a number of situations trigger anxiety. Here it is important to find out which situations are more of a problem than others. For instance, what kind of people trigger anxiety? Strangers, people he knows well, crowds, close contacts? Alternatively, what sort of 'things' does the person think might harm him? Contact with people, food, animals, toilets, dishcloths, dust? The person may experience anxiety across a range of apparently unrelated situations such as these. Anxiety may be even more generalized than this. The person might feel anxious when meeting people, when he is alone, when on buses, when in shops, when he is in his garden. Highly generalized anxiety like this is often called 'agora-phobia' or 'the agoraphobic syndrome'. Although there are common focal situations reported by a number of 'agoraphobics', all such people need not have problems with exactly the same situations. Consequently it is important to keep an open mind on what might trigger anxiety, rather than trying to diagnose 'agoraphobia'.

In this context it is worth noting that some persons report 'impressions', where their experience of the situation is more important than the situation itself. For instance, many people with a diagnosis of agoraphobia describe feeling anxious in any situation where they cannot identify 'security'. This leads to anxiety in 'public' places, which diminishes when they reach some 'private' place such as home, or even up a side-street. Other people may describe their impression of an interpersonal contact: 'My mother really stifles me'. The person's evaluation of the 'stifling presence' of his mother is perhaps more obvious than the fact that he is in the same room as his mother. He may be aware of this 'stifling presence' even when she is not present: this impression may be stimulated by familiar objects, the room or even memories of his mother.

Finally, there is the most generalized anxiety state of all: the so-called free-floating anxiety. This appears to be unrelated to any situation. Research shows that this phenomenon may not be quite as inexplicable as we once thought [10]. It may be that the experience of anxiety is related to the person's perception of events that may already have passed, may be ongoing or may be imminent. In some cases this perception may be 'subconscious' and the person may need some assistance to detect his thoughts and beliefs about himself and his situation. Even if we accept the traditional concept of free-floating anxiety we may be able to tie this to events – such as the time of day, when awakening or falling asleep, when lying down, when in the bath, while eating, etc. The anxiety may, however, be unrelated to any event. In such cases the nurse should attempt to establish when it is present and when it is absent.

Although the illustrations given of possible 'related events' are fairly classic, I hope that I have indicated the potential breadth of influence. Indeed, some precipitants of anxiety are not concrete events. For some people it may be the thought of doing something (or not having done something) that produces anxiety. This leads us to the next question.

'Do you ever feel anxious just thinking about something? Perhaps some-thing that has happened, or maybe is about to happen?'

These closed questions aim to identify any 'anticipatory anxiety'. There are a number of situations where this is likely. The person who has been in hospital for any length of time may feel apprehensive about returning home again. What is it about 'living in the community' that frightens him? Many people are apprehensive about meeting people, going to formal functions, making complaints, being interviewed for a job. All of these involve the person's expectations about what might happen. The person may be painting a vividly threatening scene, which may be more threatening than the reality. To clarify the source of his anxiety the nurse should arrange for the person to specify thoughts, images and memories that trigger anxiety. If the person finds this difficult, he might be helped by being invited to do an action replay, rerunning the situation where he last felt anxious in his imagination.

'I understand how difficult it is for you to answer these questions. Let's try a little experiment. Let's see if you can recall what you are thinking, whenever you get anxious. I often think that this is like an action replay – you know, like we see on sports programmes. Lie back and close your eyes. Now just run through, in your mind's eye, what happened the last time you felt anxious. (Pause) Let's take that incident you mentioned just now. When you started to feel tense in the sitting room, with the other people. Imagine that you are in your seat. OK? Try and picture what is going on around you. OK? Who can you see? What are they doing? How are you feeling? Are you thinking anything about them? Is anyone else about? Are you thinking anything as all this is going on? That's good. Keep it going. Just try to re-live the situation. Just like an action replay.'

The nurse should note the person's comments during this exercise. Afterwards she can clarify the relationship between what he was thinking and what was happening around him. This may reveal his 'expectation' that someone was going to say something to him, or do something. This expectation may constitute the threat.

'We have described how you feel when you are anxious, and what sorts of things appear to be related to those feelings. How do you think you handle those situations?'

Here the nurse is trying to help the person to evaluate his problem. Although we assume that the person is distressed by his anxiety reactions there may be times when he feels that his reactions are acceptable, given the pressures of the situation. In this context we are trying to get a balanced evaluation of his anxiety. We want to distinguish the times when his reactions are appropriate (when he is 'under threat') from the times when his reactions appear dysfunctional.

In discussing his reactions it is important to ask whether he ever contributes to the situation which leads to the anxiety experience.

Case illustrations
A man once described how he felt anxious each time his wife went out on her own. He was afraid that she might be seeing other men. It might be important to ask him whether he has ever done anything, or not done something, which might cause her to want to hurt him. He may have quarrelled unnecessarily with her, or failed to show her affection.

A man is frightened that people may be laughing at him; has he ever done anything to cause them to express this attitude? Is he socially unskilled in some way? Does he tend to make indiscreet remarks? In this context it is important to broaden out the assessment to include other possible deficiencies: things the person has not done, errors he has made, skills he may lack, etc., that might contribute in some way to the creation of the anxiety-evoking situation.

'What happens when you get anxious? How do you cope with it? What do others do, such as members of your family?'

Here we are looking at the outcome of his anxiety. All our actions lead somewhere. They all have some outcome, however subtle. Here we are trying to find out what happened after the onset of the anxiety.

- Does the person run home from the shops?
- Does he call his doctor and go to bed?
- Does he take medication to try to calm himself?
- How does he feel after taking such action?
- Does he feel differently after avoiding a crisis?
- Do his 'coping tactics' make him feel better or worse?
- If he feels better, does this last or is it short-lived?
- What do other people do to try to help him cope?
- Does he approve of their actions?
- Does he ask for such assistance?
- How does he feel about being helped in this way?

By the end of the interview the nurse should have a clearer idea of what the person calls his anxiety reaction. This can be summarized in terms of how he feels (physiologically), what he thinks (cognitively) and what he does (behaviourally). These three channels will be related to some situations that appear to trigger these reactions. These situations may be real, in terms of things which actually happen, or they might involve the anticipation or expectation of what might happen. Some idea of the relative severity and fluctuation of the person's reactions should also be possible. For example, is his anticipatory anxiety worse, the same or less than anxiety related to 'real events'? It may also be possible to open out this picture by inviting the person to evaluate his reactions. How appropriate does he think they are? How does he compare his reactions to those of his friends, family, etc. in the same situations? Finally, we would try to gain an insight into how he copes with anxiety. What measures does he take to resolve his difficulty? What do other people do to encourage his tolerance or avoidance of stress?

What I have described resembles a cognitive–behavioural analysis of anxiety. It provides a simple framework for exploring the person's experience of anxiety. In Peplau's view no substantial therapeutic work can be accomplished until the patient is aware of their anxiety and is able to share this awareness with the nurse. 'Helping psychiatric patients to recognize and name anxiety as such, when it is occurring, is a learning experience which psychiatric nurses can provide [11].'

I have not entertained the alternative view of anxiety as a personality trait. I assume that our purpose in assessing anxiety is to help the person overcome or come to terms with this problem. The personality model of anxiety is something of a dead end in this respect: change is seen either as an impossibility or very much a long-term venture. If our aim is to help the person in the short term, this three-channel model seems to be the most straightforward way of understanding the person's plight. More importantly, it is clear that this structure provides a comfortable working model for nurses who are unfamiliar with the analysis of complex psychological problems. One of my goals in presenting this anxiety analysis model is to allay some of the anxieties of the nurse called upon to pursue such an assessment.

The last stage of the assessment interview involves asking the person for any additional comment. Is there anything he wants to add? Does he have any questions about what has taken place? In this interview the nurse has tried to encourage the person to adopt the role of 'collaborator' rather than 'guinea pig'. It is appropriate, in winding up the interview, to invite him to comment, or perhaps make a suggestion about where the assessment might go next.

THE ASSESSMENT OF ANXIETY THROUGH INDIRECT METHODS

Much valuable information may be obtained through interviewing. In some instances this can be a lengthy and arduous process. Often important points are missed. This may be due to the person's anxiety, the pressure on time, or the nurse's lapses of memory. A wide range of questionnaires and rating scales may be used as an adjunct to the interview (Appendix B). These may help to amplify points raised in the interview or may yield wholly new pieces of information. Methods of indirect assessment have several advantages and only a few disadvantages.

In their favour is the fact that a lot of information can be obtained for very little nursing time. The person can be instructed briefly in the completion of the scale. The information is analysed at the nurse's convenience. The methods I shall illustrate here describe how anxiety may be 'revealed' within different situations and disorders. They provide a useful picture of various facets of the problem, covering areas which the nurse might not have considered in her interview. To some extent a 'good' rating scale looks like a godsend to the less experienced nurse, who may feel that she needs pointers or guidance.

However, there are also disadvantages. These paper and pencil methods rarely tell us anything like the whole truth. People are often unhappy about having to answer 'True' or 'False' to questions to which they would like to answer 'Sometimes' or 'It depends on the situation'. The situation-specific nature of anxiety is one of the main arguments against the traditional personality trait theories. These assume that the person will act in exactly the same way in any situation because of the action of his underlying 'anxious personality'. In reality people vary enormously in their reactions across different situations. This causes some problems for the more specific kinds of anxiety rating scale. The range of situations offered may be too limited to catch the person's actual response. Another problem is that although people may answer truthfully, what they say they would do is not always the same as their actual practice. Consequently it is important to be cautious about relying too heavily upon the person's reported anxiety. What the person reports on paper may be different from what he experiences in reality.

If nothing else these scales provide pointers for further questioning or investigation. For example, following the first interview the nurse might choose an appropriate scale and show the person how to complete this. She returns later to collect and score the scale, using the findings as the basis for further discussion with the person. These findings might lead to self-monitoring by the person himself or closer observation of the person's responses by members of the staff team.

What kind of method shall we use?

Many nurses use nothing other than their eyes and ears to assess people, simply because they do not know where to start in selecting rating scales or questionnaires. Even if they had access to such methods they might not know how to use them. I can appreciate their difficulties. Most indirect methods have been developed by psychologists and psychiatrists, and are often used only in research programmes. However, if a method of assessment has proved useful, then as many people as possible should learn to use it. Where would we be if only doctors used thermometers?

The methods I shall discuss here show some of the 'classic' features of a rating scale or questionnaire. Consideration will be given to their relative strengths and weaknesses.

The assessment of specific fears or phobias

The Fear Survey Schedule (FSS) has been used in clinical and research settings since 1956 [12]. In the intervening years a number of variations have been developed. The length of these various schedules ranges from the original 50 items to one with 122 factors listed [13]. A vast amount of research has been done in an attempt to identify the 'best' schedule. Sadly, no clear answer is available. As with many of the indirect measures discussed in this book, these studies have employed university students as the key sample population. The scores used represent, therefore, a biased sample: younger, well-educated, possibly more affluent individuals. As a result, the value of such 'norms' for comparison purposes may be limited.

The schedule does, however, have an important function. It can be used to screen fears or phobias in a person who is manifestly anxious. One of the most popular schedules is the one developed by Wolpe [14]. This covers 91 fear situations: 'being in a strange place', 'flying insects', 'sick people', 'a lull in the conversation', etc. The person is asked to indicate how unpleasant or upsetting he finds each situation. A five-point rating scale, ranging from 'Not at all' (1) to 'Very much' (5) is used for all items. Studies of students suggest that women score significantly higher than men, and report differences in their ratings of specific fears. Both men and women rate 'fear of failure' highest. However, women are more troubled by dead people and rejection by others than men, who rate looking foolish and seeing one person bullying another as more threatening.

Despite my scepticism about the value of norms, it is clear that we cannot accept the person's scores at face value. High scores need not necessarily indicate 'a problem', especially where such a fear is shared by most of the population. However, the scale can show how widespread the person's anxieties are. The various situations on the schedule can be grouped together under categories: fear of 'noise', 'tissue damage', 'social-interpersonal situations', 'animals', 'classical fears' and a 'miscellaneous' category. This kind of screening may be helpful in identifying a class of fears, where they are evident. Often a person presenting with a singular fear may show a range of other fears, following completion of the Fear Survey Schedule. Such findings are obviously crucial in terms of planning an appropriate anxiety reduction treatment programme.

The Fear Questionnaire is a similar schedule that uses only 23 items [15]. In the first item the person is asked to describe his 'phobia' in his own words. In the succeeding 15 items fears involving (for instance) hospitals, being watched or stared at are rated using a nine-point scale. The person is asked to indicate whether he would not avoid the situation (0) through to 'Always avoid it' (8). A total score is gained through adding items 2—16. The person then identifies any other situations that he might avoid, again using the same rating. Finally he is asked to rate how troublesome he finds various 'feelings', e.g. 'feeling irritable or angry'. Again a nine-point scale is used to rate the degree of disturbance by these feelings. This is a very useful schedule for distinguishing 'agoraphobic' problems from other common phobias: 'blood-illness-and injury' and 'social phobias'. The scale allows separate scoring for these three phobic areas. Apart from its cost-effectiveness in identifying the presence of various common fears and phobias, the schedule offers a simple yet effective way of monitoring the person's progress during treatment.

The facets of anxiety

We noted earlier that the assessment of anxiety needed to be multidimensional. William Zung, an American professor of psychiatry, noted that although there was a wide range of methods available for anxiety assessment, either as an affect, a symptom or a disorder, there was no standard method for recording and evaluating anxiety **as a clinical entity**. By analysing existing scales and noting differences between one and the other, he argued that such was the disparity between different scales that no common target was evident. The rating scale he designed was intended to meet the following criteria. He wanted to devise a scale that would assess the presence or absence of all significant anxiety symptoms, but would also quantify the amount of anxiety present by a short and simple method.

The method he finally devised is available in two formats. The first is a scale that can be completed by the person himself and the other is completed by a member of staff based upon her observation of the person in an interview. Zung's scale [16] is based upon his analysis of a range of other descriptions of anxiety disorder. These commonly refer to various **affective** symptoms, e.g. apprehension, fear, dread, helplessness. They also describe a range of **somatic** symptoms – disturbance of the:

- musculoskeletal system (tension, tremors, weakness, restlessness);
- cardiovascular system (palpitations, increased pulse and blood pressure);
- respiratory system (dizziness, choking, constrictions in the chest, paraesthesia);
- gastrointestinal system (nausea, vomiting, anorexia);
- genitourinary system (urinary frequency or urgency);
- skin (flushing, sweating, pallor);
- central nervous system (loss of concentration, poor memory, irritability, sleep disturbance, insomnia, nightmares).

The rating scale devised for use by staff is called the Anxiety Status Inventory (ASI). This covers five affective and 15 somatic symptoms. A guide is given to help the clinician to interview the person, using the same approach with each person. For example, in relation to 'mental disintegration', on the 20 items on the scale, the person would be asked, 'Do you ever feel that you're falling apart?' His answer would be rated on a four-point scale. This describes the **severity** of the symptom: How intense is it? How long does it last? How often does it occur? The scale awards a score of 1 if the symptom is not present at all, is very slight or does not last long. A score of 4 is given if the symptom is severe in intensity, lasts a long time, or is present most of the time. The following extract illustrates the use of the scale.

> **Nurse**. Have you ever had times when you felt yourself shaking or trembling?
> **Person**. Oh yes, often.

Nurse. When was the last time you felt like that, within the last week?
Person. Yesterday, when I was speaking to my daughter on the telephone.
Nurse. How bad was the trembling? (Intensity)
Person. I would say pretty bad. I could hardly get my coins into the slot.
Nurse. How long did it last? (Duration)
Person. Only a minute or so. Maybe not even that long. Till I started talking.
Nurse. Over the past week how much of the time would you say that you felt like that: having these trembling attacks? (Frequency)
Person. Oh, perhaps every other day. Sometimes twice a day.

A score (1–4) is then given which, in the judgement of the interviewer, represents the severity of the particular symptom. This judgement should try to balance what the person describes with what the person observes. For instance, the person may say that he never experiences tremors, but may be shaking visibly during the interview. In making the judgement it is clear that, if the person shows a particular symptom, describes it or acknowledges that it is a problem, then a high score must be given. If the symptom is not shown, reported or complained of, then a low score may be given. The real difficulty lies in attributing the intermediate scores.

Each of the 20 items should be considered independently. The interviewer must finish scoring one before moving on to the next. At the end of the interview a total score can be given by adding up the scores, the maximum score being 80 and the lowest possible score 20.

The same 20 symptoms are presented on a simple rating scale for completion by the person. This is called the Self-rating Anxiety Scale (SAS). For example, the symptom 'restlessness' provides the statement: 'I feel calm and can sit still easily'. The person must indicate one of four responses to this statement by circling 'None or a little of the time', 'Some of the time', 'A good part of the time' or 'Most or all of the time'. This self-report method has been worded so that some of the symptoms are phrased symptomatically positive, suggesting that 'I do not have a problem in this area'. Others are worded negatively, suggesting that 'I do have a problem here'. This is a safeguard against the person detecting a trend in his answers.

A code for scoring the scale was provided in Zung's original article. Once completed, a total score can be converted to an 'index score' by dividing the score achieved by the total possible (80) and multiplying by 100. The person's score can now be compared with those persons surveyed on Zung's original study. This can help to judge 'how anxious' the person under review is compared with other psychiatric persons. As noted earlier, there are some difficulties in comparing people in one country with a sample population in another. Of paramount importance is the fact that an evaluation of change or progress can be made using the total scores. Also, it is possible to identify specific symptoms clearly, evaluating how severe they are and how they change across time.

This is a valuable assessment method which can be used by nurses with limited experience. It provides a major advance on other existing scales and, through its 20-item anxiety analysis, provides the novice nurse with a valuable framework to dismantle the complexity of the anxiety state.

Zung's scale can be used as a short-cut to identifying exactly how the person feels when he is anxious. It can also be used as an adjunct to the identification of the situations which provoke anxiety, in these various forms. Consequently Zung's scale has widespread applicability, from specific to more generalized anxieties. For instance, a person who is afraid of going out of his house can tell the nurse exactly how he feels in a variety of situations by using the Zung scale in conjunction with the FSS. This will identify where he becomes anxious and how he feels. The combination of the Zung scale and the FSS may prove useful for a wide range of anxiety problems. However, there are other anxiety-related disorders that are more specific and require a slightly different approach.

Coping with anxiety: the obsessional individual

A common means of coping with anxiety is through the performance of 'obsessive–compulsive behaviour'. Although it is traditionally viewed as a specific neurosis, obsessional thoughts (ruminations) and actions (compulsions) are to be found in other psychiatric disorders. Here I want to discuss briefly how the presence of these dysfunctional strategies may be clarified. I call these patterns of behaviour 'dysfunctional coping strategies', since this seems to be the simplest possible explanation of their function: the person engages in obsessive–compulsive behaviour to avoid feeling anxious. Typical examples involve taking steps to avoid contamination, avoid making mistakes, etc. In keeping with our original discussion, the person anticipates some 'threat' and takes steps to avoid it. These coping strategies usually become more of a problem than the perceived threat is ever likely to be.

In line with my earlier argument about the diagnosis of disorders, I see little value in labelling the person as 'an obsessional'. It seems more important to describe in what way his behaviour reflects an obsessional state. What are the key patterns of action or thought that trouble him, or those around him? In line with the functional analysis of anxiety already described, it is appropriate to identify the situations in which 'obsessional' behaviour take place, the events that appear to make it more or less likely and what happens as a result of these patterns of behaviour. A key question to be asked is: 'How would you feel, or what do you think would happen, if you didn't perform this behaviour?' It is also important to try to gain the person's views on these thoughts and behaviours. Persons presenting with severe 'obsessional disorders' often maintain that these behaviour patterns are not a problem to them. In this context it is crucial to assess the person's view of the 'problem' and also his attitude towards change.

Screening obsessional behaviour

A number of sophisticated scales have been developed to assess obsessional behaviour. Many of these have been concerned with identifying obsessional personality traits [17]. Critics have noted that the items in such questionnaires tend to be non-specific, e.g. 'I tend to brood for a long time over a single idea'. This often means that information from such 'measures' tells us little about how the person practises obsessional behaviour. More specific and highly complex methods have been developed, such as Cooper's Leyton Obsessional Inventory [18]. This provides information about obsessional symptoms and traits. Although different questions are asked for these two categories, some questions are simply phrased differently to try to identify traits appearing in the absence of behaviour. For example, on the subject of cleanliness the person would be asked: 'Do you regard cleanliness as a virtue in itself?' (a trait question) and 'Do you hate dirt and dirty things?' (a symptom question). The person is required to answer 'Yes' or 'No' to 69 questions related to thoughts, checking, dirt and contamination, dangerous objects, personal and household cleanliness, order and routine repetition, overconscientiousness, indecision, hoarding and meanness, irritability and moroseness, health and punctuality.

Cooper acknowledged that the inventory has some problems, including the time it takes to complete, estimated at around 45 minutes. He also noted that, despite its rigorous appearance, the inventory was far from comprehensive. In particular it lacks many of the more unpleasant obsessional symptoms, such as blasphemous, obscene or violent thoughts. He also noted that the person cannot complete the inventory unaided. The person supervising the completion of the inventory must follow a detailed set of instructions in order to minimize any variations due to her participation.

From a nursing viewpoint it is clear that this method could be useful in selected cases or perhaps in the hands of certain nurses. However, a more convenient method of gaining an insight into obsessional problems may be the Maudsley Obsessional Compulsive Inventory, developed by Rachman and Hodgson [19]. Their intention was to construct a simple questionnaire to assess the presence or absence of certain obsessional rituals. The inventory carries 30 questions, to which the person has to answer 'True' or 'False', circling one or the other. They are told that there are no trick questions and that the answer should be given quickly without spending too much time thinking about the exact meaning of the questions. Typical questions include 'I frequently have to check things (e.g. gas or water taps, doors, etc.) several times' or 'I can use a well-kept toilet without hesitation'. The scores on the inventory can be collapsed into categories of different types of obsessional–compulsive behaviour, e.g. checking, cleaning, slowness and doubting.

If considered desirable, it is possible to judge 'how obsessional' is the person under review, by comparing his scores with those of the two sample populations.

The nurse in a standard clinical situation might wish to set her sights lower, perhaps using the inventory to pinpoint the extent to which the person complains of checking, cleaning, slowness or doubting. It should be noted, however, that this scale carries only two questions related to obsessional thoughts (ruminations) and is therefore not really appropriate for people who present with this kind of problem.

Other problems: other methods

The three assessment formats described above reveal the nature of the anxiety problem, the situations in which it shows itself and the kind of avoidance tactics in which the person engages. Among the many other indirect methods in use are the following:

- The Symptoms of Stress Inventory (SOS) [20] measures all types of stress symptoms. The inventory carries 94 items, which reflect physical, psychological and behavioural responses to stress. The inventory takes about 10 minutes to complete using a 0 (Never) to 4 (Very frequently) scale, usually measuring the person's experience over the past week. Total and subscale scores may be calculated allowing comparison with norms established for men and women.
- The Symptom Distress Checklist 90-R (SCL-90-R) [21] is a 90-item scale that measures the extent to which any 'complaint' bothers the person – using a 0 (Not at all) to 4 (Extremely) scale. A wide range of areas are addressed, including somatization, obsessive–compulsiveness, hostility, phobic anxiety and interpersonal sensitivity. Unlike the methods described above, this scale does not focus exclusively on anxiety but includes other related symptoms. The scale takes about 15 minutes to complete and allows three global scores across nine dimensions of psychiatric distress. An abbreviated version of this measure is also available [22].

The other key area for the exhibition of anxiety is within 'social situations'. As we have noted already, anxiety experienced in the presence of individuals or groups, or in anticipation of meeting people, is a common focus of anxiety. A number of important methods have been developed to assess this problem area. Since this overlaps with the area of 'interpersonal behaviour' I have left the discussion of these methods to Chapter 8.

CLOSER OBSERVATION

Self-study methods

Once the anxiety response is defined and some idea of the situations that precipitate attacks is clear, more detailed information can be collected. The person can also participate in this exercise, providing that he is given some assistance. Two kinds of detail can be added to the picture. The person may extend the subjective rating of the experience of anxiety to his everyday situation; or he may add more details of what he does, and what happens to him, in anxiety-evoking situations.

The self-rating of anxiety

Figure 5.2 illustrates a simple anxiety rating scale, which the person can carry in his pocket, recording his anxiety at periods during the day.

On the format illustrated the person records how anxious he feels, using a ten-point scale (0–9) every 3 hours, from rising to going to bed. This little booklet (10×15 cm) fits in his pocket, and requires only a few seconds to note his reactions throughout the day. This format has been used within a wide range of hospital and community settings with good success. Of course this format gives no information as to the situations surrounding the anxiety experience. In general, the format is most applicable to 'free-floating anxiety' problems where no specific focal situations are evident, but fluctuations in the level of anxiety do take place. Using this format, it is possible to monitor the

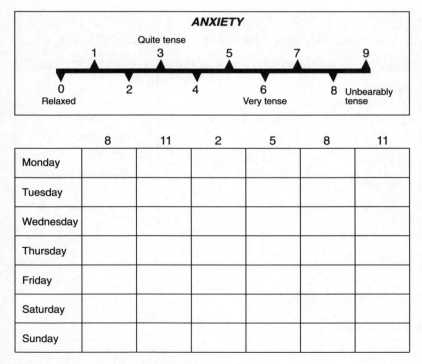

Figure 5.2 A simple anxiety rating scale.

rise and fall of anxiety during the day and across longer periods of time. The person requires little instruction and the method is highly cost-effective.

The incident diary

Figure 5.3 illustrates a diary format that can be used to collect more detailed information about the situations that provoke anxiety and how the person responds to these situations.

The record sheet is broken down into three sections: the setting, the person's reactions and the outcome. The person can summarize any critical incident in which he felt anxious, noting where he was, what was going on around him, what he was doing. These make up the 'setting' for his anxiety reaction. Next, he notes how he felt, what he was thinking and what he did next. These represent his 'reaction'. Finally, he notes what happened as a result of his reaction. What did other people do? What did they say? How did he feel? What did he think? This format can be filled in as soon as possible after an 'anxiety incident', or regularly each evening as a resume of the day's events. This format is appropriate for a wide range of anxiety situations, from the highly specific 'fear of public speaking', which might happen only once a month, to 'inter-personal anxiety', which might occur several times a day.

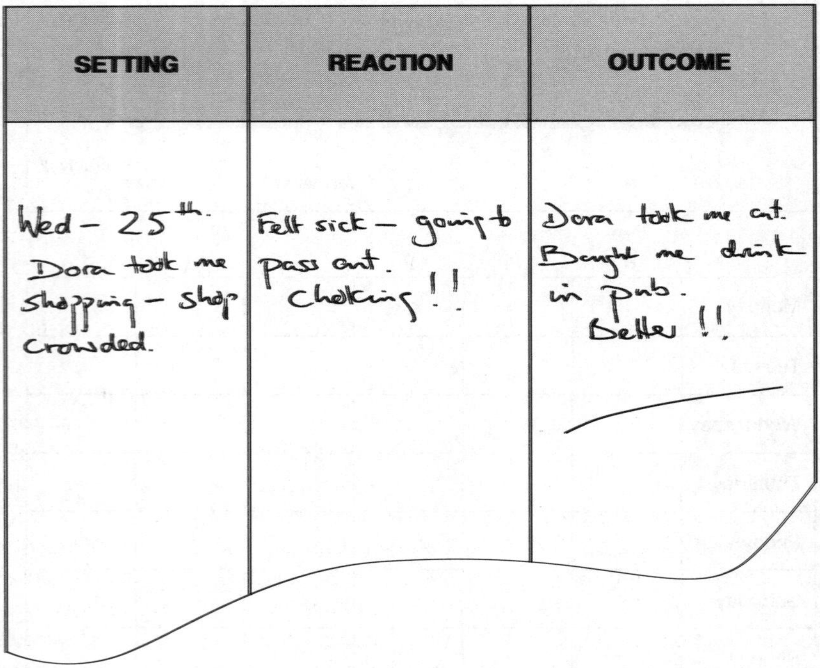

SETTING	REACTION	OUTCOME
Wed – 25th. Dora took me shopping – shop crowded.	Felt sick – going to pass out. Choking !!	Dora took me out. Bought me drink in pub. Better !!

Figure 5.3 Example of an incident diary.

Self-monitoring of behaviour

In many situations the number of times the person does something, or the length of time he spends in that behaviour, may be an important measure of the anxiety experience. For instance, the number of cigarettes smoked, the amount of food 'binged' or the length of time spent 'concentrating' on a book or television programme might help us to appreciate the level of anxiety present. This would be an appropriate procedure for someone who reported chain-smoking, binge-eating or loss of concentration as a result of anxiety. The person might also be asked to monitor 'avoidance' behaviour: the things he fails to do because of anxiety. A person who feared he was going to have a heart attack each time he experienced palpitations began to avoid activities he thought physically taxing, e.g. climbing stairs, walking long distances, sexual intercourse. He was asked, therefore, to 'tick off' each time he avoided these activities on a simple checklist. Those who are frightened of meeting people might be asked to record each time they spoke to someone, distinguishing between 'new' and 'old' acquaintances and perhaps between 'short' and 'long' interactions. Again, a simple checklist can procure this information.

Almost any kind of behaviour, either motor or cognitive, can be self-monitored. Apart from behaviours that involve 'doing' something, the person may record each time he thinks a certain kind of thought or experiences a certain 'mental image'. Anxious people often report 'self-defeating' thoughts or impressions. They may think: 'I've made a fool of myself' or 'I'm going to make a mess of this', or they may imagine that 'People are laughing at me' or 'They must think I'm mad'. Where these thoughts or impressions are regularly repeated a simple checklist may be composed and the person is asked to tick off each time he has this particular experience. A tally counter can also be used that fits in the pocket or can be attached to the wrist. The person 'clocks' up negative thoughts or impressions as they occur. A young woman who experienced high levels of anxiety related to a fear of making mistakes recorded between 150 and 200 of these thoughts each day during the assessment stage. This information proved to be more valuable than assessing the experience of anxiety that the thoughts accompanied.

There are some behaviours that it is not appropriate to self-monitor. Subtle 'displays' of anxiety such as minimal eye contact, speech hesitation, facial touching or repetitive hand movements may suggest anxiety to an onlooker but may not be noted by the person. Even if these are pointed out to him, their subtlety may render them too elusive for self-monitoring. In this context it is worth re-emphasizing that self-monitoring can be a tedious procedure for the person, especially where high levels of the behaviour are evident. This usually means that the activity quickly becomes aversive, and the person gives up the exercise. This outcome can be avoided by making the exercise as attractive as possible, which is often very difficult, and by giving the person plenty of encouragement whenever he loses interest, or especially when he completes the record.

Staff observation

Several different kinds of staff observation are possible, involving a combination of ratings and direct observation of the person's behaviour. For simplicity's sake these are divided into two categories: the 'avoidance test' and observation.

The avoidance test

The avoidance test is a format that assesses the extent to which a person is afraid to approach some feared object or situation. Although commonly used with highly specific fears, such as spiders, snakes, etc., the format can be used for almost any situation. The person is asked to approach the situation he fears. He might be asked to walk across the room to a cage with a cat in it, pick up the cat and hold it to his chest. The 'measure' of his anxiety will be based upon how far across the room he can get, or how long he can remain within a certain distance of the feared object. The person is advised that he can end the test at any time by simply asking to stop.

This assessment also provides valuable information about time tolerance. The nature of the person's anxiety would influence the organization of the test. If he was afraid of touching an animal, then the test would include this as part of the instruction. If he couldn't stay in a room with the door closed, this situation would be arranged to assess 'how long' he could remain there. Someone who is afraid of heights might be asked to climb a ladder, counting the number of steps he climbs before coming down.

The avoidance test has a number of weaknesses as a realistic assessment. Firstly, it is usually conducted under artificial conditions. In real life the person is under a range of pressures, not simply the one, single 'stress factor' we are assessing in this experimental context. Secondly, the very fact that the person is being studied, and perhaps also accompanied, makes this test markedly different from normal. Finally, the fact that the person can terminate the painful experience makes the test wholly unrealistic. In real life he would have to tolerate the distress or risk possible social sanctions by 'escaping'. The avoidance test makes it almost 'acceptable' to take this escape route.

Despite these drawbacks, this exercise can be very useful in certain cases. Providing that the same format is used all the time, it will be possible to compare the person's performance before and after treatment. The assessment experiment may also provide useful pointers for the design of an appropriate therapy strategy. In this sense the advantages may outweigh the drawbacks.

Observation in the natural environment

The problems noted above regarding the 'unreality' of the avoidance test can be overcome by transferring this assessment to the person's natural environment. The person who becomes anxious in crowds can be assessed as the nurse accompanies him down a busy shopping precinct. The person who experiences anxiety when confronted by any sharp object can be observed as he handles cutlery, needles and gardening tools at home. The person who is afraid of certain animals can be assessed at the local zoo, pet shop or in the city square, which is thronged with pigeons.

This approach is not without problems. The presence of the 'observer' can influence the behaviour of the person, usually making things easier because of assumed moral support. The nurse may find it inconvenient to take one person out on such an assessment trip. If she can afford the time she may be uncertain as to what kind of information to collect. Despite all these practical problems this *in vivo* assessment technique has much to recommend it. The nurse has an opportunity to study the person's reactions. She also has an opportunity to note facets of the problem, or his coping style, that he may have omitted. It is almost impossible to recreate an anxiety-evoking scene under artificial conditions. Perhaps the simplest solution is to head straight for the real world. Many of the situations the person describes may be near at hand, in any case. Crowds, queues, heights, animals, friends, needles, confined spaces, insects, people staring, people laughing and being alone are all situations in which people report anxiety. These situations are either naturally available in a hospital or can be organized to look natural without much difficulty. (There are of course a number of ethical issues involved in creating or simulating distressing situations for people-in-care, which are beyond the scope of this chapter.) For the hospitalized person, assessment in the natural environment may be only a few minutes' walk away.

What kind of information should be collected in this situation? My preference lies in the direction of collecting as much information as possible. Most of the direct measures of how close, how high, how many people, how long he remained in the situation can be recorded fairly easily. These can be combined with ratings, by the nurse and by the person himself, of anxiety at various points during the exercise. Finally, the nurse might make short notes on changes in the person's behaviour in response to changes in the situation, points that may not have been noted previously. For example, I was once accompanying a man who was afraid to travel in a lift when the lift jammed. I was able to study his reaction at close range and was able to compare his relatively cool response with my own near-panic reaction. This proved to be an insightful experience for both myself and the person.

Other forms of direct observation

Two other ways of studying the person's reactions are possible, both involving 'artificial situations'. In the first a **role play** is arranged, in which people act out the sequence of events that leads to the onset of anxiety. The person is encouraged to imagine that he is in the real situation, requiring him to attribute 'real' status to the other performers, usually other people or members of staff. This is usually used in social or interpersonal anxiety and will be covered in detail in the chapter on relationships. The second method involves 'representations' of the problem situation. The person who is frightened of the sound of thunder, rushing water or traffic may be assessed by studying his reactions to such sound played on a tape recorder. This approach may be the easiest or the only way to test the person's reactions. This kind of 'experiment' may be much less time-consuming than taking the person to the real-life setting. On the other hand, the sounds he is frightened by may be so unpredictable – like thunder – that planning of the assessment may be a near impossibility. Visual material, either in the form of photographs or video-tape recordings, may also be used for common fears, e.g. animals, crowds, heights. In some cases these experiments may suggest that 'no anxiety' is experienced under these simulated conditions. However, even where the person's response is 'unrealistic', these simulations can be used to help explore the kinds of feelings and thoughts the person experiences when confronted by such scenes. In this sense, the use of such aids may be indicated where the person is unable to explain exactly how he feels in such situations. Recordings, photographs or film material may help him to express his anxiety in a verbal manner.

CONCLUSION

Anxiety is probably the commonest clinical problem encountered by psychiatric nurses. It is an experience shared by highly disturbed people and the normal public alike. Anxiety can express itself through various other disorders or may be seen as a problem in its own right. In addition to people perceived as suffering from a manifest 'anxiety state' or anxiety-related disorder, it is not unusual to find anxiety reported by people with a formal diagnosis of depression, or schizophrenia: in either case this may be both focal or generalized. Older people with diagnoses of depression or dementia may also exhibit anxiety, although it may be redefined as 'agitation'.

In this chapter I have tried to talk about anxiety as something that can be a problem to the autistic child as much as the disorientated adult. In between there is a range of people who may show a highly characteristic kind of anxiety, such as the obsessional individual, or who have difficulties that are remarkable in terms of their diffuseness – free-floating anxiety. I have tried to demystify the problem by defining it in terms of the three channels of functioning involved. I have offered no more than an overview of the possibilities for nursing assessment of anxiety. As nursing develops and the contexts in which nursing is practised widens, nurses will be expected to become increasingly flexible and creative in their approach to their work. In assessing people showing any kind of anxiety nurses may need to choose between using standardized methods or creatively adapting such methods for specific contexts.

I hope that I have stimulated the reader to consider how, through developing an understanding of anxiety, we can begin to examine the relationship between the person's world and disruptions of his physiological, cognitive or behavioural state. We can also start to understand how these aspects of the person play a part in maintaining the problem.

NOTES

1. Ehrenzweig, A. (1970) *The Hidden Order of Art*, Paladin, London, p. 292.
2. Esslin, M. (1968) *The Theatre of the Absurd*, Penguin, Harmondsworth.
3. Hoad, T. F. (1986) *The Concise Oxford Dictionary of Word Origins*, Oxford University Press, Oxford.
4. Sarbin, T. R. (1964) Anxiety: reification of a metaphor. *Archives of General Psychiatry*, **10**, 630–3.
5. This view was expressed by Borkovec, T. D., Weerts, T. C. and Bernstein, D. A. (1972) Assessment of anxiety, in *Handbook of Behavioural Assessment*, (eds. A. R. Ciminero, K. S. Calhoun and H. E. Adams), John Wiley, New York.
6. Peplau, H. E. (1990) Interpersonal relations model: principles and general applications, in *Psychiatric and Mental Health Nursing: Theory and Practice*, (eds W. Reynolds and D. Cormack), Chapman & Hall, London.
7. Peplau, H. E. (1963) A working definition of anxiety, in *Some Clinical Approaches to Psychiatric Nursing*, (eds S. Burd and M. Marshall), Macmillan, New York.
8. Both these examples are taken from Peplau, H. E. (1990) Interpersonal relations model: principles and general applications, in *Psychiatric and Mental Health Nursing: Theory and Practice*, (eds W. Reynolds and D. Cormack), Chapman & Hall, London.
9. Paul, G. L. (1969) Outcome of systematic desensitisation. 1: Background, procedures and uncontrolled reports of individual treatment, in *Behaviour Therapy: Appraisal and Status*, (ed. C. M. Franks), McGraw-Hill, New York, p. 64.
10. Beck, A. T. (1978) *Cognitive Therapy and the Emotional Disorders*, International Universities Press, New York.
11. Peplau, H. E. (1990) Interpersonal relations model: principles and general applications, in *Psychiatric and Mental Health Nursing: Theory and Practice*, (eds W. Reynolds and D. Cormack), Chapman & Hall, London.
12. D. A. Akutagawa appears to have been the first to develop a Fear Survey Schedule – Akutagawa, D. A. (1956) A study in construct validity of the psychoanalytic concept of latent anxiety and a test of projection distance hypothesis'. Unpublished doctoral dissertation, University of Pittsburgh.
13. For a detailed history of the development of the Fear Survey Schedule see Tasto, D. L. (1986) Self report schedules and inventories, in *Handbook of Behavioural Assessment*, (eds. A. R. Ciminero, K. S. Calhoun and H. E. Adams), John Wiley, New York.
14. Wolpe, J. (1973) *The Practice of Behaviour Therapy*, Pergamon, New York.
15. Marks, I. M. and Mathews, A. M. (1979) Fear Questionnaire. *Behaviour Research and Therapy*, **17**, 264.

16. Zung, W. K. (1971) A rating instrument for anxiety disorders. *Psychosomatics*, **12**, 371–9.
17. Sandler, J. and Hazari, A. (1960) The obsessional: on the psychological classification of obsessional character traits and symptoms. *British Journal of Medical Psychology*, **33**, 113–22.
18. Cooper, J. (1970) The Leyton Obsessional Inventory. *Psychological Medicine*, **1**, 48–64.
19. Hodgson, R. J. and Rachman, S. (1977) Obsessional compulsive complaints. *Behaviour Research and Therapy*, **15**, 389–95.
20. Thompson, E. A. and Leckie, M. (1989) Interpretation manual for symptoms of stress inventory. Unpublished manuscript, University of Washington Stress Management Program.
21. Derogatis, L. R. (1992) *SCL-90-T: Administration, Scoring and Procedures Manual – II*, Clinical Psychometrics Research, Towson, MD.
22. Derogatis, L. R. and Melisaratos, N. (1983) The brief symptom inventory: an introductory report. *Psychological Medicine*, **13**, 595–605.

The assessment of mood: the sickness of the soul | 6

Yet there's no one to beat you
No one t'defeat you
'Cept the thoughts of yourself feeling bad.

Bob Dylan

Melancholy is a fearful gift ... the telescope of truth, which brings life near in utter darkness, making the cold reality too real.

Byron

A feeling of sadness ...
That is not akin to pain,
And resembles sorrow only
As the mist resembles rain

Longfellow

INTRODUCTION

We can find parallels to many of the experiences we associate with psychiatric disorder in the works of the great writers, poets and artists. In many ways, the experiences associated with mental disturbance are universal: features which are common to nearly the whole human race. The only difference is that in true psychiatric disturbance these experiences are exaggerated far beyond the range encountered by 'normal people'. The suffering and anguish experienced by people in depression has often been captured best by novelists and poets, the American writer Sylvia Plath, who committed suicide, being a fine example.

It was becoming more and more difficult for me to decide to do anything
.... I couldn't get myself to react. I felt very still and very empty the way
the eye of a tornado must feel ... a time of darkness, despair and
disillusion – so black only as the inferno of the human mind can be [1].

Depression is typical of a universal experience. Some people rarely experience extreme anxiety. Many people will never experience the kind of perceptual
disturbance we associate with psychotic states. How many of us, however, can
pass through life without experiencing the depths of despair, or severe unhappiness, even where such an experience is short-lived and natural, as in bereavement? The answer is, probably, none of us. The inevitability of our chance
encounters with despair led Homer to conclude, somewhat pessimistically,
that 'twins from birth are misery and Man'.

Yet, some people can be unhappy without apparently being inconvenienced
by their low spirits. We all have encountered the stereotyped pessimist, that
classic 'prophet of doom' who repeatedly moans about this or that, who never
deviates from his sober expression and who can always manage to see the black
side of any happy event. In principle, he is the classic depressive personality.
But is he? His view of the world is undoubtedly negative. Yet this jaundiced
perspective does not seem to obstruct him: he is not disabled or handicapped.
He is unlikely to commit suicide, although on the surface his life appears to
lack any real purpose and is a thoroughly joyless experience. Perhaps he enjoys
being pessimistic. Perhaps his crusade – which involves deflating egos, demys-
tifying wonders, collapsing dreams and generally bringing everyone down to
earth with a thump – should give us an important clue. Perhaps the whole
point of his life is to make the rest of us aware of the futility and pointlessness
of our life-experience. Although the pessimist shows a lot of depressive
features, he is in no way disabled by these 'abnormalities'.

In this chapter I shall discuss people who not only appear despairing,
unhappy or even ridiculously happy given the circumstances but who also are
restrained, obstructed or eventually defeated by their state of apparent, or
disguised, melancholy.

Melancholy

It is interesting to note that the term 'melancholy' has been revived in
psychiatric circles [2]. Many of our 'advances' involve moving in a full circle:
the completion of a true revolution. Melancholy is one of the four classic
humours of ancient times. In attempting to understand the role and function
of 'unhappiness' in our lives, many a philosopher or poet has compared
depression to true vision. Instead of assuming that depression is a weakness,
or in any way pathological, some have argued that the depressive sees the
world stripped of all falsehood and superficiality. However, this may become
a surreal, nightmarish vision that he cannot handle.

Lord Byron believed that 'melancholy is a fearful **gift**'. This idea is reinforced in quite a different context by those who have viewed the 'insane' as
having more insight and understanding than those who were not psychiatrically disturbed. The late R. D. Laing perhaps represented the best-known
example of someone who had witnessed the 'journey to enlightenment'
afforded by mental illness [3]. Increasingly the view is taken that people who
are depressed have a more 'realistic' grasp of 'reality'. In this sense the
experience of depression might be seen as 'enobling' [4].

The contrast between pleasurable and unhappy experiences is another
common area of interest for poets. Shakespeare, among others, noted how our
misery is heightened, rather than reduced, by our awareness of the happiness
of others. 'Oh how bitter it is to look into happiness through another man's
eyes'. The Western cultural tradition established and maintained the idea that
sorrow, struggle and unhappiness are all part of the rich tapestry of life.
Seneca, the Stoic philosopher, warned us against extremes, however: 'An
excess of sorrow is as foolish as profuse laughter; while on the other hand, not
to mourn at all is insensibility'.

From such a history of ideas has developed the traditional view that deep
and sustained despair (**melancholia**) or extreme happiness (**mania**) are distur-
bances of our normal reactions to the world and its events. In recent years the
view that depression is a 'perceptual problem' – brought about by the person's
distorted view of his world – has grown in popularity. This cognitive paradigm
involves a reworking of a theme that has intrigued the poets and philosophers
down the ages. La Rochefoucauld, in the 17th century, shared Bob Dylan's
later view that thought was a crucial factor: 'No person is either so happy or
unhappy as he imagines'. The heritage of today's cognitive theories can be
traced back even further to Dante, the great 13th century Italian poet. He
would have had little time for the lay person's 'Come on, cheer up' philosophy,
observing that 'there is no greater grief than to recall a time of happiness when
in misery'.

The recognition that our thoughts, perceptions and even our memories can
play a part in the construction and maintenance of the emotion of depression
is an important issue, and one to which we shall return over and over again
in the course of this chapter.

AFFECTIVE DISTURBANCE

The term 'mood' (or 'affect') is an umbrella expression encompassing all
emotional states. The term 'affective disturbance' is, however, reserved almost
exclusively for a depression of mood – when the person is manifestly 'low in
spirits' – or mania – where an exaggerated happiness or excitement is evident.
Since anxiety was discussed in the previous chapter, I shall restrict my discussion of mood to the presence of absence of an adaptive state of happiness or

well-being. I shall say little about 'normal affect'. As Chateaubriand, the French author and statesman, observed, when it comes to unhappiness it is very much an individual affair: 'One can never be the judge of another's grief. That which is sorrow to one, to another is joy. Let us not dispute with anyone concerning the reality of his sufferings; it is with sorrow as with countries – each man has his own'. I shall try to stick to this person-centred philosophy, while at the same time acknowledging that the use of some standardized measure to judge the relative weight of despair of all sufferers can also be helpful.

The depressions – for surely these states are many and varied – are a major problem in psychiatric practice. Apart from the significant population afflicted with affective disorder [5], there are many other groups who suffer mood disturbance as a function of some other problem of living. I have noted earlier that there is much debate over the causes and treatment of psychiatric disorders (Chapter 1). Despite these disputes there is agreement over the definition of most disorders. It would appear that this cannot be said of the depressions. We appear to be undecided as to the very nature of the problem: is it a single symptom, or is it a syndrome involving a group of disease symptoms [6]? The whole position is confused even further when we realize that not only do writers disagree about the symptoms of depression [7], but also many of these symptoms are not peculiar to depression, existing within other disorder definitions.

Traditionally, depression has been listed under a range of diagnostic headings:

- **psychoses** – e.g. involutional melancholia, manic-depressive illness;
- **psychoneuroses** – e.g. depressive neurosis;
- **personality disorder** – cyclothymia.

Commonly, a disturbance has been made between 'reactive' depression, where some external event – such as bereavement – is used to explain the disturbance of affect, and endogenous (or psychotic) depression, where no such obvious factors can be identified and the depression is assumed to arise from within the person. Recently, this distinction has fallen into disfavour. Researchers have begun to explode the myth that external factors relate to one group and not the other. Some writers have suggested that the best way to look at the problem is to use a three-way classification.

- In the first class we could include problems such as 'normal grief'.
- In the second class we include depression that is secondary to some other problem, such as agoraphobia.
- We reserve the third class for 'primary' affective disorders, usually referred to as 'unipolar' or 'bipolar' disorder. In the first of these disorders only depression is shown. In the second, depression and mania are commonly present.

Despite the practical, common-sense appearance of this classification system, it is clear that severity is the most commonly used way of classifying the problem. Close behind is the presence of accompanying, non-depressive symptoms, and the attitude of the clinician, especially his attitude towards the assumed 'cause' of the problem. I recognize that psychiatric nurses are not (generally) expected to 'diagnose' depression, or any other disorder. I offer this crude summary of the diagnostic classifications simply to draw the reader's attention to the fact that depression is a complex phenomenon, which can mean many different things to different clinicians.

Depression is a major problem that manifests itself in a variety of guises. Common to all these subgroups is a common group of symptoms. This depressive thread is highlighted by many of the assessment systems, which we shall discuss in a moment. In view of the confusion that exists in the field at present, it is important that nurses are confident about what they want to study, to understand the person's disturbance of affect. In this chapter I offer some suggestions that might encourage just such an orientation.

The assessment targets

The present state of depression research has two important messages for nursing.

First, we should understand that a generally accepted classification does not exist. Consequently, we should acknowledge that we may well not be dealing with a single problem. The 'depressed person' could be suffering from any one of a number of disorders, none of which are defined unequivocally.

Second, the term 'depression' is a classic 'umbrella' concept, embracing a wide range of symptoms, behaviours or aspects of the person's functioning. As we have noted already, when one person talks about depression, he need not necessarily embrace the same group of symptoms as the next person.

In the light of these observations, nurses should concentrate more upon the study of 'what the person complains of' (i.e. his reports of his experience), paying less attention to the study of his assumed disorder. This might help them to appreciate more fully the relationship between the person's problems of affect and other facets of his life-experience. In this sense we are trying to follow Chateaubriand's advice by accepting the person's reality of his own suffering.

The term 'target' means an aspect of the person's functioning singled out for close attention in the assessment process. Despite the disagreements over the definition of depression, there is some agreement about the kinds of phenomenon that characterize the disorder and should therefore be the focus of the assessment process.

Overview of the assessment targets

A complete nursing assessment of the person with a suspected mood disturbance would include the collection of information in the following areas:

- **the person's perception of himself** – how does he compare himself (as he sees himself now) with how he thinks he should be?
- **the person's goals or expectations of himself** – what goals does he set for himself, how realistic might these be and how likely is he to achieve them?
- **the person's strengths and potential** – what are his 'good points'; what has he achieved in his life; what opportunities might be open to him?
- **the person's manifest mood state** and (especially) his risk of self-harm.
- **the person's available (and potential) support systems** – do his family and friends have realistic or unrealistic expectations of him [8]?

The above represents the skeleton of the assessment process. Here we examine some of these dimensions of assessment goals in more detail.

Mood

Disturbance of mood (or affect) is central to depression. The person may complain of feelings of sadness, loss of enjoyment or loss of feeling itself. He may report losing interest in things, feeling apathetic and bored with life. He may also complain of anxiety, which can be either psychic (worrying thoughts) or physical (tension). Not all persons will complain of all, or indeed any, of these problems. Some will report feeling well, despite appearances to the contrary. Others may emphasize physical distress, such as pain, at the expense of reporting their mental symptoms. Such persons may only admit to feeling sad, unhappy, tense, etc. if asked directly. Indeed, some persons find it easier to report 'physical' symptoms where psychological problems either embarrass or confuse them.

Behaviour

Change in the person's observable behaviour is commonly observed. He may show a marked reduction in activity, doing less, saying less than is habitual or routine. In parallel with these behavioural deficits may emerge certain excesses. He may complain more: about financial worries, problems at work, lack of affection, etc. He may also lose his temper more often, become upset more quickly or spend more time checking pieces of work – displaying his indecisiveness. These behaviour patterns are observable to friends and family and may be the first signs that 'something is wrong'.

Physical state

The person may also complain of certain somatic problems. These are related to disruptions or dysfunctions on a biological level. Pain, tiredness, loss of appetite, urinary disturbance, sleep disruption and loss of sex drive may all be reported. Occasionally, he may report chest pains and tachycardia, similar to the experiences of the anxious person.

Thinking

Three main kinds of cognitive, or thought, disturbance are possible. The person may experience low self-esteem: his overall evaluation of himself may be poor; he may think that he is a failure, hopeless, inadequate or in general 'powerless' to control his situation. Second, he may have negative expectations. He may see only the gloom ahead. He may see no light at the end of the tunnel when things go wrong, thinking that things will never improve. Lastly, he may blame himself for things that are not his fault, 'accepting' blame that should be attributed to others. Or he may severely criticize himself for things he has done, perhaps in the distant past; or for things he believes he has done, or has failed to do.

Motivation

Finally, the person may be unable to tackle things he 'needs' to do, or seems unwilling to try things which might – in the views of others – make him feel better. The person may see no point in doing anything, believing that he will get no enjoyment out of it, or that he hasn't got the energy, or that he couldn't do it even if he tried.

The assessment interview

Although not all depressed people are reluctant to be interviewed, the withdrawn or uncommunicative person poses the biggest problem for the nurse. For this reason I shall take this individual as the model for our hypothetical interview. How does the nurse cope with a person who appears unwilling or unable to provide the information she needs? There is no simple solution. In the following notes I merely make some suggestions about how the interview might be structured to some advantage.

The beginning

The person should be given some simple outline of the nurse's intentions. These should be offered in a confidential and confident manner. She should try to suggest that she is there to help the person express how he feels, not to diagnose, judge or otherwise label him. If her aim is to help amplify a medical assessment, she should say so. If the aim is to provide guidelines for the nursing team, this should also be indicated in a simple straightforward manner. These proposals should be put forward in the form of suggestions, which the person may reject if he so wishes. By doing so the nurse is trying to establish some collaboration from the outset.

'Hello, John. Do you mind if I sit down and talk with you for a few minutes? I wanted to have a word with you about how you're feeling. Do you feel up to that just now? I know that you've been quizzed quite a bit already, but I haven't got a long list of questions. I just wanted to find out how you are feeling ... so that I can get some idea of what is bothering you ....any problems you may have which I might help you with. OK?'

Labelling

I have already begun this chapter with a prejudice. I have mentioned 'depressed' people a number of times. I hope that you accept that as a convenient hunch or hypothesis, which will be investigated in the assessment. This raises an interesting point. Often we check the person's notes on admission or following an interward transfer, to see 'what he is suffering from'. We cannot close our eyes to such diagnostic criteria. However, if we begin our assessment with a label in the forefront of our minds we may only look for – and find evidence to confirm – someone else's diagnostic prejudices: the self-fulfilling prophecy. If we stick to the person-centred approach described in the early chapters, existing diagnoses may prove to be less of a filter of our experience of the person.

Structuring the questions

If the person finds it difficult to answer questions, the nurse should take a more active role. At least initially, the line of questioning should be more direct, perhaps using closed questions that are short and well punctuated to help the person concentrate and absorb their meaning. Where the person fails to answer, the question should be rephrased or another topic should be selected. Silences should be avoided. It is now generally accepted that where the person is passive or withdrawn the nurse should become more active to compensate for this. Silences serve only to allow the person more time to reflect upon his inability to answer simple questions [9]. He may also attribute (incorrectly) negative attitudes to his interviewer: '(Thinks) I can't even answer a simple question. This just shows how far gone I am. She must think that I'm hopeless. That's it. I'm hopeless. What's the point any more?'

The general picture

Our first step is to establish an overview of the person's problems as he sees them. We begin by asking how he feels? This can be extended to cover other facets of his experience: How is he getting on with others? How is he sleeping or eating? Can he concentrate at work, television, etc.? Is he still going out or doing the sorts of things which are part of his routine? Many people volunteer such information. They have already judged that 'something is wrong' because of changes in one or more of these areas. Where the person is more withdrawn it may be helpful to structure the questions around the kind of 'problem list' shown in Figure 6.1.

NAME .... WARD ....

DATE OF ASSESSMENT .... ASSESSMENT No ....

PROBLEM LIST
AFFECT
       Sadness
       Anxiety
       Guilt
       Shame
       Other (specify)
MOTIVATION
       Avoidance
       Dependency
       Reduced activity
       Other (specify)
COGNITION
       Indecisiveness
       Self-criticism
       Overwhelmed
       Concentration loss
       Memory loss
       Absolutist thinking
BEHAVIOUR
       Passivity
       Coping deficits
       Social skill deficits
PHYSIOLOGY
       Sleep
       Appetite
       Sex

Figure 6.1 A problem list for establishing an overview of a person's problems.

This can act as a cue, ensuring that none of the typical problem areas are omitted from the discussion. The nurse should review her information at intervals, allowing the person to add or withdraw comments as he desires. Giving feedback like this can also help ensure that the person is 'tuned in' to the interview: is he taking part, or merely 'sitting in'?

'From what you have said you seem to have some problems with sleeping – mainly getting off at night. Occasionally you wake early, but not every morning? You are also having trouble at home. Your eldest son has been taking drugs and you are worried about him. You also worry a lot about your wife. She isn't sleeping with you any more. You feel that this may be your fault. How do you feel about that? Is that an accurate reflection of what we have discussed so far? Have I left anything out? Is there anything you want to change?'

'We have talked a bit about your problems. How you feel about various things. Trying to get things into perspective. Do you think that you could summarize the points I have made so far? Just to see if you and I are in agreement?'

In the first example the person is given a potted summary of the interview, to check and modify if he wishes. In the second example he is asked to evaluate the discussion that has just taken place. If he can do this, it shows that he has been participating fully. If he gets lost, it may be an indication that the nurse needs to adapt her style slightly, perhaps asking shorter questions and summarizing points as she goes along. This procedure also has a therapeutic value. By discussing, defining, clarifying and then summarizing the whole conversation, the person may begin to see his problems more clearly. This may offer him some relief.

Support and stress

The level of support and stress present is crucial in most psychiatric disorders. In depression the role of such life events may be even more significant. The nurse should ask detailed questions about the significant people in the person's life. What role do they play in supporting him? The relationship format discussed in the next chapter may be helpful in this respect. The nurse should ask about his family, friends and other people in his life. Are they close confidantes? Or are they the kind of people who avoid or resent such disclosures? This part of the interview establishes the level of support present. Who can the person depend on, in what way and to what extent?

It is also important to establish the role of any significant stress factors. Is he in any debt? Threatened with divorce or separation? Is he experiencing any interpersonal conflict – with family, friends, employer, etc.? What about his home? Does he have problems with repairs, electricity, troublesome neighbours, etc.? Here the person should be encouraged to identify features of his life that are causing distress, or that he perceives as distressing, as well as the existing supports he draws upon to reduce this.

Coping and self-esteem

The person who is depressed will find no difficulty in listing his faults and inadequacies. For this reason it is important to restore some balance. What does the other side of this 'personality coin' look like? What are the person's assets? What sort of coping skills are evident? To establish this, the person might be asked to describe how he deals with difficult situations, no matter how inadequately.

'You have been under a lot of strain recently. You moved house and then found that it had dry rot. Then your wife fell ill and you had to look after her when she came out of hospital. That was a very bad time. How did you cope with all of that?'

The person may be unaware of his coping abilities. He may see himself as a complete write-off. Where this may be the case the question may be framed in a different manner.

'I can appreciate how you feel. You feel that you buckled under the strain of all that upheaval and illness. You may be right in saying that you didn't cope at the end. You failed to some extent to hold your own. What made you seek help? At what point did you realize you needed some help? How did you have the presence of mind to look for assistance?'

Where the person feels defeated and hopeless he may toy with the idea of suicide. He may comment upon the pointlessness of his existence. He has no assets. He is worthless. In such cases it might be worth asking what is preventing him from committing suicide right now? This question might elicit some comment about religious beliefs, loyalty to family, or the chance that 'something might turn up' – the Micawber syndrome. These replies may reflect the values or ideas that help him to continue living, fighting or trying to avoid further descent into depression and suicide. These are also important assets in his overall self-concept. They also serve a critical function in the therapeutic process to follow: these serve as the basis of the person's recovery.

On a similar level, what is the person's view of himself? There is a temptation here to invite the person to comment upon his successful job, the success of his family, his qualifications and various other 'merits', in an attempt to correct his negative view of himself. The assessment is a premature place to do this: the person may 'accept' the argument presented simply to escape from further discussion. Instead of trying to correct his style of thinking, the person should be encouraged to acknowledge – however reservedly – his assets. 'Are you punctual?' 'Do you talk about people behind their backs?' 'Are you loyal to friends?' 'Have you ever made anything with your hands?'

These questions are carefully phrased to elicit a Yes/No answer, in which the chances are that 'Yes' will occur more often than 'No'. By such a line of questioning, a picture of the person's present – or recent past – assets is possible. The nurse may then ask the person to 'tell me a bit more about that'.

Translation of problems

The interview may produce a list of vague problems: 'I just can't cope any more. Life is pointless. I'm all washed up'. At the end of the interview it may be worth trying to re-define these vague problems more clearly. What does the person feel that he cannot cope with any longer? Arguments at home? His job? His weight? The size of his overdraft? In some cases he may say 'Everything', which may reflect the way he feels. However, it is important to check that some problems are not more acute and troublesome than others. Where the person feels that life is pointless, he may be ignoring – or minimizing – the importance of some things. Does he feel that everything is pointless? Or are some things more important than others, no matter how small? In translating the problem, the nurse should try to define, using the person's own words, the affective difficulties he is experiencing.

Presentation and appearance

The final task in the interview is to summarize the appearance of the person. Many of the points covered in the next chapter will be of relevance here. How is the person dressed: is he untidy or poorly groomed? Does he appear to have made an effort with his appearance? How long does he take to answer questions? Does he appear hesitant in his replies? Does he avoid eye contact, stare or frequently close his eyes? Does he sit facing the nurse or turned away from her? Does he use gestures, making use of his hands to express himself, nodding appropriately? Or does he appear rigid, frozen, perhaps clasping himself tightly? At the end of the interview it is important to summarize the non-verbal qualities of the person, as a back-up to the verbal information that has been collected.

At the end of the interview, or perhaps series of interviews, a picture of how the person is functioning across the various areas of behaviour, emotion, physical and psychological states will be available. This will be based mainly upon what he has reported. However, the nurse's close observation of his appearance and behaviour during the interview may indicate levels of pain, discomfort, restlessness, loss of concentration, etc. that he fails to report or perhaps wishes to keep a secret.

STANDARDIZED METHODS

Self-report

A number of self-report methods have been developed to help people describe their experience. This allows their distress to be measured in some way.

The Beck Depression Inventory (BDI)

One of the earlier self-report methods, the BDI is still viewed by many as the best available measure of the severity of depression. The scale covers 21 items, which are presented in the form of four statements. The person is asked to read through the statements, circling the one that most closely corresponds with his present experience. The BDI covers various facets of affective disorder, e.g. feelings of sadness, shame, guilt and disappointment, as well as thoughts about appearance, decision-making, work, etc. A number of physical factors are also included, such as eating, sleeping, weight loss and sex. A typical item looks like this:

0 = I don't feel that I am worse than anybody else
1 = I am critical of myself for my weaknesses and faults
2 = I blame myself all the time for my faults
3 = I blame myself for everything bad that happens.

The inventory is scored simply by totalling the scores circled by the person in his replies. Research has produced norms that allow us to judge the severity of the depression by comparing the person's score with various gradings of mild, moderate and severe depression. The BDI may be used as a screening assessment to establish whether a 'clinical depression' exists. It may also be used as a pre- and post-treatment measure to evaluate the effect of different therapies. Where the person has been depressed for some time, the scale may be administered at regular intervals to monitor changes in mood. The scale is simple to administer and can be completed by the person in a matter of minutes. Where the person is more severely depressed it may be more appropriate for the nurse to read out each of the statements slowly, asking the person to indicate which response best reflects how he feels [10,11].

The Zung Self-rating Scale

Developed in 1965, this scale comprises 20 self-statements [12]. The person is required to rate each one using a four-point rating scale. Two items deal with affect, eight with physiological and ten with psychological equivalents of affect. Typical examples are:

I get tired for no reason (physiological);
I still enjoy the things I used to (psychological).

Each statement is rated on a scale ranging from 1 = 'A little of the time' to 4 = 'Most of the time'.

The statements are balanced between negative and positive expressions. This is shown in the two examples above: the first is negative, the second positive. This format is used to avoid stereotyped answers where the person simply scores each statement in the same way. Because of this positive/negative balance the scores run 1–4 for negative items and 4–1 for positive items. The higher the final score, the more depressed the person.

Zung designed this scale to provide a brief yet valid assessment. He felt that existing scales were too time-consuming for staff or too demanding for the person, especially if he was having psychomotor problems. The scale has gained some popularity as a convenient tool for assessing the general level of depression. However, some concern has been expressed about its lack of sophistication from a psychometric perspective.

The visual analogue scale

Several studies have used a simple visual analogue scale to measure the general feeling of depression. A line 100 mm long may be used to gauge the severity of depression. The person marks a point on the line to indicate his perceived level of depression. It has been argued that this method is sufficient for most clinical purposes and is almost as accurate as much more detailed and sophisticated interview methods [13]. From my research with women with depression I developed a similar format where the person selects a rating from a visual analogue (Figure 6.2). This little booklet can be carried in the person's pocket and allows regular monitoring of mood levels throughout the day.

The value of self-reports

As I have noted previously, some concern may be expressed over the value of self-report information. There is a concern that what the person 'says' on such paper and pencil tests may not be an adequate reflection of his situation. For instance, a person may record that he finds great difficulty in sleeping. Staff may report that this is not the case – he sleeps soundly every night. Surely this illustrates the weakness of the scale? However, this is to misunderstand the nature of the problem. Depression often involves a 'distortion' of the person's experience, at least from our perspective. The very fact that the person complains of sleep disruption, which he thinks is a problem, qualifies this as of interest to us. The problem involves the person's perception of his sleeping behaviour, not the behaviour itself.

This point requires emphasis since there may be a temptation to conclude that because reports on a scale like the BDI do not correspond to the staff's observations, either the person is being dishonest or the scale is faulty. These two self-report methods only assess the problem of depression from the

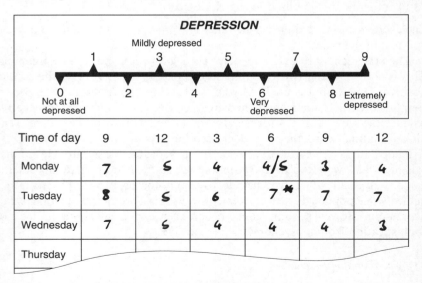

Figure 6.2 A visual analogue scale for measuring depression.

person's perspective. They are not 'objective' measures of reality. Rather, they are measures of the person's 'construction' of his own reality, as it is perceived – and experienced.

Interview methods

A number of scales exist to help us assess the depth of depression during an interview with the person. The BDI was designed originally for this purpose, but gradually developed into a self-report instrument. Here I shall discuss briefly two of the more popular methods for assessing depression within an interview format.

The Hamilton Rating Scale [14]

This scale can be completed during the course of an ordinary interview, although supplementary information is often required from staff or relatives. It aims to assess the person's condition over one or two weeks prior to the interview. It cannot, therefore, be completed any more frequently than this. The scale consists of 17 items covering the symptoms of depression reported most frequently by persons. Each of these symptoms is rated on a three- or a five-point scale. Cognitive, behavioural and physiological symptoms are included along with less usual symptoms such as depersonalization, derealization, paranoid and obsessional symptoms.

This scale was designed first in 1960 and was revised slightly in 1967. Although the scale is popular, it is thought that it has some psychometric weaknesses. It has been noted, for instance, that items often mix what the person **thinks and says** with his **actual behaviour**. The suicidal intent item mixes 'feels that life is worth living' (a cognitive–verbal expression) with 'attempts at suicide' (which denotes actual behaviour). From this perspective, the scale, although a helpful guide, may be structurally weak.

The Montgomery and Asberg Depression Rating Scale

The Montgomery and Asberg Depression Rating Scale (MADRS) [15] has attracted considerable attention over the past decade. This scale includes ten items related to sadness – apparent and reported, tension, sleep disruption, appetite, concentration, lassitude, loss of feeling and pessimistic and suicidal thoughts. All the items are rated on a 0–6 scale: 'Not apparent or in keeping with present circumstances' to 'Extreme, continuous or highly explicit'. Each of the items carries a guidance note on how to rate the presence or absence of the factor.

'Tension'
Representing feelings of ill-defined discomfort, edginess, inner turmoil,

mental tension, mounting to either panic, dread or anguish. Rate according to intensity, frequency, duration and the extent of reassurance called for.

0 = Placid. Only fleeting inner tension.
1
2 = Occasional feelings of edginess and ill-defined discomfort.
3
4 = Continuous feelings of inner tension or intermittent panic which the person can only master with some difficulty.
5
6 = Unrelenting dread or anguish. Overwhelming panic.

This scale is designed to be sensitive to change, especially as an evaluation of treatment. The scale appears to provide a useful assessment of the various facets of severe depression, which might require an assessment from the clinician's perspective. There are indications, however, that unsophisticated raters tend to score lower than those who have formal training in the administration of the scale.

Comment

Interviewer rating scales are used where the information cannot be collected by any other means. In some cases these ratings will be completed only by psychiatrists. In other settings nurses may apply such measures routinely. The interview rating may be used where the person is unable to complete a self-report scale. Where this is the case it may be more appropriate to interview the person using the BDI or Zung as a guide, rather than switch to the interview format.

It is often argued that self-report methods are unreliable. We have discussed this point already. Even where the person's ability to answer the self-report is in question, or the person is unable to answer the self-report, his family or significant others might be able to help complete the BDI or Zung. In the case of the hospitalized person, the nursing staff could do this. It could be argued that these significant others can draw on a wide experience of the person, and may offer a more valid rating than is possible during a brief clinical interview.

Self-report methods are best suited to evaluate the person's thoughts and perceptions – his verbal–cognitive behaviour. Where other aspects of his functioning are thought to be important, such as overt behaviour, these are best measured directly, through observation. The value of the interview rating scale is probably restricted to situations where the person cannot be observed closely in his natural habitat. Of course there are some persons who may respond to neither, such as people who are withdrawn, perhaps to the point of muteness.

CLOSER OBSERVATION

General activity measures

The Behaviour Rating Scale (BRS)

Where the person is hospitalized there is an opportunity to study his behaviour directly. This kind of closer observation may be most appropriate for withdrawn persons such as the one mentioned above. One of the few standardized methods described in the literature is the BRS, developed in the early 1970s [16]. This scale looks only at observable behaviour, ignoring all subtle behaviours, speech and estimates of affect. The four areas defined on the scale are as follows.

1. **Talking**: verbal behaviour towards another person.
2. **Smiling**: facial movements in which the corners of the mouth turn up. The teeth may not show.
3. **Motor activity**: the following are activities:
a. Person in room with visitor
b. Person at card table talking, reading or sewing; dressing, taking a shower, watching TV, playing cards, drinking coffee. N.B. Behaviour such as lying down or looking out of the window is not counted as an activity.
4. **Person out of the room**.

Using such operational definitions nurses observe the person at random intervals, on average every 30 minutes. The observations are taken between 8 am and 4 pm, resulting in 16 observations over this 8-hour period. In the original study of this scale comparisons were made between the scores of the people-in-care on the BDI and the Hamilton with scores obtained from these behavioural observations. The authors concluded that these behavioural samples were one way of verifying self-report ratings or interview ratings. A small follow-up study suggested that changes in overt behaviour were a more reliable way of predicting improvement once the person had left hospital. Readers may find the strict 'behavioural' definitions offered in this scale somewhat restrictive. This method does have some advantages, which can be summarized as follows.

- Since the behaviours are defined precisely, staff need not make complicated decisions. The person is or is not engaged in the behaviour.
- Staff require little training to make such observations.
- The observation format does not interfere with the person's care.
- This kind of careful observation may enhance the quality of nursing care.
- Interview scales, such as the Hamilton, are usually done by a psychiatrist. This is not only a more expensive method, but describes the person only at a certain point in time, in a given situation (the interview). If such scales are given repeatedly, they may interfere with the person's care routine.

- Behavioural measures overcome the problem of people who cannot or will not complete self-report or interview methods.
- Taken over a period of time, behavioural measures provide an accurate record of behaviour change during the course of a period of depression. Such day-to-day observations can identify crises and may be compared with more stringent measures of the person's physical state – such as biochemical measures.

Increasingly, the only people who receive treatment in hospital are those with more serious (especially life-threatening) forms of psychiatric disorder. Nurses in acute settings invariably find that they have less time to devote to ongoing assessment than they would like. Brief observational rating systems of this sort may prove attractive under these conditions.

The Pleasant Events Schedule

Most depressed people report a lack, or a loss, of pleasure or satisfaction. They may have lost friends, pets or treasures. Or they may simply see their lives as being low in satisfaction. The behavioural treatment model of depression emphasizes the role of reinforcing or pleasurable events, planned as part of the person's life. Even if we do not accept this theory it is clear that nurses do try to engage people-in-care in activities of a therapeutic nature. We might improve this procedure if the activities selected were the ones that the person used to enjoy, or that still offered some satisfaction. The Pleasant Events Schedule [17] is a 320-item rating scale that lists a range of activities, from walking around naked to talking with friends. The person is asked to read through the statements, indicating how often he has engaged in each activity over the past 30 days. A three-point scale is used for this purpose. He then goes through the scale again, indicating how pleasurable he finds, or found, each of the activities.

Although this schedule, with its 320 items, may appear rather exhaustive (if not exhausting), American nurses have used it routinely with people-in-care in Oregon, where it was developed, for many years. British nurses intending to use the schedule may need to translate some of the American phraseology for the British context.

The Activity Questionnaire

Several authors have pointed out that depressed people tend to be slow and confused in their thinking. For this reason the lengthy Pleasant Events Schedule may prove to be too arduous. It is important, however, to try to find out which kinds of activity might help to restore the person's mood to something near a 'normal' level. The following activity questionnaire should indicate the kinds of activity that might be included in the care plan [18].

Introduction: You're feeling pretty depressed at the moment. You feel that you can't be bothered doing anything. Nothing gives you any satisfaction any longer. You don't see the point of trying to do anything. Maybe we could spend a few minutes talking about the kinds of thing you used to enjoy doing?

1. What sorts of thing did you use to enjoy doing before you became depressed?
2. Did you enjoy learning new things – like new sports or crafts – before you became depressed? What sorts of thing?
3. Did you enjoy going places: to the beach; up into the hills; visiting stately homes? Where did you like going?
4. What sorts of thing did you enjoy doing on your own: reading; playing solitaire; doing jigsaws?
5. What sorts of thing did you enjoy doing with other people: playing sports; talking; chatting on the phone; having a drink?
6. What sorts of thing did you enjoy doing that didn't cost anything: going to the library; watching pigeons in the square; walking the dog?
7. What sorts of thing did you enjoy doing that were inexpensive: having a snack in a cafe; going to the cinema; buying a magazine?
8. What sorts of thing did you enjoy doing at different times of the year: sunbathing in summer; walking in the woods in autumn; feeding the birds in winter; watching bulbs grow in spring?
9. What sorts of thing did you enjoy at different times of day: reading the newspaper in the morning; listening to the lunchtime news; watching the sun set?
10. What sorts of thing might you enjoy doing if you didn't have inhibitions: learning to paint; jogging; dancing?

	Monday	Tuesday	Wednesday	Thursday	Friday	Saturday	Sunday
7 - 8	Ded		AWAKE SINCE 3	B/FAST			
8 - 9	"		WASHED	TIDYING UP			
9 -10	coffee		CALLED TOM	STILL TIDYING			
10 -11	TV		"	UP !!			
11 -12	TV						

Figure 6.3 A typical activity schedule for a depressed person in hospital.

In addition to identifying the activities that the person might enjoy doing again, some record of his present activity is also necessary – if only to serve as a comparison. In Figure 6.3 I have illustrated a typical activity schedule belonging to a depressed person in hospital.

The person is asked to make a brief note of what he is doing at each hour of the day. If the person is unable to do this, staff may sample his behaviour every hour, noting the prevailing activity.

Comment

These three methods all look at activity, but have different functions. The BRS provides a specific measure of the person's behaviour from random samples throughout the day. High levels of activity may suggest that he is 'less depressed', low activity levels that he is 'more depressed'. Although I have noted the usefulness of this measure, it should be clear that such a method would tell us little about the 'masked depressive', who may appear happy, smiling and active but he may be deeply depressed. The Activity Questionnaire is designed simply to help the nurse draw up a list of activities that might be included in the person's care programme. Such a list is also possible from the Pleasant Events Schedule, but this can also tell us something about his present activity level and his potential for gaining satisfaction in the future. The assessment of activity may not only tell us something about the person's current affective state, but may help us plan how to raise this by arranging the occurrence of more pleasurable activities.

EXPLORING THE PERSON'S THINKING

We have discussed ways of assessing the person's emotional state through self-reports and a few days of assessing his behaviour patterns. The person's thinking style is the next key area to which we need to turn our attention. We need to collect information about how the person thinks about events in his life, and how these thoughts might relate to his affective level.

The triple-column technique

The 'triple column technique' has been popularized by the psychotherapists Albert Ellis and Aaron Beck, both of whom acknowledge the role that thinking plays in the generation of mental distress. In this method the person is asked first to identify a negative emotion experienced recently. How did he feel? Angry? Hurt? Jealous? He is also asked to rate – on a 0–100 scale – how unpleasant the feeling was. This is written down in the first column.

The person is then asked to identify the situation he was in at the time of the emotion. This is written down in the second column. The person is then asked to do a 'mental replay' of the scene, noting the events that led up to the unpleasant feeling. If nothing of any consequence happened, what sorts of thoughts were in his head just before the feeling occurred? These events, or his 'stream of consciousness' are written down in the first column. He is then asked to specify the emotion. How did he feel? Angry? Hurt? Jealous? He is also asked to rate – on a 0–100 scale – how unpleasant the feeling was.

Finally, he is asked to try to pick out the kinds of thought that occurred to him at the time of the incident, or within his daydream. These are called 'automatic thoughts' because they simply 'pop' into the person's head. These are also written down in the form that they 'appeared' to the person, e.g. 'I'm all washed up; everyone's against me; there's no point in trying'.

The exercise is completed by asking the person to rate the extent to which he believes the automatic thoughts, again using the 0–100 scale. Figures 6.4 and 6.5 illustrate the use of the triple-column method, along with a simpler questionnaire method, both aimed at identifying these thinking styles.

Thinking errors

A wide range of cognitive distortions has been described by some of the important figures in depression research [19,20]. Their view is that certain

DATE	EMOTIONS	SITUATION	THOUGHTS
	How did you feel ? How bad was it ?	Where were you ? What were you doing? What were you thinking ?	What thoughts popped into your head ?
Mon 25ᵗʰ Oct	Anger – 70 Jealous – 80	In town. Thinking of going to Job Centre. Saw old friend.	Why does he have all the luck ?? My life is a mess. I'll never get out of this !!

Figure 6.4 The triple-column technique for identifying automatic thoughts.

IDENTIFYING YOUR NEGATIVE AUTOMATIC THOUGHTS

We have discussed how the way you feel is influenced by the way you think. I want you now to practise finding out what sort of thoughts you have when you feel bad. Think about the last time you felt bad; you might have felt sad, or angry; guilty or frightened. Try to remember how you felt and what was happening around you and answer the following questions :-

Feelings

How did you feel ?   JEALOUS

How bad was the feeling - measure it by using a scale of 0 - 100
(where 100 is the very worst)

Score   80

Situation

Where were you ?   IN HIGH STREET

What were you doing ?   WINDOW SHOPPING

What was going on around you ?   SAW OLD FRIEND IN CAR

Were you thinking about anything in particular ? THINKING ABOUT GOING

TO JOB CENTRE - SEEING BANK MANAGER

Automatic Thoughts

What thoughts just 'popped into your mind at the time ?

GOD, HE'S DOING WELL

MY LIFE IS IN A MESS

WHY DO SOME PEOPLE HAVE ALL THE LUCK

Did you believe those thoughts ? Measure to what extent you believed them using a scale 0 - 100 (where 0 means you did not believe them at all; 100 means you believed them completely).

Score   90

Figure 6.5   A simple questionnaire method for identifying automatic thoughts.

thinking errors play a large part in triggering or maintaining painful affect. Among the thinking errors described by Beck and Ellis are:

- **all-or-nothing thinking**: the person sees things only in terms of black and white, rather than shades of grey – 'You're either a total success or a complete failure';
- **over-generalizing**: assuming that because a bad experience happened once, it will always happen in similar circumstances – 'I was unhappy the last time I saw him. It will be the same next time';
- **exaggeration**: reacting to a difficult situation as though it were a major disaster; blowing events out of proportion;
- **catastrophizing**: assuming that something terrible will happen as a result of the way the person coped with a difficult situation, e.g. fearing that because he has had a row with his wife she will leave him, he will lose contact with his family and his whole life will collapse;
- **discounting the positive**: overlooking the positive aspects of any situation; assuming that they 'don't count' for some reason; thinking that he is all weaknesses and failings, with no strengths or assets;
- **jumping to conclusions**: coming to a conclusion without recourse to any obvious facts to support this view, e.g. deciding that someone doesn't like the person because she has not come over to introduce herself – often called 'crystal ball gazing';
- **shoulds and musts**: the person feels extremely anxious if he does not live up to some very high standard of social or ethical behaviour: 'I must always be nice to people, or they won't like me'; 'I should always be on time or people will think that I am lazy'.

Although there is some dispute as to the significance of these thoughts in the production of mood disorder, it is often easier to understand the person's state if his major thinking errors are identified. The idea that these thinking styles are a barrier to effective problem-solving or coping is a very plausible one. By asking the person to make a note of the kind of automatic thoughts he has in 'depressing' situations, we can draw up a list of his typical thinking errors. This may help us understand at least one of the reasons why he becomes depressed.

The assessment process grows with the passage of time. Initially, the nature of the nurse's inquiry may be relatively superficial. With time, the degree of exploration will become more focused and more revealing of the nature and function of the person's mood problems. The exploration of the person's thinking and belief systems occupies the middle and later phases of the assessment process. By this time the person will be receiving different kinds of help and his depression may be beginning to lift a little.

Assessment should not, however, be restricted to the beginning of the person's period of care and treatment. Assessment should be contiguous, opening out different facets of the person's functioning, enlarging upon existing pieces of information. This process is most evident in mood disturbance, where the person's ability to participate in the assessment process is very much a part of the disorder itself.

Case illustration

Marion is a 28-year-old dentist. She is unmarried and lives alone. She was admitted to hospital after a drug overdose. This is her fourth admission, the first occurring when she was a student. On admission she is withdrawn and uncommunicative. Staff feel that she is unable to complete the BDI, which is routine after 3 days on the ward. The registrar completes the Hamilton. Marion is thin and pale in appearance. Her eyes are dark, adding to the gauntness of her appearance.

She is weighed on admission and daily thereafter. Staff begin the Behaviour Rating Scale observation on the third day, following a case conference. Ratings of her sleep are also kept by night staff. Over the first few days these observations are monotonous: Marion rarely stirs from her chair where she sits, curled up, only occasionally getting up to look out of the window. She comes for meals when encouraged by staff, but eats little. On day 4 a food and fluid intake record is started. On the same day a nurse completes the BDI by reading out the statements. Marion simply answers 'the first one' or 'that one'. Her voice is weak and thready. She avoids eye contact and sits turned away from the nurse during any interaction. The nurse notes these features and draws up a short checklist covering these key verbal and non-verbal behaviours. On day 5 the staff rate the level of appropriate eye contact, orientation to the nurse, gestures, volume and tone of voice during each interaction. Staff also note her predominant activity on the activity schedule, hour by hour. At the end of the day they total the number of hours spent in different activities. By the middle of the second week Marion has become a little more active. However, she does not volunteer any information or start any interaction with staff or persons. Staff hold regular short conversations with her to try to gain a more detailed history of the events leading up to her admission. All the questions are 'closed', eliciting only 'Yes/No' answers. Her mother is interviewed on day 8, having flown from Australia. On day 10 Marion is able to complete the BDI with a little help from the nurse. On day 12 she begins to talk a little to the nurse who handled her admission. This nurse is identified as the 'keyworker' and begins to extend the range of the short interviews to cover Marion's thoughts about work, friendships and her overdose. On day 19 she completes the Activity Questionnaire interview, and a list of preferred activities is drawn up. On day 21 she begins to keep her own activity schedule. By day 25 the interviews with the nurse have progressed to analysing her thoughts about some of the unpleasant events in her recent past, using the triple-column technique.

Discussion

Marion's assessment is a fairly typical example of the assessment of a depressed person. Initially, various physical observations are made – weight, pallor, etc. In some settings these might include various blood analyses. Close observation of her behaviour begins early on and is maintained for the duration of her stay, expressed through the Behaviour Rating Scale, activity schedules and sleep record. Close observation is also maintained on her food intake due to her wasted and undernourished appearance. Her affective level appears to be very low on admission, but can only be assessed indirectly through the Hamilton. Later the BDI gives a rough estimate of her actual mood state, and is eventually done weekly through to discharge. The nurses use a range of interviews – some formal, others less so – to monitor her verbal and non-verbal behaviour and also to collect some information about her expressed emotions and beliefs.

As her depression appears to lift, the intensity of the assessment increases. She begins to monitor her own activity, draws up a list of possible 'pleasurable' activities and starts to evaluate her thinking style. By this stage treatment is well established, but the assessment is ongoing. This kind of assessment is typical because it reflects the need for assessment to build up gradually. It should be geared to the actual presentation of the person. By closely observing the person, the nurse will know when she might be ready to move on to a new 'level' of assessment. In this sense assessment and treatment run together, although it is to be hoped that the assessment done at the beginning will influence the choice of care and treatment methods. In some situations it is possible to arrange that all the assessment takes place at the beginning, using this information to plan the treatment, then following up with evaluations of progress.

In this example we see the need for 'staging' assessment, building it up, layer upon layer, in order to collect more elaborate descriptions of the person's state or information about different aspects of his problem.

ASSESSMENT OF THE PERSON WHO IS SUICIDAL

Intentional death

Man has exercised a fascination with his ability to kill himself since the earliest recorded times. The writings of philosophers, from Marcus Aurelius and Seneca to Albert Camus, and writers, from Virgil to Sylvia Plath, have all made great contributions to our understanding of the phenomenon of suicide. Rational study has, however, been obstructed greatly by religious taboos, which prevail across all cultures. At the same time, the confusion over the definition of 'self-destructive' behaviour has often diminished our appreciation of the nature of suicide itself. People who – for example – 'drank themselves to death' may (or may not) have committed suicide.

It seems clear that 'true' suicide is dependent on **intention**. If this can be established, then the legal definition of 'accidental death' may be ruled out. The obligation – or temptation – to define an apparent suicide as accidental, however, leads to under-reporting, estimated to be in the region of 50–100%. Suicide is the situation where someone brings about his own death, the assumption being that he did so knowingly. This separates it from accidental death – death by misadventure. Where someone makes a non-fatal suicide attempt – often called parasuicide – this usually involves drug overdose. I mention parasuicide here because there is evidence that 1% of those admitted to hospital after parasuicide will commit suicide within one year. It is also known that 20% of parasuicides will make another attempt within one year. This risk factor remains at a high level for about 10 years, with the result that about one half of the people who commit suicide have made earlier attempts [21]. These findings slay the myth that suicide is always unexpected, or that parasuicide is a trivial issue, which never leads to the 'real thing'.

Women and men

Throughout the world, the 'successful' suicide rate for men is approximately three times that of women, although women make more suicide attempts. How men and women kill themselves also differs greatly. Men adopt more violent methods from which there is 'no turning back' – shooting, jumping, poisoning – while women tend to use drug overdoses.

Age differences

Differences exist also between men and women with respect to age. The suicide rate for men increases steadily with age until the mid 80s, with a peak during the period 50–65. The rate for women levels off during the ages 40–55 and again around the seventh decade. The belief that suicide increases during the menopause has not, however, been supported by research [22]. Suicide in younger people is very low for children under 10 but rises during the pubescent period and increases rapidly almost tenfold between the ages of 15 and 19.

Circumstances

There is much evidence that suicide is commonest during the depressive phase of manic-depressive psychosis, often triggered by bereavement, although a history of alcohol abuse is also a common factor. Across both these groups social isolation greatly adds to the likelihood of suicide. Suicide rates are four times greater for single, divorced or widowed people. In the case of widowed people, the first year represents a high risk period.

The risk of suicide increases if the person is manifestly depressed – especially when vegetative signs are present: problems in sleeping, early morning wakening, appetite or weight loss, decreased energy or libido. However, the expression of feelings of hopelessness and general pessimism are the most significant indicators of suicide risk. Indeed, suicide risk is associated more with feelings of hopelessness than depression alone [23].

Suicide – myths and realities

It has been estimated that more than 1000 people in the world commit suicide each day. In Britain there are over 3000 deaths each year from suicide with parasuicide being ten times as common. Suicide is a highly emotionally charged subject. It is also one surrounded by myths. There are well-established beliefs, even in professional circles, that suicide happens most often without warning; that those who threaten suicide rarely carry it through; that all attempted suicide is attention-seeking or trivial; and that all people who kill themselves must be mentally ill. All such beliefs are false.

The suicide myths

- **People who talk about suicide never do it**. Repeated threats of suicide suggest that the person is having suicidal thoughts, which should be addressed seriously. The threat of suicide should be taken as a sign that something is wrong in the person's life. Failure to acknowledge the threat may only confirm the person's fear of failure or sense of worthlessness.
- **Elevation of mood following a period of depression suggests that the threat of suicide has passed**. An improvement in mood often occurs prior to a suicide attempt. A cheerful disposition may even reflect the person's relief that they have finally come to a decision to commit suicide.
- **Suicide is more likely in the winter – when the weather is gloomy**. Although some forms of mood disturbance occur in poor light conditions, the suicide rate peaks in the spring.
- **The shame and pain associated with suicide will deter people from attempting to commit suicide a second time.** Having attempted suicide once, the person is more likely to try again, if his life conditions do not change. Four out of every five 'successful' suicides have made at least one previous attempt.
- **Suicide usually takes place at night.** The professional belief that suicide is 'a cry for help' is supported by the fact that many suicides occur between 3 pm and 6 pm. Attempts during daylight hours may, therefore, be viewed as at least an unconscious cry for help.
- **Discussing suicide with the person will 'give them ideas'.** It is clear that the truly suicidal person already has the idea. Talking, at any level, may actually help focus on the problems that make suicide an attractive proposition.
- **If there is no suicide note, it is not a 'proper' suicide.** Only a small proportion (15%) of people who commit suicide leave notes.

- **Once someone has decided to commit suicide, nothing will deter him.** Providing that the problems that precipitate the decision are addressed, many suicide attempts can be prevented. It is important to recognize that the attempt, even when it appears 'final', is a communication – or signal – of the person's despair. All who 'receive' that communication need to respond appropriately [24].

The nursing assessment of suicidal intent

People may kill themselves most often when we consider them to be 'of unsound mind'. It is also clear that many people kill themselves when in a highly rational frame of mind. We do such people a grave disservice by suggesting that everyone who kills himself is unbalanced [25]. Suicidal thoughts are commonly expressed by depressed persons and, as the figures show, may be crucial signals of a potential death threat. For this reason the assessment of suicidal intent is a crucial issue in the assessment of the depressed person.

There are, however, many dimensions to the nursing assessment of suicidal intent. This includes the following.

- **The history of suicidal behaviour**. The person may have made previous attempts on his life. If so, what was involved: chosen methods, circumstances, etc.?
- **Family history of suicide**. Values about 'the meaning of life' are often modelled within families. Is there any family history of suicide that might provide important pointers for later exploration?
- **The person's view of the future**. Suicidal intent is assumed to be grounded in a sense of hopelessness. Exploring the person's short- and medium-term plans is important. To what extent has he 'given up on life'?
- **Mental health status**. Suicide is more likely if the person is depressed, has a serious alcohol abuse problem, suffers from bipolar disorder or has a diagnosis of schizophrenia. If the person carries any of these diagnoses, how serious is his 'primary disorder'?
- **Withdrawal and social isolation**. Social support – or more importantly its relative absence – is a major factor in suicide. To what extent has the person retreated from social supports, or to what extent have others abandoned him?
- **Behaviour suggestive of suicidal intent**. Suicide is rarely an impulsive act. Preparation is often necessary – gaining access to medication, sharp instruments or firearms. The person may also begin to put his affairs in order – preparing, revising or checking wills, or advising family members about finances. Is there any aspect of the person's behaviour that suggests that such preparations are ongoing or imminent?

Talking to the person

Staff often avoid talking to people-in-care about suicide. A commonly expressed fear is that this will 'put the idea of killing themselves into their heads'. Most authorities believe that nothing could be further from the truth [25]. By asking about suicidal thoughts, or even past attempts, we may offer a degree of relief, providing that the subject is handled in a non-threatening or non-judgemental manner. In this sense the suicidal intent assessment can be therapeutic. It is clear that many nurses are alarmed, however, by the prospect of talking to people at any length about suicide. We should not underestimate the degree of skill and courage that is needed. Both are often only acquired through painstaking training and experience.

Choosing the moment

Information about suicide is often collected when the person is communicative or when an attempt has just been made. In the former he may not feel suicidal. In the latter his faculties may be blunted by the emotional or physical effects of the attempt. The best time to discuss suicide is when he is highly suicidal. This is, of course, the most difficult time. The threat to the nurse is greatest here, especially if she fears she may make matters worse. Yet this is perhaps the only time when a realistic picture of his despair or commitment to dying can be assessed. Here we can find out what is motivating him to take this action, how he might go about it and what might be deterring him, even temporarily.

When the person does not feel suicidal his views may be more carefully judged, even academic. When he is toying seriously with his 'final solution' a more accurate evaluation of his position may be possible. Contrary to popular myth, many suicidal persons plan their exit down to the last detail. In many senses it is an affront to their integrity to classify all suicides as 'of unsound mind'.

The interview with a suicidal person can be a chilling affair. It is not for the faint-hearted and clearly is not a job for the novice. We should be aware of other factors that might influence the person's report on his feelings. He may exaggerate the seriousness of his intent to increase staff or family support. Although we may suspect this, we may not dare risk doubting the person's word. In other cases the person may reduce the emphasis of his true feelings. He may have high moral principles or may feel guilty about harbouring such thoughts. In some cases he may simply fear being labelled as a suicide risk, perhaps resulting in compulsory detention under the Mental Health Act. On the other hand he may not wish to lose the respect of staff for whom he has some affection. Any of these factors may encourage him to conceal his intentions, or inflate or play down the seriousness of his feelings.

The high-risk scenario

By assessing the person at the height of his suicidal risk we may identify the factors of most significance. We should not forget that such information may also be 'news' to the person. He may get a chance to look more objectively at what is driving him to his death. Paradoxically, this may help him come to terms with his situation. The suicide assessment may have a vital therapeutic value.

Discussion with the person at other times is also important. Where the person is thought to be a suicide risk, persistent monitoring is indicated, increasing this at times of obvious crisis. Like many of the other problems we have discussed, suicide is a continuum. At one extreme is the strong desire to go on living, at the other the clear intention to kill oneself. Attitudes towards living and dying change as one progresses towards either end.

It is possible to assess suicide risk using the linear analogue method mentioned earlier in the chapter.

'Tell me how you feel about life generally. (Drawing line on paper) Let us say that here (pointing) you feel that you have everything to live for ... and here (pointing to the other end of the line) you feel "what's the point, there is nothing to live for?" Where would you say you are now between those two points?'

Parasuicide

The person who jumps from a high-rise building or leaps into a deep river is taking an irreversible course of action. Other death games may carry risks but may be less absolute. Russian roulette is an experiment in mathematical probabilities. An overdose, taken in the knowledge that someone might find him, is also an experiment in the schedules of fate. In both cases, if the experiment is done often enough, the odds will eventually be loaded against the person. Even if the person 'expects' to be found, the risk remains, and will increase with each attempt.

Where an apparent example of 'parasuicide' is involved, we need to ask the question: 'Why should he take such a risk?' It is well known that certain life events – like bereavement – can decide the person in favour of suicide. Other events, such as the arrival of a friend, or the anticipated forfeiture of his wife's insurance claim, may act as a deterrent, at least temporarily. Let us now consider two factors that play a part in the creation of suicide, factors that need to be identified in the assessment.

The escape solution

Suicide can be seen as a means of escape. It can solve what is seen as intractable distress. This distress may be real, as in bankruptcy or bereavement; or perceptual, where the person feels that something is insoluble though others might not agree. Either way the person feels hopeless in the face of adversity. He may even show a disturbingly calm acceptance of the pointlessness of his existence. The 'best' solution – under the circumstances – may be to commit suicide. He may even suggest that this is the best solution for all concerned, reducing the burden on family, friends and even staff. Often the action taken may be absolute. Although rare – and most likely in the case of men – violent means may be used by the person who feels hopeless and wishes to guarantee his escape.

The change effect

The person may try using suicide as a solution to a problem in a less dramatic fashion. He may be trying to make others realize how desperate he is, or may be trying to force them to give him more support. As noted earlier, this is often called the 'cry for help'. It has been suggested that more than half the persons hospitalized for suicidal attempts tried to kill themselves to escape what they saw as intolerable situations. A smaller proportion tried to manipulate others in the way described here, and a third had mixed motives [26]. Those who take the escape route may be much more seriously depressed than those who are trying to influence others. The 'escapers' feel hopeless. The 'influencers' are by definition hopeful of some change.

Clues and cues

A number of factors may make suicide more or less successful. We need to identify these to reduce the risk. People who talk a lot about death or dying, even obliquely, may be signalling their future actions. They may be fairly explicit: 'I don't see the point in carrying on any longer', or 'This is the only way out for me'. In other cases the message may be less clear: 'Things aren't going to get any better', or 'I know that I'm just a burden on everyone'. Some people may let slip their intention to kill themselves by saying 'Goodbye' instead of 'Goodnight', or saying 'I don't suppose that I'll see you again'. These 'slips' are not always indicative of suicide intent. The rule is, however: 'Better safe than sorry'.

All such comments should be recorded *verbatim*, as part of the overall assessment of the person. The discovery of stockpiles of drugs or potentially harmful objects may also be important clues, which should be noted. The same is true of sudden decisions, such as changing a will or getting rid of pets. Where the person is extremely agitated, he may become very calm before committing suicide. This calm may be interpreted as a sign of progress and may lead to a slackening of observation. Although these 'clues' may lead to nothing, there is no harm in being suspicious.

Significant features

Our assessment should attempt to judge the degree of risk involved. As I have noted already, there is always some risk. In time all attempts, no matter how abortive, may acquire significance. Positive answers to the following questions may help identify attempts that already indicate seriousness and might herald a final suicide attempt.

In assessing the previous suicide attempt:

- Did the person commit the act in isolation, where he was unlikely to be found?
- Did he fail to summon help?
- Did he develop a pattern of missed appointments or general 'unreliability' before the attempt? Did he apologize for his lateness or bad organization?
- Did he make any 'final acts' – making a will, arranging insurance cover for his family or settling finances?
- Did he ensure that he had ample means to complete the suicide?
- Did he leave a suicide note?

The empathic assessment

In assessing suicidal intent we must try to see his situation and his actions from his perspective. Staff and families are often stunned by suicide. They cannot understand why he should want to die. 'He had everything to live for – a lovely family, nice home, good job'. Although apparent to us, such 'realities' may not be so clear to the person. He has his own way of construing reality.

Alternatively, he may appreciate that he is fortunate but may believe that he does not deserve such good fortune. His unworthiness, coupled with his well-endowed status, may be the provocation for his suicide. We need to see things through the person's eyes. We must be open to what he sees as missing from his life, and why he feels that life is not worth living. Both viewpoints may illustrate his distorted vision. They may illustrate how he evaluates his own worth or his life in general. We should try to see his problems as he sees them, at least at first.

It is very tempting to reassure the person: 'Don't worry, you'll get over this. Lots of people feel like you do. They get over it.' This temptation should be resisted. We need to know why he thinks that he won't get over this. The nurse needs to find out what kind of beliefs might serve as the basis for killing himself.

Alternatively, he may not face any tangible problem, but may find his life a vacuum – devoid of any pleasure or meaning. Again it is important to establish why he thinks this is so, instead of trying to point out all the things he might do to restore his reason for living. In some cases the person may have real problems. He may be in financial difficulties; he may live in bad housing;

he may have terminal illness. He should be given the opportunity to express his feeling about these 'trials' before any attempt is made to soothe his distress or to help him adjust to these problems. We try to see his problems through the person's eyes. At the same time we try to retain our objectivity. Where the person has experienced major trauma or is massively disadvantaged it is difficult to avoid feeling for him. This is to be avoided wherever possible. The person may interpret such emotion – especially sympathy – as further indication of the hopelessness of his situation.

So how should the nurse respond to the person who has much to be suicidal about? She should show concern, empathy and a willingness to allow the person to express his feelings to the full – at least for the moment. I suppose I am advocating a sensitive, controlled show of **grave concern**. Grave enough to show the person that he is being taken seriously yet not so grave that he interprets this as a sign of the futility of his situation.

The Hopelessness Scale

Although much of the information we need about suicidal intent can be obtained from interviews and observations, a specific scale has been developed to help enhance the assessment of this key area [27]. The person's confessed 'hopelessness' is a better predictor of suicide than his level of depression. The Hopelessness Scale tales only minutes to complete and may be given to the person at regular intervals to monitor the risk of suicide.

Hopelessness is defined as the person's negative attitude towards himself and the future: he does not expect any change. The scale carries 20 items, which are scored in a straightforward 'True or False' format. Although of special relevance to suicide and depression, it has been suggested that this scale is relevant to other forms of psychological disorder, such as psychosis, physical illness and drug abuse.

Case illustration
Just before Christmas 1962, Sylvia Plath moved from Devon to London with her two young children. She rented a flat in Primrose Hill in which the Irish poet W. B. Yeats had lived as a child. By now she was estranged from her husband, the English poet Ted Hughes, who, having helped her find the flat, visited the children weekly. Although she had never previously written to her, she tried to keep up appearances by writing to her mother: 'I have never been so happy in my life'. When she was visited on Christmas Eve by a friend he found '[her hair] hung straight to her waist like a tent, giving her pale face and gaunt figure a curiously desolate, rapt air …. [It] gave off a strong smell, sharp as an animal's' [28].

Sylvia Plath had written extensively of her suicide attempts. She had attracted much hostility for this, being called at one point the 'Judy Garland of American poetry. If you want to kill yourself, you don't make an attempt; you do it …. Writing poems about your suicide attempts, is pure bullshit' [29]. She was a complex character, who empathized with all manner of tragic figures – from the victims of the Nazi holocaust to Lazarus. In a BBC reading of her poem 'Lady Lazarus' she acknowledged that 'one pays dearly for immortality: one has to die several times while still alive' [30].

After 10 years of suicide attempts Sylvia Plath found herself 'betrayed' by her husband; confined with her small children to her flat by the deep snow and frozen streets of the coldest winter in 150 years; pipes frozen; roof leaking; power cuts rendering the flat dark and icy. She felt guilty for having criticized her family and friends in her novel *The Bell Jar*. She also feared another major breakdown, more ECT and (perhaps) permanent insanity. Individually, she might have dealt with these pressures. Overall the cumulative effect was overpowering and she eventually gassed herself on 11 February, having made arrangements for her children's breakfast, as they slept.

Had she survived, the circumstances of her latest attempt might well have proved the classic case of attempted suicide. She was depressed, following the breakdown of a relationship with a man she adored. She was bereft of a confidante, with two small children dependent on her for all their needs. She felt guilt about her past actions towards her friends and family. She felt ambivalent: neither the criticism nor the praise heaped on her was justified. She was weakened, physically and psychologically, by the terrible cold and isolation caused by the weather. She could see no way that things could improve; things could only get worse. In a macabre recreation of the death of the Jews whom she so admired, she put her head in the gas oven, having made all the necessary preparations for her children.

Plath has become (probably) the most famous suicide of the century, if not of all time. Debates still rage in academic circles over the circumstances of her death: was this another 'cry for help'; was this only another example of her 'art of dying'? Like many other cult figures of her generation and since, her death guaranteed her immortality, far more of her work being published since her death than during her lifetime.

Jeffrey Meyers notes that poets like Sylvia Plath are icons of all our self-destructive urges:

Our age is obsessed by its own capacity for self-destruction: by pollution, drugs, AIDS, poison gas, radiation, terrorism, genocide, death camps and nuclear war. The manic poets who enriched our lives as they ruined their own, symbolize individual examples of this destructive impulse. We are fascinated by their suffering and see it as a vicarious substitute for our own [31].

The nursing assessment of people with a mood disturbance, especially those who are suicidal, can present grave threats to the psychic welfare of the nurse. Where the assessment of the suicidal person is concerned, nurses have an opportunity to confront their deepest fears. The person who is suicidal may offer the nurse his own 'tragic gift'. He may help her appreciate something of (both) the inestimable value and futility of life.

NOTES

1. Plath, S. (1971) *The Bell Jar*, Harper & Row, New York.
2. The term 'melancholy' is experiencing something of a revival, in an attempt to distinguish severe depression from other affective disorders. See Mendels, J. (1970) *Concepts of Depression*, John Wiley, New York.
3. Laing, R. D. (1985) *Wisdom, Madness and Folly: The Makings of a Psychiatrist 1927–67*, Macmillan, London.
4. For a fuller consideration of the 'sadder but wiser' hypothesis, see Layne, C. (1983) Painful truths about depressives' cognitions. *Journal of Clinical Psychology*, **39**(6), 848–53; Barker, P. (1992) *Severe Depression: A Practitioner's Guide*, Chapman & Hall, London.
5. Beck, A. T. (1972) *Depressions: Causes and Treatment*, University of Pennsylvania Press, Philadelphia, PA.
6. Mendels, J. (1970) *Concepts of Depression*, John Wiley, New York.
7. Hamilton, M. (1982) Symptoms and assessment of depression, in *Handbook of Affective Disorders*, (ed. S. Paykel), Churchill Livingstone, Edinburgh.
8. Norey-Whiteside, P. (1988) Depression and suicide: a response to loss, in *Applied Psychiatric-Mental Health Nursing Standards in Clinical Practice*, (eds M. J. S. Krebs and K. H. Larson), John Wiley, New York.
9. Beck, A. T., Rush, A. J., Shaw, B. F. and Emery, G. (1979) *Cognitive Therapy of Depression*, John Wiley, New York.
10. Beck, A. T., Ward, C. H., Mendelson, M. *et al.* (1961) An inventory for measuring depression. *Archives of General Psychiatry*, **4**, 561–71. Beck has since developed a further version of this inventory, which is illustrated in Beck, A. T., Rush, A. J., Shaw, B. F. and Emery, G. (1979) *Cognitive Therapy of Depression*, John Wiley, New York.
11. Beck, A. T. (1972) *Depressions: Causes and Treatment*, University of Pennsylvania Press, Philadelphia, PA.
12. Zung, W. K. (1965) A self rating depression scale. *Archives of General Psychiatry*, **12**, 63–70.
13. Aitken, A. C. B. (1969) Measures of feeling using analogue scales. *Proceedings of the Royal Society of Medicine*, **62**, 989–93.
14. Hamilton, M. (1967) Development of a rating scale for primary depressive illness. *British Journal of Social and Clinical Psychology*, **6**, 278–96.
15. Montgomery, S. A. and Asberg, M. (1979) A new depression scale designed to be sensitive to change. *British Journal of Psychiatry*, **134**, 382–9.
16. Williams, J. C., Barlow, D. H. and Agras, W. S. (1972) Behavioural measurement of depression. *Archives of General Psychiatry*, **27**, 330–3.

17. MacPhillamy, D. and Lewinsohn, P. M. (1971) The Pleasant Events Schedule. Unpublished manuscript, University of Oregon. This schedule is available from Peter Lewinsohn at the University of Oregon. See also MacPhillamy, D. and Lewinsohn, P. (1974) Depression as function of levels of desired and observed pleasure. *Journal of Abnormal Psychology*, **83**, 651–7.
18. This questionnaire derives from the work of Beck, A. T., Rush, A. J., Shaw, B. F. and Emery, G. (1979) *Cognitive Therapy of Depression*, John Wiley, New York.
19. Beck, A. T. (1972) *Depressions: Causes and Treatment*, University of Pennsylvania Press, Philadelphia, PA.
20. Ellis, A. (1961) *Reason and Emotion in Psychotherapy*, Lyle Stuart Press, New York.
21. Kreitman, N. and Dyer, J. A. T. (1981) Suicide and parasuicide. *Nursing*, **30**, 1310–11.
22. Weissman, M. M. and Klerman, G. L. (1977) Sex differences and the epidemiology of depression. *Archives of General Psychiatry*, **34**, 98–111.
23 Beck, A. T., Steer, R. A., Kovacs, M. and Garrison, B. (1985) Hopelessness and eventual suicide: a 10 year study of patients hospitalized with suicidal ideation. *American Journal of Psychiatry*, **142**, 559–63.
24. Lester, G. and Lester, D. (1971) *Suicide: The Gamble with Death*, Prentice Hall, Englewood Cliffs, NJ.
25. Beck, A. T., Rush, A. J., Shaw, B. F. and Emery, G. (1979) *Cognitive Therapy of Depression*, John Wiley, New York.
26. Kovacs, M., Beck, A. T. and Weissman, A. (1975) The use of suicidal motives in the psychotherapy of attempted suicides. *American Journal of Psychotherapy*, **29**, 363–8.
27. Beck, A. T., Weissman, A., Lester, D. and Trexler, L. (1974) The measurement of pessimism: the hopelessness scale. *Journal of Consulting and Clinical Psychology*, **42**, 861–5.
28. Adapted from 'Epilogue: Sylvia Plath' in Meyers, J.(1987) *Manic Power: Robert Lowell and his Circle*, Macmillan, London.
29. *Ibid.*
30. *Ibid.*
31. *Ibid.*

The assessment of relationship problems: from intimacy to isolation

7

Tell me with whom you live and I will tell you who you are.

Spanish proverb

Before we can ask such an optimistic question as 'What is a personal relationship?', we have to ask if a personal relationship is possible, or, **are persons possible** in our present situation?

R. D. Laing

INTRODUCTION

The child is father of the man [1]

Modern psychiatry has paid much attention to the issue of relationships. All the 'psychoanalytic' models of mental disorder suggest that the person-in-care's distress arises from dysfunctional relationships with significant others in his environment, either past or present. These relationships feature, although at times obliquely, in the psychotherapeutic process. The interpersonal relations model of mental disorder took those considerations a significant stage further and, by virtue of its consideration of how people are largely a function of their relationship with others and their culture, has much to offer us today [2]. The interpersonal psychiatry of Harry Stack Sullivan (1892–1949) emphasized communication, interaction, interpersonal relationships and other aspects of what might be called 'social psychology' [3]. His emphasis on these interactive elements led many of his critics to suggest that he had lost sight of the personality itself [4]. Ironically, he may have been the first important figure in modern psychiatry to recognize that mental disorder of all kinds – rather than simply the neuroses – derives from the person's engagement with the world and those within it.

In Sullivan's view, the 'self' was made up of 'reflected appraisals', brought to bear on the child by parent figures and other significant others. He believed that from birth onwards every individual interacts continually with and absorbs attitudes from reacting to other people. These multiple experiences are the shaping of the 'force of life' [5]. As a person develops from infancy through childhood and adolescence to adulthood, other relationships may be established, which will have a profound influence on who the person is. Because a person is so enmeshed in such relationships Sullivan believed that the concept of the 'self' was deceptive. It was more accurate, in his view, to think of the 'self' as an 'envelope' that encloses the person's whole experience, and that 'envelope' originates and functions interpersonally. Sullivan's ideas paralleled those of the social psychologist George Herbert Mead, who described the 'mind' as a continually changing dynamism, and also many modern philosophers who have rejected the concept of self on the grounds that it is the last vestiges of old-fashioned mind–body dualism [6].

Sullivan could hardly be called a key figure in late 20th-century psychiatric or psychotherapeutic theory. However, his theory that the person's view of himself derives from the views constructed in the relationships of childhood was an important influence on Laing's interpretations of psychosis and is to be found today in the 'cognitive therapies'. In particular, it is recognized that the dysfunctional schemas that support self-defeating thinking styles – related, for example, to depression – arise from the 'construction of the self-view', which begins in childhood [7].

Sullivan's view of interpersonal relations was provocative to say the least, when he suggested that, if his theory was to be in any way successful,

> it will finally have demonstrated that there is nothing unique in the phenomena of the gravest functional illness. The most peculiar behaviour of the acutely schizophrenic patient, I hope to demonstrate, is made up of interpersonal processes with which each one of us is or historically has been familiar. Far the greater part of the performances, the interpersonal processes of the psychotic patient are exactly of a piece with processes which we manifest some time every twenty-four hours [8].

This view has always made 'common sense' to me. Sullivan's dictum that 'we are all more alike than different' seems eminently sensible. Sadly, some nurses take the view that Sullivan's theory is no more than 'untestable ramblings' [9]. This could hardly be further from the truth, as Peplau illustrated with her development of his theory of interpersonal relations within nursing [10]. In particular, her description of how nurses might explore the relations that go on within the person, which will be alluded to in Chapter 8, have major implications for the kinds of relation that go on between the person-in-care and others, which will be addressed in this chapter [11].

It is not, however, my intention to discuss relationships in this highly specific way here. I note only that we should not make the mistake of assuming that any of the relationship problems we shall address exist in any kind of a human vacuum. If the reader is not already acquainted with the significant and sizeable literature on interpersonal relations within nursing, I hope that these introductory comments will encourage them to become so [12].

Our relationships play a central role in shaping the direction of our lives. However, this constitutes a vast canvas, too great for either the space available or my own experience to do justice. Instead I shall discuss the role that relationships play in our lives at present: the relationships we have with people in general, from our intimate contacts through to the more general context of our place in society. I shall focus on only some of the different kinds of interpersonal problem that are commonly presented within the nursing situation, and how nurses might go about assessing these.

Human relations

It is a cliche to acknowledge that people are social animals. Yet this is where we must begin: at the banal end of the spectrum, looking at the individual's place in a social world that differs only from that of our animal cousins in its complexity. If we can fit into our society we may be called adaptive or adaptable. If we do not, history tells us that we are likely to be labelled a deviant, a misfit, an eccentric or some kind of inadequate personality.

There is great pressure to conform to society's rules and regulations. Those who decide to flaunt them must be brave indeed – or may simply be incapable of keeping up with the standard. One of these rules is that people should have relationships. The man or woman who has no friends or acquaintances is viewed with suspicion. 'What is he hiding? Why do people not want to know him?' we may ask. Apart from the fact that 'having relationships' expresses the fulfilment of a convention, they serve other important functions. As Aristotle noted, 'in poverty and other misfortunes of life, true friends are a sure refuge'. Those characteristics of a true relationship were echoed by Oliver Cromwell when he said that 'the light of friendship is like the light of phosphorus, seen plainest when all around is dark'. And from Plato we derive the idea of a relationship which is genuine because it is freed of passion and instinct, a relationship that Plato thought would be long-lasting since it was based upon more elevated forms of choice. The 'Platonic' relationship would help each person aspire to new heights rather than simply meet basic needs.

The idea that our relationships might also serve an 'elevating' function was expressed also by Confucius: 'Never contract friendship with a man who is not better than thyself'. Here also is found the idea that relationships can be a means to an end: the enrichment of the individual through positive association with others. However, not anyone can provide this growth function for us. As the old saying goes: 'Never become the fourth friend of a man who has had three before but lost them'. Most of us know the pitfalls as well as the heady heights of the relationship game. Perhaps one of the most significant comments on the subject comes again from Dr Johnson: 'A man should keep his friendships in good repair'. When we come to consider the relationship problems of the psychiatric person, the need for repair is often all too obvious.

I said at the start that I would also try to cover (wo)man's place in society. This is a vast topic, which I shall not do the injustice of considering here. What I mean is that, through our discussion of certain kinds of interpersonal difficulty, I hope to shine some light on our wider role as members of a society: a society that indirectly fabricates the interpersonal rules and regulations that people find awkward. In this sense we are citizens first and individuals second. This can present a significant conflict for many of us, a conflict we often cannot resolve.

Relationship problems

In order to simplify matters a little, I shall classify problems which involve relationships under five main headings:

- **the person who experiences interpersonal anxiety** – the person who can't;
- **the person who is unable to assert himself** – the person who doesn't;
- **the person who finds the mechanics of interaction difficult** – the person who doesn't know how to;
- **the person who believes that he is isolated or alienated** – the person who doesn't think he can;
- **the person who is isolated or alienated** – the person who doesn't have a chance to.

These are rather simple, non-exclusive categories. A person with 'relationship problems' may show two, three or perhaps all of these problems. However, it is important that we identify in which way these subgroups of relationship problems may be evident in the case of the person concerned.

In Figure 7.1 I have tried to illustrate how relationship problems might mirror varying degrees of social incompetence.

At one end of this figure we have the 'social masters': those people who are active in a wide range of social arenas and who cope successfully with all manner of social problems. Because of their 'master' status, making and maintaining relationships presents no problem. As we move further along the base of the figure, we encounter people who are progressively less masterful. At first we meet people with single problems: teachers who find it difficult to 'relate' to large classes; party-goers who find it difficult to relate to strangers. Then we meet people with a few such problems: the worker who cannot keep his emotions under control when in conflict with colleagues, especially if they are relative strangers to him. Or the young man who finds large groups of

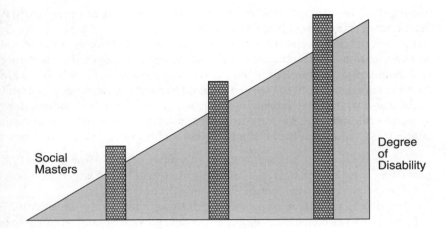

Figure 7.1 Relationship problems and social competence.

people threatening and is uncomfortable when required to discuss personal material in a 'one-to-one' interaction. As we progress further along the figure, the nature and scale of people's social interaction problems increase, making them more and more socially incompetent. At the furthest end of the figure we would probably meet some of the very withdrawn people whom we today call those with a 'serious or enduring mental illness': people who may avoid almost any kind of relationship.

This model of social competence can be misleading. A person might have a single relationship problem, which differs according to his situation. A 'shy' person in a small community might be liked and respected for his 'sensitive nature'. In a bustling metropolis he may be ignored or alienated by people used only to the pressures of the concrete jungle. Although the person is the same in both situations, the problem can vary enormously. It hardly needs repeating that the 'meaning' of any pattern of human behaviour is context-bound: it depends where and with whom the behaviour takes place.

ASSESSING SOCIAL AND INTERPERSONAL FUNCTIONING

The relationships interview

Most people discuss their relationship problems in terms of their reactions to others: feelings of depression, agitation, embarrassment, anxiety, etc. Many people who complain of these problems may, in effect, be complaining about their relationships. Our first task is to gain some idea of how the person developed his current 'social skills'. This is a study of the development of his ability to relate to others. We need to ask about how he formed relationships with people as he was growing up. Was he a shy child? Did he have many friends? Did he tend to fight or get bullied? When did he have his first 'relationship', whether platonic or sexual?

From this brief review the nurse might move on to look at some of the typical situations that might present any of us with difficulties. This is hardly an example of a 'diagnostic' interview. All of the situations in which we are interested are common: they are problematic to most people in general, if not to the nurse who is interviewing in particular. Despite the 'common' nature of these situations, the answers to these questions may provide important information about who the person is, in terms of his relations with others.

'Tell me a bit about how you get on with other people. How do you find starting conversations?' (Does he find it easier to talk to strangers, acquaintances or groups? Why does he think this is the case?)

'How do you feel about asking people for things – like doing you a favour?' (Under what circumstances might he do this, how often, and with whom?)

'How do you feel about expressing your opinions?' (To what extent is he 'his own person': can he disagree with people, especially with those who are in some position of authority?)

'What do you do if someone appears to be making unreasonable demands on you?' (Does it make any difference if they are friends, family, strangers or colleagues?)

'How do you feel about paying people compliments?' (How difficult or easy would he find that and why?)

'How do you find making arrangements with people?' (How easy or difficult is it for him to make 'dates' with women (or men), or to 'negotiate' meetings with friends or colleagues?)

'Speaking of "negotiations" ... how do you handle your relationships? (Can he 'give and take' or does he always have to 'have his own way'? Can he compromise? Does it make any difference if this involves family, friends, colleagues or relative strangers?)

'If you feel you are in difficulties, would you ask for help?' (If not, why not? If so, from whom and why?)

'How do you feel when you are applying for jobs or "putting yourself forward" in some way?' (Does he think he can 'present' himself? When he stands back from himself, what does he 'see'?)

'When you have something to complain about, can you do that without losing your temper? (To what extent would his response be influenced by who was involved, or what were the circumstances?)

'People will often try to put pressure on you to do things against your better judgement? How do you handle that?' (Can he stick to his beliefs, values or whatever when 'under pressure'? What kind of 'pressures' are imposed on him? Does he feel obliged to drink, have sex, take drugs or give information about others, etc.?)

'How do you feel about telling people how you feel about them?' (Can he express both positive and negative feelings or neither? How does he feel about that?)

'We have talked about your "relationships" with others in great detail. Looking back on all of what you have told me, what do you think all of that says about you? What do you think that says about [name]?'

These examples no more than scratch the surface of the person's relationships with others. They may, however, provide a relatively non-threatening means of encouraging the person to reflect on his relationships with others. Such 'reflections' may provide him with a useful introduction to identifying his difficulties in relating to others. As noted earlier, these situations – and the problems associated with them – are common to most people, including ourselves. In this sense these questions are as relevant to someone with a diagnosis of 'schizophrenia' as they are to someone who is ascribed any kind of neurotic diagnosis. Much mental disorder involves a re-enactment of relationship problems from the past or is in some way influenced by our relationship history. We often pay people with more 'serious' mental illness a great disservice by **not** asking them this kind of question. We do not do so on the assumption that their problem somehow lies within them. We might care to consider how their present difficulties exist between them and the significant others in their lives.

A general social skills questionnaire

In Figure 7.2 I have illustrated a short questionnaire which may help identify the areas of the person's life that are a problem to him.

This covers many of the areas we have already covered in the relationships interview. This kind of approach provides the person with an opportunity to decide for himself, at his leisure, which interpersonal situations are the most or least problematic. This sort of scale might help the nurse identify some of the 'kinds' of relationship problem discussed in this chapter. This might be used as a formal measurement tool, although it was not designed for this purpose. Its main purpose is to provide pointers toward more specific areas of assessment.

Following on

Once we have some idea of the situations that cause the person some difficulty, we need to establish more clearly what these situations mean to the person. He might complain of anxiety in public. What does he do in such situations?

- Does he feel unable to speak?
- Does he talk incessantly or excitedly?
- Does he stammer or stutter?
- Does he feel deficient in some way, but is unable to specify this clearly?

NAME .... DATE ....

Please read each of the following statements. Rate how you handle each of these situations using the scale below:

1 = I have NO DIFFICULTY doing this
2 = I have a SLIGHT DIFFICULTY doing this
3 = I have QUITE A BIT OF DIFFICULTY doing this
4 = I have GREAT DIFFICULTY doing this
5 = I NEVER do this or would AVOID the situation

CIRCLE THE NUMBER WHICH MOST CLOSELY REFLECTS YOUR REACTION

TALKING TO PEOPLE
1. When I meet people I can start a conversation with them.   1 2 3 4 5
2. I can start talking about something and carry on a conversation.   1 2 3 4 5
3. When others are talking I can join in.   1 2 3 4 5
4. When someone is talking to me I can appear interested.   1 2 3 4 5

SAYING HOW YOU FEEL
1. When a person has done well I can compliment them.   1 2 3 4 5
2. If someone does something for me I can thank them.   1 2 3 4 5
3. I am able to encourage others.   1 2 3 4 5
4. If I care about someone I can show them how I feel.   1 2 3 4 5
5. I can tell someone that I am angry without losing control.   1 2 3 4 5

EXPRESSING MY NEEDS
1. I can put my point of view in an argument without losing control.   1 2 3 4 5
2. I can give people instructions without feeling embarrassed.   1 2 3 4 5
3. I can ask to see the person in charge if I am making a complaint.   1 2 3 4 5
4. I can tell people exactly what I want (e.g. in shops)   1 2 3 4 5

DEALING WITH OTHERS
1. I am able to understand how other people are feeling.   1 2 3 4 5
2. I can listen to what a person has to say.   1 2 3 4 5
3. If I fall out with someone I can work out what went wrong.   1 2 3 4 5
4. I can deal with someone who is angry without becoming upset.   1 2 3 4 5

FRIENDSHIP
1. I can talk to people I have met for the first time.   1 2 3 4 5
2. I can talk to people in a group.   1 2 3 4 5
3. I can make dates to see people.   1 2 3 4 5
4. I can take the initiative to make a friendship.   1 2 3 4 5
5. I can go to a new place in order to meet new people.   1 2 3 4 5

DEALING WITH MYSELF
1. If I am upset I can calm myself down.   1 2 3 4 5
2. I can control my temper before it gets out of hand.   1 2 3 4 5
3. I can make plans and stick to them.   1 2 3 4 5
4. I can negotiate with people.   1 2 3 4 5
5. I can work out how I feel and how I should deal with it.   1 2 3 4 5

Figure 7.2 A short social skills questionnaire.

GOALS

Read over the scale again and pick out the situations which you would like to be able to deal with better. Make a list of these below.

1. _____
2. _____
3. _____
4. _____
5. _____
6. _____

Figure 7.2 Continued.

- Why are any of these things a problem to him?
- How does he think he should behave?
- What does he think is wrong with his performance?

THE PERSON WHO CAN'T

The person who **can't** presumably **could** if something wasn't stopping him. The question is: what? In this first class of relationship problems we are dealing with people who know what they would like to do but are prevented from carrying this out for fear of what might happen. This fear may have some history. The person may have had a bad experience with people in the past. Or it may be based entirely in his imagination. Either way, this fear hinders the creation of effective relationships. In some cases this may be made worse by friends telling the person: 'It's all in your mind ....you only think that you've got a problem'.

This interpersonal anxiety is a variant of the generalized anxiety discussed in Chapter 5. Here the person feels distressed whenever he plans or is required to meet with people. In some cases he may have no problem with strangers. In others, he may be comfortable with friends but awkward with everyone else. He may say that he 'doesn't know what to say' when meeting people for the first time, or feels uncomfortable 'talking about myself'. He is rarely ever unskilled. He may doubt his ability, but he does know what to say. He is prevented from putting this knowledge into practice by his anticipation of what might go wrong. This leads to an avoidance of social contact, or very superficial relationships. In some cases he may break the contact in mid-sentence to escape from his distress.

Usually, we talk about these interpersonal functions as 'social skills', although this classification does tend to underestimate what is involved in such encounters. The ability to communicate information, show interest in others, establish rapport, take risks in self-disclosure, and say and do 'the right things' are complex interpersonal skills. For many people this is a tall order. Situations play an important part in deciding what constitutes appropriate interpersonal conduct. For example, appropriate behaviour on a first date, when making a complaint or when paying a compliment are all variations on a theme. They all require the use of gestures, speech, facial expression and the use of what actors call 'timing'. However, if the way these actions are performed didn't vary from one situation to another, we would not be able to tell a complaint or a compliment from hesitant love-making. Those who are 'social masters' often find it difficult to imagine how complex such interpersonal behaviour can appear to the socially anxious.

The person who finds such interactions threatening may be overwhelmed by their inherent complexity. It appears so complicated that he can never imagine himself getting it right.

Who experiences interpersonal anxiety?

Most of us have felt uncomfortable in the presence of someone, at some time. This may be someone of high status, such as a supervisor or dignitary, or someone to whom we attribute importance, such as a bank manager or a 'blind date'. In such situations our anxiety centres upon our ability to handle the situation correctly or successfully.

The person with interpersonal anxiety feels much the same. He is apprehensive about the situations we all take for granted. He might be the 'shy young man' who fails to grow out of his adolescent lack of confidence. Or he might be the older person who has never felt comfortable with people. Such people lack the social contacts most of us use as the base for our lives. Or they may be unable to use such contacts to their satisfaction. People who are interpersonally isolated – lacking friends and 'confidantes' – are psychologically vulnerable. Their interpersonal anxiety may be a harbinger of more serious psychological distress. In other cases it may coexist with an established psychiatric disorder, where it is difficult to say which came first.

Case illustrations

Roger works in a small electronics firm on an assembly line. He is in his early thirties, unmarried and living with two friends in a flat in a large town. He used to be a drummer with a rock band that split up some years ago. Despite his experience 'on the road' Roger has always had difficulties in dealing with people. He appears 'normal' but confesses to considerable inner anxiety. He has several friends and regular relationships with women. He retains a great fear of meeting new people, entering new situations and talking to women. Surprisingly, he has no problem with sexual relationships. His anxiety centres upon simpler things like eating in restaurants, holding hands in public and expressing his feelings.

Harry is 50 and is diagnosed as a schizophrenic. He lives with his wife in a council flat and attends hospital each day for 'day care'. As a young man he was an art teacher and retains an interest in cultural pursuits. His wife says he was a quiet young man, who mixed well and played the organ in church. He was also secretary of the local art club. Harry confesses that he finds any interaction with people difficult. 'I've lost all of my confidence. All those years in hospital have just chipped away at me.'

Roger and Harry have similar problems. Their ability to socialize is limited by anxiety. Both men have grown up acquiring at least a modicum of social skills. However, Roger does not appear to have gained the confidence to be himself. Harry once had this to some degree, but has lost it with the passage of time. Both men could do the things they would like to do, but their faith in themselves does not match their technical ability. As a result they become the 'people who can't'.

Assessment of interpersonal anxiety

The social anxiety shown by Roger and Harry can lead to avoidance of almost any kind of social contact. The person may feel that he will make a fool of himself; embarrass others; lose control; or 'go mad'. Often he will scrutinize himself closely – and objectively – during each and every social interaction, becoming like a 'spectator' in his own life. This preoccupation with his performance reduces his chances of behaving normally, leading to even greater anxiety and further avoidance. The person's 'problem' is very similar to the anxiety problems discussed in Chapter 5 and might be assessed by any of the approaches discussed there. Interpersonal anxiety is special in that the person may only experience anxiety in general social, or specific interpersonal situations. Or his anxiety may be far more severe in such situations. This suggests that there is something 'special' about the interpersonal context that generates such anxiety responses.

In the assessment the nurse is interested to know:

- in which situations the anxiety response occurs or is more marked;
- how severe the anxiety response is, in specific situations and overall.

Although the context is different the same format may be used here, stressing interpersonal relationships.

The Social Anxiety and Distress Scale (SAD)

Developed in 1969 by Watson and Friend [13], this scale measures the tendency to avoid or feel anxious in social situations. The questionnaire deals directly with individual interactions, e.g. 'I usually feel relaxed when I meet someone for the first time'; and with groups – 'Even though a room is full of strangers, I may enter it anyway'. The scale carries 28 items, which are scored True or False. Some of the statements are worded positively, such as those above. Others are negative, such as: 'I try to avoid people unless I know them well'.

After completion the scale is scored by counting the number of times the person gave a negative reply to either positive or negative statements.

The scale has been well researched and has been shown to be reliable and consistent in a number of studies. This is a popular scale in work with people showing social anxiety of an interpersonal nature. To use this assessment the person needs little preparation. The scale can be completed in a few minutes and scored just as quickly. Studies indicate that changes in the level of interpersonal anxiety and distress are reflected in a change in the total score. This emphasizes its value as an evaluation tool.

The Social Situations Questionnaire

This method was developed and published by Trower, Bryant and Argyle [14]. The questionnaire comes in two parts. The first part deals with the person's feelings in various situations. He is asked to rate his degree of difficulty on a five-point scale. He rates how difficult he finds the situation now and how he felt approximately one year ago. The scale includes general social situations, e.g. 'going into shops', as well as the more specific 'being in a group containing both men and women of roughly the same age as you'. It also includes some highly specific social behaviours, such as 'looking at people directly in the eyes'.

The first part includes 30 such statements. In the second part the person is asked to rate how often he has performed various social activities, this time using a seven-point scale, ranging from 'Almost every day' to 'Never'. In this section there are 22 items, including, once again, 'going into shops' as well as more specific items such as 'making the first move in a relationship'. The person is asked to rate the relative frequency of each action over the last 3 months, and a similar period a year ago.

Although this scale covers many more areas of behaviour it is no more difficult to complete than the SAD. The statements are clearly presented and clear instructions are given in the use of the ratings. The scale has obvious uses in the evaluation of progress. It may also prove very helpful in selecting specific treatment goals, such as 'anxiety in groups' or 'talking to people'.

THE PERSON WHO DOESN'T

The person who doesn't is in many ways like the person who can't. He fails to do things he knows are appropriate and regrets this for a long time afterwards, the man who would like to pay his wife a compliment or tell the office grouch to stop complaining but who 'chickens out' being typical examples. We might call him **unassertive**. The unassertive person has become almost a vogue problem ever since Alberti and Emmons highlighted various methods for solving such problems a quarter of a century ago [15]. Often seen as a

branch of the West Coast American obsession with 'personal growth', assertion deficit has always been a bigger problem than we have cared to admit.
Often it is overlooked because such people merge into the background. They
make few demands. Society even encourages unassertiveness as a way of
maintaining control, or resisting political change.

The unassertive person is often described as lacking in spontaneity, emotionally inadequate, inhibited or otherwise constricted. Some people have
argued that assertiveness is the open expression of practically all feelings with
the exception of anxiety. Anxiety seems to inhibit the show of other emotions.
However, there is some dispute over the definition. It might be useful here to
try to draw together some of the key descriptions in the pursuit of simplicity.

Dictionary definitions are often conflicting. Some define assertiveness as
'imposing one's proper authority' and would include 'domineering'. Perhaps
it can be defined simply in terms of 'standing up for one's rights; exercising
the right to say no, to tell the truth, to stand one's ground, to refuse to be
manipulated'. The assertive person carries out these various actions without
infringing the rights of others. Assertion may be seen as the midpoint between
aggression and passivity, perhaps even as the neutral pivot between these two
extremes of emotion and behaviour. The assertive person won't allow himself
to become downtrodden; neither does he trample on others.

Assertive behaviour

Contrary to popular belief, assertiveness is not a personality trait. It is a skill
that may be exercised in some situations but not in others. The managing
director of a large firm may be a forthright leader in the boardroom but a
'henpecked' partner at home. A small number of people are unable to assert
themselves anywhere. More commonly the problem is situation-specific. For
instance, men find it easier to be assertive towards women; and both men and
women can be assertive with people they know well rather than with strangers.
This tells us that we should avoid looking at assertiveness as a global construct.
It is a facet of individual functioning that can vary from one situation to
another.

Not all unassertive people appear meek and downtrodden. In some cases
the person may be a mixture of very passive and highly aggressive reactions.
The two cases here illustrate this dichotomy.

Case illustrations
Sally is a clerk in the civil service. She is in her late twenties and has just
returned to her old job after a period in a travel agency. Attractive,
intelligent and sociable, she was the picture of health when she married
Dick, a self-employed printer. She began to feel the pressure at work about
2 years ago. Her office is very hierarchical. She is still a junior clerk,
because she broke her service, and as a result she gets most of the work

to do. Most of the staff feel overworked, but don't complain for fear of recrimination. Sally began to dread going to the office. She hated the pressure, the fear of making mistakes, meeting the deadlines. One Sunday night she resolved to resign. She told Dick, who at first supported her. They would manage. She felt a wave of relief. By the end of the night Dick had confessed that the business wasn't going too well and would she reconsider? In a fit of despair she locked herself in the bathroom and took an overdose of sleeping pills.

Alex is 25 and is married with a young daughter. For the past 2 years his GP has been treating him for depression. He complains of headaches, listlessness and anxiety about going out. He has a long record of convictions for assault and has been in prison several times. His record of violence dates back to his youth. He has had a number of psychiatric admissions, all involving overdoses or mild self-injury. Each admission relates the catalogue of violence and ends pessimistically with the diagnosis 'severe personality disorder'. Alex is very soft-spoken, almost inaudible at times. Although heavily tattooed, and with a scar across his cheek, he appears shy and retiring. He tells his story with much embarrassment. He describes all his 'outbursts' as situations where he gets frustrated or annoyed or when people disagree with him. He simply 'flies off the handle' and feels better for this release of emotion, but suffers regrets later when he sees what he has done.

Could these two people be more different? Different classes, different capabilities and different presentation. Yet they represent the same core problem. They are unable to solve their interpersonal problems without using some coping mechanism that works to their ultimate disadvantage. Sally plays the 'neurotic female' and Alex the 'aggressive male'. Although Sally is a 'doormat' at work, at other times she is seen as witty and strong-minded and certainly no 'loser'. Alex is at the other extreme. He swings markedly from being shy and retiring to violent, almost homicidal, behaviour. He can also be tender, especially with his family. Like Sally, his problem is situation-specific.

Both these people show complex human problems, which function on various levels. Under such complex circumstances we might prove most helpful by focusing on very specific aspects of their problems. In so doing we may help them begin to construct the 'bigger picture' of their life problems, their basis and possible solutions. In the examples illustrated here, we might begin by assessing the person's behaviour and the situations in which it takes place. Given that the person assumes that how they behave is unacceptable, we need also to ask: 'What might be appropriate responses in these situations?' How might Sally have dealt with the pressure at work? How might Alex have dealt with his frustration? The answers to these questions represent alternatives. They are not the only options open to them, but might form the basis for them deciding alternatives for themselves.

The assessment of assertion

A number of methods have developed to study assertiveness. Most follow similar lines to that developed by Rathus, the designer of probably one of the earliest and best-known scales.

The Rathus Assertiveness Scale

The Rathus Assertiveness Scale [16] covers 30 items. The person is asked to rate how characteristic these are of his behaviour in various interpersonal situations. A six-point scale is used which ranges from +1 ('Somewhat characteristic of me') to +3 ('Very characteristic of me'). Negative ratings of –1 to –3 are used to suggest how 'uncharacteristic' of the person is each statement.

Two typical examples are as follows.

- I am careful to avoid hurting other people's feelings, even when I feel I have been injured (unassertive).
- If someone has been spreading false and bad stories about me, I see him as soon as possible to have a talk about it (assertive).

All 30 statements reflect these negative (unassertive) and positive (assertive) qualities and are arranged randomly to reduce the risk that the person will answer in a stereotyped way to each statement.

Norms developed by Rathus show that men tend to score more highly than women. Using these norms it is possible to judge, crudely, how assertive the person is. However, we need to be cautious about accepting these scores (and normative values) at face value. These assume that North American patterns of interpersonal behaviour are exactly the same as those found in other cultures. It has been reported, for instance, that even within the USA there are differences between 'White' and 'Black' populations. Common sense would tell us that great differences might exist between the kind of interpersonal behaviour that is regarded culturally as 'assertive', 'unassertive', 'hostile' or downright 'aggressive'.

The value of this kind of scale is to offer a standardized format for evaluating the progress of the person. The 30 items may be used as a useful means of helping the person appreciate which aspects of his interpersonal behaviour are problematic, in which way. The ratings provide a simple means of helping him judge how such problems change, across time or in response to some intervention.

The Assertiveness Inventory

The Assertiveness Inventory [17] focuses on the person's emotional response to given situations. The scale covers 40 items on which the person is asked to judge:

- how anxious he would feel about doing something;
- what the likelihood is of him performing this particular behaviour.

A five-point scale is used to assess each item with 'None' (1) and 'Very much' (5) used for the anxiety rating and 'Always do it' (1) to 'Never do it' (5) for the probability rating. The following represent typical items from the scale. The person is asked to judge: 'How anxious would you feel about ... and how likely is it that you would ...

- give a friend a compliment;
- cut short a telephone call when you are busy'.

This scale has the advantage that it judges what the person might do as well as how he might feel: both are usually considered important in the initial assessment and ongoing evaluation of an interpersonal problem. This kind of scale helps us judge whether a change in the person's level of anxiety influences his behaviour and *vice versa*. This scale also helps pinpoint areas in which the person thinks that he needs some help.

The scale may also be used as a basis for goal-setting. Once he has scored the scale the person is asked to go through it again, circling those statements that represent areas in which he would like to change. As we have noted earlier, covering all of these 40 areas in an interview might well be exhausting, for the nurse as well as the person-in-care. It might also become extremely boring. The use of self-report methods such as the two noted above has obvious advantages in covering a wide area of interpersonal functioning in a relatively short period of time. They are appropriate, however, only for some people, perhaps similar to the two people illustrated. Someone who is poorly educated might feel threatened by the scoring system and this might well compound his difficulties. This kind of scale could be used, however, in an adapted form as the basis for a structured interview, the nurse using the questions and ratings as the basis for her questions.

THE PERSON WHO DOESN'T KNOW HOW TO

In this situation the problem is functional: the person has not acquired the ability to handle certain social situations, or his skills may be limited in some way. Social behaviour is a complex activity, combining speech pattern and content with body language. Some people fail to develop these skills beyond a basic level. If they are not painfully aware of their shortcomings, we can be sure that their gaucheness will not escape the notice of their peers.

We usually acquire much of our social skill from our parents, or whoever rears us. We look to these early 'role models' for guidance in the art of growing up. Peers at school or play influence further development. We learn to express ourselves at a primitive level in the home. We then use these skills to adapt ourselves to a variety of social situations. Where children grow up alone, or in an isolated area, or separated from their parents, their social development may be impaired. It is possible to repair such damage in adulthood, but some people fail ever to redress such impairments.

The importance of social skills in mental health was once summarized by a colleague who used a motoring analogy. The person who is socially proficient can handle any situation with self-assurance. He may have had good role models and a wealth of experience as a child. He merely needs to accelerate a little to respond to any new challenges. His sophisticated abilities make the fast lane his natural place on this motorway, where he speeds past those who are less proficient. The less sophisticated person may have had poor role models, lack of practice or a learning disability. As a result he is ill-equipped to face the stresses of the road ahead. He is suffering from a 'primary handicap', which is like driving a car with poor brakes or faulty steering. At the first hazard a crash is probable. People with underdeveloped skills often fail to deal with the pressures of the world. Such failures may herald the onset of a psychiatric disorder.

Other 'drivers' on this social functioning motorway once had social skills but have lost them. One example might be the person with an enduring mental disorder whose social functioning has been eroded by years of institutionalization, or the cumulative effects of his illness. This is often called a 'secondary handicap'. It follows rather than precedes the psychiatric disorder. His lack of social skills may be much greater than the person with a primary handicap. He may have lost the ability to communicate altogether. This person has moved into the deceleration lane, or on to the hard shoulder. He is leaving the motorway to look for some assistance.

It is important that we do not misrepresent social skills as mere 'cocktail party behaviour'. The ability to establish a social identity and to cope in society does involve us in playing roles. To assess social skills we need to study the way the person uses his body and his voice to project an image: to play a part. When people are required to be sympathetic or assertive, to handle a drunk or pay a compliment, they need to play special roles. Our assessment of their social skills focuses upon the specifics of their ability to play these roles.

Case illustrations

Jill is 20, with a history of manic-depressive disorder dating back to the age of 14. She also is described as having a mild learning disability. She is notable for her apparent indiscretion and lack of tact. She is overtly explicit when discussing personal material and openly gives away family secrets. Her awkwardness extends to a rather wooden posture: she is slightly stooped and she rarely gestures. She smiles in almost all interpersonal encounters, even when telling a sad story.

Derek was in hospital for more than 20 years, where he worked in the stores department. Now he lives in a hostel with other 'former patients' and has no employment. He was a civil servant before his admission with a severe depressive disorder. He rarely mixes with other people-in-care and spends most of his time walking around town. He is quietly spoken, but tends to be rather verbose, taking a long time to explain what he wants to say. He rarely looks at others when in conversation, rarely smiles or shows any emotional expression.

Derek and Jill are both ill-equipped for their role in wider society. Within the shelter of the hospital they had few obvious problems. In society at large they are manifestly handicapped, although perhaps for different reasons. Jill has failed to develop her skills to the full; Derek's may have been eroded. The distinction is largely academic. Their present difficulties are our main concern. We need to know in what way they are unable to fulfil some of the commoner social roles. Most successful interpersonal relationships depend on three features. Each party:

- is able to say what he thinks and feels – to be direct;
- is able to be honest;
- knows when and where such directness and honesty is appropriate.

We noted above that Derek tends to be rather verbose. This lack of directness may become a problem, especially if the other person becomes impatient. Jill, on the other hand, tends to be too direct, often failing to allow conversations to 'warm up' before she starts to become intimate. In the same vein she is too honest about what she thinks and feels, which earns her the label of being indiscreet. In her case she does not know whether this is appropriate. Derek seems to have similar problems. He treats everyone much the same; he doesn't discriminate between friends and workmates and rarely lets people know how he feels or what he thinks.

Assessing the mechanics

The assessment of social skills can be done in the natural setting, but this often poses difficulties. Perhaps such an assessment is easiest done under role-play conditions, especially if the person shares a care setting with others, such as a day hospital or residential setting. In this context the person is asked to act out a scene from his life: standing at a bus stop, making a complaint to the hostel manager or telling someone that he likes her. The situations selected must be relevant to the problem in hand and the people who would probably make up the situation should also be appropriate: e.g. staff or other people-in-care; friends or workmates.

The role play aims to evaluate some of the mechanics of social interaction, knowing full well that the person's behaviour under these artificial conditions may be quite different to that which prevails in 'real life'. Such an assessment will, however, provide a useful indication of how the person might perform under similar conditions.

Verbal behaviour

Four areas of verbal behaviour are usually seen as important in determining whether or not someone is socially skilled or unskilled [18].

- **Volume**. Does he speak too loudly or too softly? In some situations a soft voice is appropriate (confidentiality). In others a louder voice is more appropriate (making a complaint).
- **Tone**. The resonance of the voice communicates a great deal. If it is too sharp he may sound helpless or frightened. If it is flat, he may sound bored or depressed. Where his voice sounds 'thin' he may appear weak or submissive. If it sounds 'cracked' – breaking between fullness and threadiness – this may be interpreted as anxiety.
- **Rate**. The speed at which the person speaks may suggest his emotional state: anxious, angry or excited (too fast); or depressed or disgusted (too slow). Again appropriateness varies with situations. A person telling a story in a fast, breathless manner may sound excited or happy, which may be seen as appropriate. A person telling a workmate how to work a piece of machinery in the same fashion may sound impatient or anxious.
- **Interruptions**. Any breaks in speech may also be significant. Some people 'um' and 'er' incessantly, as though they are uncertain of what they are trying to say, or are bored. Where long pauses occur between sentences, this may be interpreted as anger or irritation. In this category we might also include stammering and stuttering, which tend to reflect anxiety, although all three could reflect this.

Body language

Of course people communicate much – if not most – of what they have to 'say' through their body language. Among the various patterns of non-verbal behaviour that are common, the following are important.

- **Eye contact**: The extent to which people look at each other during conversation varies. It is even influenced by the sex of the speakers. It has been suggested that people might spend as much as 75% of the time looking at the other person when listening, but only 40% of the time when doing the talking. In the assessment we might detect low levels of eye contact – which might be interpreted as embarrassment or lack of confidence – or staring – which might suggest hostility or confrontation.
- **Interpersonal distance**: The space between speakers is important. In a confidential exchange closeness is appropriate. Where conflict exists, the parties will be wider apart. In assessing this we need to ask: 'Is he standing too close or too far away for this situation?'
- **Gestures**: The person might use gestures that are descriptive, nodding his head to indicate 'Over there', opening his arms to suggest 'This big'. He might also use gesture to add emphasis to what he is saying, nodding or

shaking his head in agreement or disagreement; pointing in an aggressive display; putting his hands up to suggest 'No way'. He might also give away signs of emotion: touching or scratching his face – self-doubt; tapping his feet or picking at his clothing – impatience; picking or biting his fingernails, moving around in his seat – anxiety.

- **Facial expression**: Usually we 'accompany' the words we are saying with different facial expressions. If something is said to be disgusting, we screw our face up; if something is said to be funny, our face creases in smiles; if something is deadly serious, we hold a deadpan expression. Of particular importance here is the need for appropriate partnering of speech and facial expression. Does the person's face communicate the same thing as his words?

The content

The elements of interpersonal behaviour noted above address how the person communicates. Let us now consider the nature of what he says.

- **Length**. The length of any communication says a lot about the person. Too short and it may suggest lack of interest, anxiety or depression. Too long and it suggests dominance or aggression.
- **Appropriateness**. The appropriateness of the person's speech depends very much on the situation. Does he disclose too little, or too much, about his personal life? Does he answer the questions asked? Is what he talks about relevant to the conversation and the context?
- **Quality**. Finally, we might wish to evaluate the quality of the content. Does it contain appropriate humour? Is the content varied and interesting? or boring and monotonous? Is the material too vague or too specific?

Rating the role play

A role play of a common interpersonal situation might be assessed in many ways. The focus and the amount of detail included depend upon the aims of the assessment, the skills of the observer, the time at her disposal and the specific problems of the person.

Figure 7.3 illustrates how some of the facets of social behaviour already noted might be assessed. The nurse might choose to use this kind of format when the person's social functioning appeared to be significantly impaired, and is thought to be a significant contributor to his difficulties.

Short role plays would be chosen that address the situations which appear to cause the person most difficulty, e.g.

- holding casual conversations;
- asking for help;
- accepting a compliment;

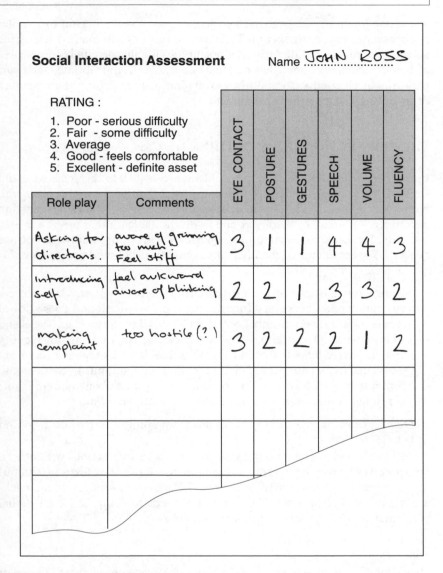

Social Interaction Assessment   Name JOHN ROSS

RATING :

1. Poor - serious difficulty
2. Fair - some difficulty
3. Average
4. Good - feels comfortable
5. Excellent - definite asset

Role play	Comments	EYE CONTACT	POSTURE	GESTURES	SPEECH	VOLUME	FLUENCY
Asking for directions.	aware of grinning too much. Feel stiff	3	1	1	4	4	3
Introducing self	feel awkward aware of blinking	2	2	1	3	3	2
making complaint	too hostile (?)	3	2	2	2	1	2

Figure 7.3 Assessment of social behaviour.

- disagreeing with people;
- making a complaint.

The role play context would be described briefly on the form and ratings are given for the person's performance of each of the eight facets. Ideally, the assessment would be conducted jointly with the person-in-care; each offering their ratings of the person's performance and using these as discussion points.

The nurse might also engage in the role play, inviting the person to rate her performance. Such mutuality might reduce some of the discomfort felt by the person and might provide further opportunities for sharpening his awareness of how his behaviour and that of others compare. If appropriate, such role plays might be conducted and assessed within a small group, each member contributing to each other's assessment.

THE PERSON WHO DOESN'T THINK HE CAN

In the three examples above all the problems are visible. In this sense we could say that they are real problems. In this category the problem is more ephemeral, but no less disabling. The person believes that he cannot or does not function effectively. This may be wholly at odds with the evidence that meets our eyes and ears. Here, the assessment of the person's behaviour is only part of our concern. We are interested mainly in his thoughts, beliefs and perceptions.

Case illustration
Dick is an architect with the local council. He is married with two children. He is a member of Rotary International, plays squash and does a lot of charity work. He is a member of the golf club, where he goes each weekend with his wife. Over the past 2 years Dick has been having 'an identity crisis': 'I have been looking at myself and I don't like what I see. I am weak, ineffectual and superficial. Sure, I go out a lot, but I don't seem to communicate with people. I'm so boring, going on and on about the same old things. I just seem to struggle to be with it all the time'.

Dick is feeling depressed, but hides this from family and friends, who find little to fault in him.

Although Dick's problems are still focused on his interactions with others, they involve the way he interprets these relationships. They are a product of his perception and judgement of his own behaviour, seen against the background of his 'perfect self'. The assessment needs to compare Dick's actual performance with the way he thinks he functions.

The interview

Dick's interpersonal alienation might be viewed as stemming from a range of thoughts he has about himself. Indeed, his fears may be more tightly focused than the vague social anxieties we have discussed already in this chapter. We might care to ask him:

- How do you feel about being rejected?
- How do you feel about being criticized?
- How close do you feel to the people around you, your family, friends, colleagues?

- How do you feel when other people show their feelings towards you – anger or affection, for example?

If Dick has any fears in any of these areas they may block the establishment of open relationships. Perhaps he is constantly setting rules, restricting his relationships, blocking his actual contact with others. He may also be unable to discriminate between the way he should act towards different groups of people. He appears to be something of a politician, always showing a friendly face, which may not reflect his true feelings. He may be dissatisfied with his life because of this lack of genuine closeness.

We might go on to ask:

- How do you feel about trusting people with your worries or anxieties?
- Do you ever feel that you must smile and be happy for everyone?
- What part do you think other people play in your present problems?
- If you disagreed with someone, or they obstructed you in some way, whose fault would that be?

Finally we need to consider Dick's expectations of his social relationships.

- What are you looking for in your relationships?
- Tell me how you see yourself.
- Describe the kind of person you would like to be.
- How do you guarantee that your relationships with people turn out well?

Fear of Negative Evaluation (FNE)

The person who feels isolated from others may appear to lack genuineness. He may hold distorted beliefs about his own ability and may be uncertain about the kind of relationships he wants to have. He may experience apprehension about meeting and dealing with people. He may appear, like Dick, to operate effectively but may be troubled greatly. Watson and Friend [19] developed a questionnaire which is a partner to the SAD scale mentioned earlier. The Fear of Negative Evaluation (FNE) scale is a 30-item True/False inventory which assesses the extent to which the person fears a hostile reaction in some social setting. This anticipatory anxiety is different from the anxiety experienced in the situation. A typical item is: 'I am usually worried about the kind of impression I make (Yes/No)'.

People who score highly on the FNE tend to become nervous in situations where they think that others will be evaluating their behaviour in some way. As a result they work harder to avoid disapproval or to gain recognition.

Listening to the internal dialogue: looking at thoughts

We have assumed that many of Dick's problems lie in his perception of his own behaviour. It may be appropriate, therefore, to look more closely at what he thinks about the situations in his life. Figure 7.4 illustrates a simple format

IDENTIFYING YOUR NEGATIVE AUTOMATIC THOUGHTS

We have discussed how the way you feel is influenced by the way you *think*. I want you now to practise finding out what sort of thoughts you have when you feel bad. Think about the last time you felt bad; you might have felt sad, or angry; guilty or frightened. Try to remember how you felt and what was happening around you and answer the following questions.

Feelings

How did you feel? _____

How bad was the feeling – measure it by using a scale of 0–100 (100 is the very worst)

Score _____

Situation

Where were you? _____

What were you doing? _____

What was going on around you? _____

Were you thinking about anything in particular? _____

Automatic thoughts

What thoughts just 'popped into your mind' at the time? _____
_____
_____
_____
_____
_____
_____

Did you *believe* those thoughts? Measure to what extent you believed them using a scale 0–100. (0 means you did *not* believe them at all; 100 means you believed them *completely*.)

Score _____

Figure 7.4 A simple format for recording thoughts and feelings.

for helping the person to reflect on his thoughts and feelings in any given situation [20].

The person is encouraged to recall a recent situation when he 'felt bad'. Having identified the situation he is encouraged to label his recollection of the feelings – using his own language – and to rate the severity. Then he is encouraged to relate the feelings he experienced to the situation he was in:

where exactly was he; what was he doing; what was going on around him, etc. Finally he identifies the thoughts he had in the situation: the thoughts that seemed, in some way, to be related to the situation, and the demands it made on him. Some people do not recall obvious 'thoughts' but can recall 'images' which they had at the time: 'Everyone seems to be laughing at me'; 'I seem to be shrinking!' Finally the person is asked to judge to what extent he believed the conversation that was going on 'in his head' at that time.

This simple examination of Dick's thoughts may clarify further the process by which he develops and maintains the difficulties in his relationships with others. The 'internal dialogue' in which he engages during such situations may involve 'replaying' some of the critical interpersonal experiences from his past. The adult who fears that others may judge him harshly may have been reared by parent figures who said 'Don't do that, people don't like it when you do that!' What 'that' was may have become obscured by time, but the fear that people might not like him for doing **something** may lie at the heart of his interpersonal difficulties. The assessment needs to explore, at some stage, what exactly Dick says to himself about himself, others and the situation. This dialogue may hold the key to his resolution of the problem.

THE PERSON WHO DOESN'T HAVE A CHANCE TO

This final group of interpersonal difficulties covers a range of people. This might include the person who has few relationships of a casual or meaningful nature. He has no supportive contacts, no one to share his troubles with. He may even have little contact with 'secondary groups': the news vendor on the corner or the assistant in the corner shop. Why he avoids even these non-threatening contacts is not clear.

The person who doesn't have a chance may be everyone we have already met rolled into one. He becomes anxious in any contact situation and resolves this by avoiding meeting people. When he can't avoid them he may feel that he can't communicate his feelings adequately. Such unassertiveness may be made worse by a lack of social skills. He may also be afraid that others will notice his awkwardness. Finally, he may exaggerate the importance of all of these factors. He may believe that he is worse than he really is. Others may find his company acceptable, even enjoyable. Due to his distorted perceptions he may be unable to appreciate this. If we ask the person why he has so few friends he might proffer the old cliche: 'Who would want me as a friend?'

This may be an accurate reflection of his predicament. If he is unaware of his problems, this may be an obstacle to forming new relationships. If he is aware of his shortcomings, he may predict his own repeated failure. The person who thinks that no one wants to know him will be unlikely to make an effort to establish new or rekindle old relationships.

The social context

In all the examples considered so far we need to see the person against the social backdrop of his life. We might wish to quantify the number of contacts he has and their role in his life. Sociologists tend to split such associations into two groups.

- **'Primary groups'** are those relationships with family or friends where we can disclose intimate details, gain support and encouragement: the fulfilling relationship.
- **'Secondary groups'** are more fleeting and superficial – people we speak to on the bus, staff who serve us in shops, colleagues we chat to idly in the lunch queue. These relationships rarely extend to anything beyond superficial conversation.

In assessing the person's social context we need to explore the dimensions of his primary and secondary group contacts. We need also to explore the meanings of such contacts for the person.

Case illustration

Mark is a lecturer in English at a university. He has published a number of books of poetry and is working on his first novel. He is of a classically asthenic build, with a beard and close-cropped hair. He is slow and methodical in his speech, as though considering every word. Neighbours find him 'a bit strange'. He lives alone, following the break-up of a long-standing relationship. He occasionally has a lunchtime drink with colleagues from his department, and dinner with the departmental head every month. Beyond this he sees no one. Mark is the classic 'garret artist', eking out a painfully remote lifestyle. Others see him as a highly committed individual who has settled for a private life devoted to his work. The impression is deceptive. Mark has begun drinking heavily in secret. He ruminates constantly about his social isolation, but feels unable to change it. He blames himself for his lack of social contact. In his view he is painfully uninteresting.

The effects of loneliness can hardly be overstated. People with inadequate or unsatisfactory relationships are prone to psychological disorder, which often ends in suicide. The abuse of drugs and alcohol is among the other common solutions used to blunt the pain of absent friends. Not everyone with poor relationships will become similarly afflicted. Some people enjoy isolation. However, the absence of confiding relationships can play an important part in the generation of psychiatric disorder.

Some of the people considered here may never have had satisfactory relationships. In others the person may be responding to what has been called an unresolved relationship problem. He may have had an involvement with a partner, family, etc. that went wrong in some way. This failure is taken as an indication that he should not, indeed cannot, get involved with others for fear of a similar ending. Such experiences are often taken as a reflection of the old adage: 'Once bitten, twice shy'.

Another group is those who interpret the breakdown of a previous relationship as a weakness on their part, or an illustration of their unattractiveness or unsuitability to others. This may lead to a succession of transient relationships. Contacts are made, often on an intimate level, but without any commitment. The person may be waiting for the relationship to collapse again, as others have in the past. Consequently he is unprepared for anything other than a brief contact.

Assessing the social network

Our first task is to assess Mark's social network. What relationships does he have at present? What do they mean to him? An important assessment goal is to describe his present social context. We might also retrace his steps to a time when his relationships were different, perhaps in his view 'healthier'. This might offset some of the gloom generated by a blank record sheet. This kind of assessment of his social network might be structured in a variety of ways. I offer here only one example, which maps his relationship to those closest to him (perhaps including old friends and family), through to newer contacts.

'I'd like to discuss your situation in more detail now. We have discussed how you feel isolated and alienated from everyone?' (Mark nods) 'OK. Now I'd like to look closely at your relationships – as they are now, and how they were in the past. Perhaps we could talk about your family first. Do you have any brothers or sisters?' (Mark nods) 'Tell me a bit about them. How did you get on together as children? How often do you see them? How do you feel about them?'

Mark is given a free rein to discuss his family relationships. The nurse prompts him with the odd word or phrase to give details about how often he sees them and what sort of 'things' they do together. How does he feel about them? Does he trust them? feel affection? animosity? jealousy? Does he get any support from them? Do they look to him for anything? Finally, a distinction is drawn between 'the relationship' as it is now and how it was in the past.

You feel that you and your brother have drifted apart, then? So you were close once, were you? In what way was the relationship different then?

Using a similar approach, the following areas would then be investigated:

- old acquaintances;
- friends from the past;
- neighbours or regular casual contacts;
- organizations to which he belongs: clubs, church, etc.;
- recent friends or acquaintances at work or in the neighbourhood;
- recent acquaintances gained through associations: clubs, societies, etc.

In taking this relationship history it is important to identify the people and to describe their role relationship to the person. This can be used to plot ways of reopening such relationships or using the experience gained to develop new ones. It might also be used as 'evidence' to show that once he had relationships that were at least mildly satisfying. Figure 7.5 illustrates a format for collecting this kind of information in a more organized manner [21].

The person is asked to detail all his contacts, whether brief or long-lasting, beginning with the most recent. He is asked to name the person, using an alias if he wishes. The relationship is then examined as follows.

1. When did you first meet Charlotte?
2. How did you come to meet her?
3. Did you spend a lot of time together? (A scale is used to rate this: 0 = Not at all; 1 = Once a month; 2 = Fortnightly; 3 = Weekly; 4 = Several times a week; 5 = Lived together.)
4. To what extent were you able to share your feelings with Charlotte? (A similar scale is used: 0= Not at all; 1= Rarely/superficially; 2= A little; 3= To some extent; 4 = A lot; 5= To a great extent.)
5. To what extent do (did) you think that you can (could) trust Charlotte, especially when you need(ed) support? (Same scale as 4. above.)
6. Did you have a physical relationship? To what extent was that satisfactory? (Same scale as 4. above.)
7. How close would you describe your relationship with Charlotte? (Scale: 0= Extremely casual; 1= Barely friends; 2= Friends; 3= Good friends; 4= Very close; 5= Inseparable.)
8. When did the relationship end? (If appropriate)
9. Why do you think it came to an end?
10. How did you feel about that then, and now?

Using this format, it is possible to describe and evaluate various facets of the relationship. We may then know how long the relationship lasted, how it began and ended and the person's perception of the nature of that relationship.

The spectre of loneliness

Loneliness has been described as 'the absence, or perceived absence of satisfying social relationships, accompanied by symptoms of psychological

	HENRY	SUZANNE
Began	AUG '93	1990 (?)
How	Net at club	COLLEGE
Time	4	3
Sharing	3	3
Trust	3	2
Intimacy	O	O
Closeness	3	2
Ended	Jan '95	SUMMER '96
Explanation	left town	QUARRELED
Feelings	Bitter never said he was going	UNCERTAIN HURT

Figure 7.5   A format for collecting information on past relationships.

distress'. Some people might admit to being lonely and might visibly be lacking in social contacts. Others might complain of loneliness but be seen by others to be sociable. Finally, there is a group that appears to have relationship problems but does not admit or complain of being lonely. Young has developed a self-rating scale that assesses some of the aspects of social relationships. His Loneliness Scale [22] assesses the person's attitude towards his relationships. This looks at the presence or absence of someone who cares for, or understands, the person, someone to whom he can disclose important feelings and share problems. It also looks at membership of groups, the availability of people to share values, interests, love and activities, as well as the availability of trust, enjoyment and physical intimacy.

The Loneliness Scale carries 18 items, each of which covers four points: for example, item 12:

> 0 = I can usually talk freely to close friends about my thoughts and feelings.
> 1 = I have some difficulty talking to close friends about my thoughts and feelings.
> 2 = I feel like my thoughts and feelings are bottled up inside me.
> 3 = I cannot seem to communicate with anyone.

The person circles the number which best describes his feelings or situation at that time. Young has collected norms to help classify different levels of loneliness. However, within nursing this scale might be used to monitor any change in the overall loneliness score, during treatment or rehabilitation. A score obtained on entry to a service might be compared with scores at discharge or following some specific therapy aimed at enhancing relationship-formation. Gains on the scale, though hardly a concrete illustration of actual change, would serve as indication of progress.

ASSESSING PROBLEMS WITH RELATIONSHIPS

Indirect measures: advantages and disadvantages

The methods of assessment discussed here rely either upon self-report or ratings by staff under role-play conditions. Both approaches have disadvantages, but the self-report methods may present more problems. Self-report scales are very economical, as they do not take long to fill in and the nurse need not be present. Where the method has been tested for reliability and validity (Appendix A) meaningful comparison between people sharing similar problems is possible. Such measures can also help prepare for further assessment. Finally, those methods that produce a total score can allow evaluation of progress across time.

However, the person may be unwilling to fill in such scales. He may feel threatened by questions about his relationships and may also find it difficult to distinguish different aspects of his behaviour. Even the simplest social interaction involves a complex of responses. Faced with this complexity, the person may be unable to distinguish (for instance) his aggression from assertiveness. Some others may have little awareness of the effect of their behaviour on others. To use a term very loosely, they may lack insight. Similarly, the person-in-care may be unable to judge or evaluate the behaviour of the person with whom he is interacting. When a person is 'justifiably angry' he has to be able to judge his partner's behaviour. What did he do to justify his anger?

The final problem is a technical one. Many of the scales mentioned are scored True/False or with some scale of relative frequency. Most people do not behave, or feel, the same across all situations. Therefore, their score is a kind of 'flattened average'. Not only do the scales lack specificity in describing the situation that the person finds difficult, but they also give an unrealistic report on his behaviour overall.

Direct observation

The ideal assessment takes place in the real world. In Jill's case we arranged a role play to look at her social skills. Ideally, we would have liked to be 'a fly on the wall' when she talked to her neighbours in the corner shop. In Dick's case we would have liked to monitor his thoughts as he arranged seating at one of his charity functions. The information collected in role play or drawn from memory can be misleading. Yet, fly-on-the-wall observations are often impossible. We may study the interaction of people-in-care on a hospital ward or in a day-care unit, but in most other situations direct observation is contraindicated. However, some people may be able to collect information about their own functioning, the value of which can never be overemphasized.

Self-monitoring

Most of the methods discussed in Chapter 4 can be used here. Roger has a basic fear of dealing with people, especially where he is required to be himself. The fact that he is competent when playing the role of 'the lover' seems to reinforce this. Although it is not mentioned in our brief sketch, we might expect him to avoid situations where his fear might overwhelm him.

Frequency measures

He could be asked to log in his diary, in a notebook or even on a scrap of paper each time he 'opts out' of meeting someone. Over weeks or months this would give us valuable information about his avoidance behaviour. He could also rate his anxiety, using the kind of scale shown in Chapter 4, making a note of the situation and its demands upon him. On the positive side, he might count the number of times he talks to people at work, goes out into company, meets someone new.

Similar measures might be taken by Sally: how often was she frightened of making a mistake? How often did she make a mistake? How often was she afraid of not meeting a deadline? or failed to complete work in time? We could extend these frequency counts to include the number of times she did speak up for herself, stood her ground, responded to criticism without tears. Ratings similar to Roger's would also be important here. Again there is no need for fancy record forms, providing that the information is collected consistently and the person knows what he is meant to be monitoring.

In Alex's case, measures of the number of times he loses his temper are obviously important. We also need to know what triggers this. He could simply write down in a notebook 'what happened', 'how I reacted' and 'what happened next'. In Dick's case the scene changes from overt behaviour and emotions to a focus on his thinking. He could count the number of times he has a certain 'negative thought' in the course of a day: 'I'm no use; I'm a bore; people must be fed up with me'. He could record these in the little notebook illustrated in Chapter 4, or even by tallying these up in his diary or on the back of a cigarette packet. It would also be important to ask him to make a note of the things he does, such as organizing meetings, taking his wife out for a meal. The kind of activity schedule illustrated in Chapter 6 might be useful here. Although this activity is not a problem, such information may be helpful later to act as a mirror to his perception of his self.

In Mark's case the frequency measure could be refined a great deal. Instead of just counting the number of times he meets people he might distinguish different kinds of conversation. He could count the number of casual remarks he made – 'Hello, good morning'; asking questions – 'Can you tell me the way to St James's Park?' and expressing opinions or talking about himself – 'I really admire women who are single parents'; or 'I used to play truant when I was at school'. Mark might be encouraged to 'brainstorm' ways he might monitor his performance in a range of social situations.

Time measures

Some of these aspects of the person's life could be studied in terms of time. It is unrealistic to expect him to carry a stop-watch to work or dinner parties. However, we might ask him to rate conversations in terms of length: brief (only a few words); short (one or two sentences); medium (giving a short commentary); long (speaking for several minutes).

Quality

The content of the person's interactions with others might also be monitored. To ease the strain, and embarrassment, of analysing social behaviour the person might award themselves points (in the manner of judges at figure skating or gymnastics) for different patterns of interaction. Different weightings can be attached to asking a question, giving an opinion, offering instructions, speaking in public, etc. Most, if not all, of these methods may be used by other people, such as staff or members of his family, to help add to the assessment of the person.

CONCLUSION

Relationships have always played an important part in the explanation of psychiatric disorder. However, 'relationships' in psychiatric nursing are often thought to be bound up in the rather vague dynamics of the therapeutic community or the magical interaction that takes place between nurse and person, which neither can explain. I have not dealt with these rather ephemeral aspects of relationship formation. As I noted at the beginning, these broader issues were not my concern and may be beyond my comprehension. Instead I have taken a fairly direct line, trying to collapse a wealth of relationship problems into a few categories. I would emphasize that these are in no way mutually exclusive. Some people may have two or more of these problem areas. Although these may be very disabling when they occur at great intensity, what is most interesting is that we can see ourselves in all of them. For me, this is an encouraging sign. Even where the person is allegedly 'different' from me – suffering from some alleged mental illness – we have something in common: a difficulty in maintaining our social competence.

In this chapter I have tried to emphasize a number of points. First of all, by focusing attention on specific aspects of the person's functioning we can help see his strengths and weaknesses through lists of different patterns of behaviour, emotions or thought processes. This takes him at least one stage forward from his rather vague 'relationship problem'. By specifying the different aspects of social functioning clearly, we can help him learn to distinguish his different roles, one from another. He is able to discover that he has several 'selves', some that might be useful to him and others that are less so. In this sense the assessment provides an educational facility. By trying to measure his social functioning we begin to understand a little of what the problem means to the person or those who interact with him. By studying his thoughts and beliefs – where appropriate – we can extend his understanding of how he functions and how he relates to others in terms of his own value system. Finally, the various strands of information drawn together from self-reports, casual observation, notes made on the back of cigarette packets or detailed ratings taken from video-tapes all add up to a multifaceted picture of a social animal. In some cases that picture needs to be complex, drawn from painstaking observation and thoughtful evaluation. In most others the information can be collected simply, using simple materials, most often of a 'home-made' nature. Either way, the picture should enlighten staff and person-in-care about the nature of his relationship problem and should open the door towards its resolution.

NOTES

1. Wordsworth's wisdom might appear sexist to today's audience. It remains wisdom nonetheless.

2. We have been rushing, at least since the 1960s, towards greater preoccupation with the 'self', 'self-centredness', if not 'selfishness'. Some of these concerns may account for the worldwide epidemic of depression, and the general air of anomie in postmodern culture. At the time of writing a friend from Australia sent me a note concerning Aboriginal art and culture. 'In Aboriginal cultures' wrote Jon Chesterson from Canberra, 'mental illness and causality is believed to be attributed to fate and events external to the individual and thus explained by supernatural forces, beliefs and customs. Traditional rites, our relationship with the land and other living species play an important role, often symbolically depicted in Aboriginal art and the Dreaming'. As Aboriginal people are increasingly 'integrated' into our postmodern society, they too might become obsessed with internal human attributes, be they physical or genetic, as a means of explaining the mysteries of mental illness.

3. Perry, H. S. and Gavell, M. L. (eds) (1955) *The Interpersonal Theory of Psychiatry*, Tavistock, London.

4. Ehrenwald, J. (ed.) (1976) *The History of Psychotherapy*, Jason Aronson, London, p. 304.

5. Devine, E., Held, M., Vinson, J. and Walsh, G. (eds) (1985) *Thinkers of the 20th Century*, Firethorn Press, London, pp. 550–1.

6. *Ibid.*

7. Beck, A. T., Rush, A. J., Shaw, B. F. and Emery, G. (1979) *Cognitive Therapy of Depression*, John Wiley, New York.

8. Sullivan, cited in Ehrenwald, J. (ed.) (1976) *The History of Psychotherapy*, Jason Aronson, London.

9. Gournay, K. (1995) What to do with nursing models. *Journal of Psychiatric and Mental Health Nursing*, **2**(5).

10. Peplau, H. E. (1988) *Interpersonal Relations in Nursing*, Macmillan, London.

11. Peplau, H. E. (1990) Interpersonal relations model: theoretical constructs, principles and general applications, in *Psychiatric and Mental Health Nursing: Theory and Practice*, (eds W. Reynolds and D. Cormack), Chapman & Hall, London.

12. Robinson, L. (1983) *Psychiatric Nursing as a Human Experience*, W. B. Saunders, London.

13. Watson, D. and Friend, R. (1969) Measurement of social-evaluative anxiety. *Journal of Consulting and Clinical Psychology*, **33**, 448–51.

14. Trower, P., Bryant, B. and Argyle, M. (1978) *Social Skills and Mental Health*, Methuen, London.

15. Alberti, R. E. and Emmons, M. L. (1970) *Your Perfect Right*, Impact, San Luis, CA.

16. Rathus, S. A. (1973) A 30-item schedule for assessing assertive behaviour. *Behaviour Therapy*, **4**, 398–406.

17. Gambrill, E. D. and Richey, C. A. (1975) An assertion inventory for use in assessment and research. *Behaviour Therapy*, **6**, 550–61.

18. This format is influenced strongly by Trower, P., Bryant, B. and Argyle, M. (1978) *Social Skills and Mental Health*, Methuen, London.

19. Watson, D. and Friend, R. (1969) Measurement of social-evaluative anxiety. *Journal of Consulting and Clinical Psychology*, **33**, 448–51.

20. Young, J. E. (1981) Cognitive therapy and loneliness, in *New Directions in Cognitive Therapy*, (eds G. Emery, S. D. Hollon and R. C. Bedrosian), Guilford Press, New York, ch. 8.
21. This format is influenced strongly by the work of Young (*ibid.*).
22. *Ibid.*

<table>
<tr><td>**8**</td><td># The assessment of the experience of psychosis: tales from the underworld</td></tr>
</table>

All are lunatics, but he who can analyse his delusion is a philosopher.
                                                            Ambrose Bierce

If one thinks about what is the case or is not the case seriously, intensely, and long enough, one seems either to drive oneself insane or to come to the conclusion that almost everyone else is or that we all are ....
                                                            R. D. Laing

INTRODUCTION

So far we have discussed ways of looking at people who behave in some disordered way. I have tried to keep as open a format as possible, eschewing wherever possible the labels which might lead us merely to confirm our prejudices about 'what is wrong with the person'. In this chapter I am faced with a dilemma. I wish to discuss people who have extraordinary experiences, and who appear to be affected by these both in the present and in the longer term. Such people have commonly been referred to as 'psychotics' [1]. In our postmodern and politically correct culture we now talk of 'people with an experience of psychosis'. I am reluctant to use the term 'psychotic', since it might suggest that I have made up my mind as to the nature of the person's presentation before beginning the assessment. I shall however use the term since I simply cannot think of an alternative way to discuss such experiential phenomena, and the resultant problems of living, without risking oversimplifying or devaluing such manifestly extraordinary experiences. I note here, however, my recognition that this is an illustration of my own deficiency; no more, no less.

In this chapter I shall discuss the kinds of experience that are called 'psychotic' and the patterns of behaviour commonly associated with 'people with an experience of psychosis'. Since I believe that it is (currently) neither the nurse's responsibility nor right to diagnose, I shall not discuss the diagnosis of psychotic disturbance.

The kind of personal maladaption that we call psychosis might be categorized in two ways. First, we might study the behaviour of the person: how the person appears and/or the experiences reported by the person. Second, we might classify the person on the basis of the (hypothetical) cause of his disorder, its prognosis and recommended treatment. Since the first option involves assessment, and the second diagnosis, I shall emphasize the former. I recognize that information collected by nurses may be used at a later stage by their medical colleagues to arrive at a diagnostic classification.

In this chapter we shall look again at the way the person perceives himself and the world around him. In the case of the person described as psychotic the kinds of experience we can expect to find will be of a different form or content from other problems of living. In some cases the content may be bizarre or unusual. Or it might take a more extreme or sustained form of usual experience. Taken together, the kinds of experience we shall discuss represent the more outstanding, outrageous and disturbing forms of psychological disturbance. In the second part of the chapter we shall look at ways of measuring such phenomena, as well as the general behaviour patterns of people who have presented with such disorders for a long period of time; those who are, increasingly, called 'people with serious and enduring mental illness'.

Lunacy

Although the layperson has little idea of what mental illness is, he is likely to proclaim that he knows one (i.e. a madman) when he sees one. The 'psychotic' is the caricature of psychiatric disturbance: the person who is out of touch with reality, believing perhaps even that he is answering his mother's instructions to kill (as in Hitchcock's classic film *Psycho*). At a less sophisticated but no less influential level, the lunatic appeared regularly in children's comics, harmlessly proclaiming his belief that he was Napoleon before being carted back off to the asylum. The layperson might be forgiven for believing that all people with a psychiatric diagnosis are homicidal maniacs or immersed in some delusion. Traditional media often proclaim this in dangerous isolation from reality. The reader will be well aware that not all people in receipt of psychiatric care are mad in the sense depicted above. They may also be aware that not all 'psychotics' are wholly out of touch with reality.

It is commonly accepted that the psychotic has experienced some loss of his reasoning power. Dr Johnson believed that 'all power of fancy over reason is a degree of insanity'. Today, we believe we have discovered the roots of 'madness' within various brain dysfunctions. We have long assumed an association between insanity and the function of the brain. The novelist George Moore observed that his: 'wretched brain gave way, and I became a wreck at random driven, without one glimpse of reason or of heaven'. The traditional failure to discriminate between the inability to reason – which might be shown by the intellectually impaired – and real madness was pointed out by the philosopher John Locke: 'A fool from right principles draws wrong conclusions, while the insane person draws a just inference from wrong principles'.

There has long existed a great reluctance to acknowledge that mental disorder is in any way simply an exaggeration of normal behaviour. The nearest we get to this historically is a recognition that great men are close to madness. Shakespeare observed that 'the lunatic, the lover and the poet are of imagination all compact', while John Dryden remarked that 'great wits are sure to madness near allied, and thin partitions do their bounds divide'.

An incomprehensible problem?

In keeping with the other chapters I shall consider briefly the reasons why we identify certain patterns of behaviour as deviant, unacceptable or pathological. I shall also consider ways of measuring what is clearly a complex problem. Before beginning to discuss these two concerns I should say what I do not intend to cover. I have expressed an interest in trying to understand the meaning of the person's behaviour. However, there is clearly much dispute as to anyone's ability to explain psychotic phenomena, far less mine. Laing suggested that there was no 'fact' of psychosis (or rather schizophrenia – the commonest form of such disturbance). He argued that we diminish the human context of the experience of psychosis by reducing it to mental pathology. We might also 'miss the point' of such experiences:

> To regard [such] gambits ... as due **primarily** to some psychological deficit is rather like supposing that a man doing a handstand on a bicycle on a tightrope 100 feet up with no safety net is suffering from an inability to stand on his own two feet. We may well ask why these people have to be, often brilliantly, so devious, so elusive, so adept at making themselves unremittingly incomprehensible [2].

Laing believed that to understand 'psychosis' we need to ask why such people are obliged to make themselves often brilliantly elusive. It is not my intention to explore anything like Laing's territory of interest. Although such enquiry might also be defined as 'assessment' it pertains more to therapeutic enquiry and, by consequence, does not rightly belong here. I shall merely try to remind the reader of the criteria by which we arrive at the assessment of personal maladaption. I shall leave the reader to explore the available literature and to construct her own understanding of the term 'psychosis'.

THE INTERVIEW

The basic interview format was discussed in Chapters 2 and 3, where some of the kinds of behaviour we might associate with psychosis were also mentioned. In this section I wish only to amplify some of the points made in Chapter 3.

Three major areas are the focus of our attention in the interview with the person with an experience of psychosis. These are the person's reports of:

- anomalies of general experience;
- anomalies of perception;
- disturbed or disturbing beliefs or value systems.

We are interested to know in what way the person is ill-at-ease with himself and/or to what extent others are ill-at-ease with him.

In interviewing the person we must take care not to lead him unduly. It would be inappropriate, for example, to use a checklist of all the possible hallucinatory, delusional or experiential problems he might experience, as this might distress the person or represent a threat. More importantly, it might lead him to consider or report experiences he might otherwise have ignored. The most appropriate approach is to follow the kind of general 'life-history' interview format described in Chapter 3. If the person introduces descriptions of problematic experiences – for himself or others – that might be viewed as exemplary of 'psychosis', then we might pursue the kind of 'problem-orientated' interview illustrated.

By inviting the person to discuss general aspects of his life that are presently a problem, we give him an opportunity to report whether he has ever felt strange, whether he has ever thought that people were conspiring against him, has ever heard voices, etc. The nurse's task here is to encourage the person to describe any such experiences more clearly, without appearing either to disbelieve or be in collusion with him. The nurse's attitude should be one of respectful curiosity and genuine interest. In the sections below I shall try to suggest the sort of phenomena we might be interested in reporting, phenomena that are commonly associated with psychotic disorder. Before proceeding, I should emphasize, however, that we should help the person enlarge upon these phenomena, should they appear, but that we do not go looking for them!

Anomalies of experience

Being ourselves is something we take for granted. We need to be ourselves to relate to the outside world: to attend, register and memorize information and to use this store of experience to determine our relations with the world and its relationship to ourselves. We cannot be aware of these various functions of the self. Such awareness might be more of a hindrance than a help. As long as we are untroubled by our awareness of ourselves we have no real difficulty. Many people do experience different kinds of self-awareness, which they find disturbing.

When we talk about 'ourselves' we recognize our whole nature. The self – as Peplau has observed – is 'an abstraction; it is a convenient way of describing a function of the total person. It is not a thing, nor a body part, nor a place in the mind. The self is a function of the mind – which is a more comprehensive function of the entire human organism' [3].

I have acknowledged several times that assessment should be undertaken with care. When we are assessing people whom we believe are 'experiencing psychosis' we need to take special care. The nature of psychosis involves and influences the person's whole lived experience [4]. The person who appears to be experiencing difficulties with the whole of himself may present us with more difficulties than the person who is (merely) having 'difficulties with anxiety' or having 'difficulties with his relationship with others'. Psychosis has always occupied a special position in the history of psychiatry, perhaps denoting for most of us the absolute definition of 'madness' [5]. The experience of madness represents the communication from the very edges of human experience; where consensual reality meets the 'Underworld' [6].

In this section I shall attempt to summarize some of the possible permutations of these difficulties involving the 'self'. In interviewing the person with an experience of psychosis we are collecting information which suggests that all is not well in his relationship with himself. But just what is the nature of that relationship?

The experience of self

Reed described four main disorders of experience involving the 'self' [7]:

- the self and the outside world;
- personal attribution;
- the united self;
- contact with reality.

The self and the outside world

Some people are unable to distinguish between themselves and their outside world. The person may report that people or objects are inside him, or that he is a part of them. He may suggest that things that are happening to the environment – such as walls being painted or carpets beaten – are happening to him. He may report feeling the effects of these environmental experiences on or in his body. This suggests that the person's self-concept is faulty: he appears unable to separate himself from the outside world. Often this is referred to as the blurring of ego boundaries. Although it can occur in a number of illnesses (such as delirium) or in drug-induced states, where it occurs in a person whose consciousness is clear and unimpaired, it is often seen as a separate disorder. Comparisons have been made between such psychotic experiences and psychedelic experience. However, the two are different for the reason given. Indeed such psychotic experiences are more like self-induced mystical states, where consciousness is not impaired. Yet the person experiences a blurring of his own boundaries and a merging with the world or the infinite.

Flying in the face of traditional psychiatric opinion, Reed suggested that such ego boundary blurring is not of itself pathological. It is a phenomenon determined by the cognitive labels that are applied by the person. A person who is delirious or suffering some pre-epileptic aura may describe such experiences as frightening. The person experiencing psychosis may also be frightened by his experience. Both these 'groups' of people attribute a negative meaning to the experience. However, where such experiences occur in a religious or mystical context they may be viewed as blissful or wonderful. As I have noted in previous chapters, such reports have often been made by people of an artistic or poetic nature. We need to ask ourselves why this might be the case?

When we interview someone who reports any kind of difficulty in his relationship with his world, it may be helpful to ask him how he feels about the content of his experience, rather than spending too much time concentrating upon the 'form' of the experience – how it happened.

Person: 'They started this morning, doing the whole place … everywhere …. I could smell it … taste it … all over me … slimy, slipping … painting me.'

Nurse: 'You feel that you are being painted? Tell me more about that.'

Personal attribution

Concern with the influence of the outside world is often extended to cover the belief that the person's actions are controlled by some outside agency. Normally, we cannot divorce our thoughts and behaviour from 'ourselves'. Although we might appreciate how a person who was controlled or manipulated in such a way might act – like a puppet or a zombie – we have little idea of how he would feel. Where the person confesses to such a loss of personal control, this is often thought to be indicative of schizophrenia.

A number of variations of this kind of experience are commonly reported. The person might say that his thoughts are alien to him. He might suggest that his thoughts are not really his own. At a more complex level he might explain away his 'problems with his thoughts' by attributing influence to some outside agency: secret police, communists, religious groups, etc. He may describe how such groups exert their influence: through hypnosis, telepathy, X-rays, etc.

The person may also believe that his thoughts are drained away by this outside power. This is often associated with the concept of **thought blocking**: the person appears to stop thinking, shows a lapse of concentration and suddenly stops talking or working. Or he may describe experiences that sound like **thought broadcasting**, believing that people are able to tune in to, or listen to, his thoughts. Often such listening implies a criticism of what he is thinking.

In all these examples the person is apparently a passive recipient of such interference: controlled by some outside force. He may specify the nature of this influence, as in the power of the secret police or Venusians. This is usually called **delusional passivity**. Where no specific mention is made of the nature of the external influence, it is simply called a passivity experience. The person may report motor and emotional passivity, as well as thoughts, believing that his actions and feelings are similarly controlled.

We need to question the nature of these experiences. Why or in what way are they pathological? The answer is a complex one. Unlike the disorder of self-concept these passivity experiences are not unusual or pathological in their content: it is their form that is so unusual.

Experiences that possess such unusual form are not exclusive to the province of psychiatry. Many people report situations where they believe that their thoughts are controlled, or that they are the agent of some superior or supernatural force. Not all of them would be described as psychiatric cases. This is true of those who profess to contact much more bizarre characters than those cited by the 'psychotic' – establishing links with Red Indian chiefs, or ancient Egyptians, or even God(s). The Pope believes – like most religious leaders – that he is God's emissary. Many other people have had revelations – a divine insight of a religious nature, which is allegedly put into their minds by God [8]. The same is true of all those who believe that they have had some kind of 'extrasensory' experience: the increasingly popular ESP movement. If we wished to be pedantic we would say that all these people were suffering from delusions of passivity. However, depending on our attitude, we might take the view that the form of their experience is quite different from that of those who are (genuinely) deluded.

In the interview with the person assumed to be having a psychotic experience we want to know:

- how often they have had such experiences;
- how long such experiences lasted;
- to what extent they occupy the person's everyday thinking.

The form of experience is more important than the content.

The united self

The two experiences listed above are unusual. The next two, although reported by people with a psychotic disorder, also occur in the normal population.

Under normal stress conditions people may experience emotional disturbance: an exaggeration of anxiety to panic proportions or a depressing despair. In some situations this emotional exaggeration does not take place, being replaced by an eerie sense of calm. Reed suggested that this can take place in a variety of situations: e.g. in fierce wartime combat or when being ravaged by a tiger. Instead of the manifest fear we would expect, a slow-motion, blunted calm occurs. Where such experiences occur in everyday life, this is called a **dissociation of affect**. The person is, quite literally, cut off from his feelings.

In many settings we can see how useful this might be as a biological defence against overwhelming emotion, as in bereavement. Where no obvious stress is evident, or there is a general background of disturbance, the phenomenon assumes quite different proportions. It can extend under some situations to what is called **ego-splitting**, where the person feels as though he is physically outside of himself. Again this is common in bereavement or severe depressed states.

In the interview it is important to find out whether such experiences are generalized, occurring in a wide variety of situations, or specific to certain stressful events. In the former they may suggest a highly unusual state of affairs, whereas in the latter this may be a natural defence against major emotional disturbance.

Contact with reality

We take reality for granted. We do not analyse it or note any change in it except under the influence of some drug. However, some people report unusual experiences of reality without any obvious influence. They may also be bemused by the experience. Two distinct forms are possible. In the first the person may feel that some change has occurred within himself. This may heighten his awareness of reality. Commonly this is called **depersonalization**. He may detect some change in his total self or in a part only. He may believe that his bowels are rotting away, or that his body is swelling to an enormous size. Such experiences may even be culture-specific: some Chinese males report a fear that their genitals are shrivelling away into non-existence by disappearing inside themselves. At an even more extreme level the person may harbour the nihilistic delusion that he no longer exists.

In the second form (**derealization**) the person remains the same but detects some change in the world around him. The world may become flattened, vague or misty. The root of these experiences may have something to do with the acute focus or emphasis of the person's thoughts. Typically we are a global whole: we function as a coordinated whole. Where the person begins to focus closely upon himself, or a part of himself, some breakdown in the usual mechanics of self-concept may occur.

In interviewing the person, information about what he experiences is obviously crucial. It may also be helpful to find out whether he has a tendency to be introspective, analysing himself, ruminating on his 'self' or some specific aspect of his experience. It will also be necessary to establish whether such experiences are continuous or related to any specific situations. The interviewer is interested in establishing not only the content of the person's experience of reality but also the form it takes.

Judgements and beliefs

The assessment of the person's values and belief systems is a tricky area, for we are obliged to judge the significance of the person's conviction or faith in a certain set of ideas. Although we tend to discriminate between so-called 'real' and 'false' beliefs (delusions), the situation is more complex than this. Two main classes of idea may be evident: over-valued ideas; and delusions.

Over-valued ideas

Where a person has a firm, extreme, conviction based upon personal experience, we call this an over-valued idea. The road safety campaigner or the political activist are typical examples: both hold views that society might view as extreme. The value aspect of this title illustrates how our view of any belief system is influenced by normative considerations. An over-valued idea is one that is not greatly appreciated by the majority of the population, or some subculture of the population. Indeed the person who holds such 'extreme' views may be perceived quite differently by different clinicians, who will be influenced by their own values and beliefs. Someone with conservative views may find the person extreme, whereas someone else with more liberal leanings may find him 'almost normal'. The standard of 'normality' that is being used to evaluate the person belongs to the individual clinician and is a reflection of his value system.

In general, over-valued ideas are seen as a problem only when they tend to dominate the person's life. In the interview we should be interested, again, in the form that the value system takes: to what extent do the person's beliefs influence the day-to-day running of his life? We should also ask: 'who determines what is or is not an "over-valued" idea?'

Delusions

Although we commonly refer to a delusion as a false belief, this is woefully inadequate as a definition. What we refer to as 'fact' is no more than a convention. Many primitive cultures – and increasingly various 'new age' groups – believe that rocks and trees possess spirits. Many contemporary religions hold similar views about the existence of souls, heaven or the coming of Christ. These are all 'facts' to them. In this sense it may be more appropriate to relate delusions to faith rather than belief. Delusions have much in common with religious faith, since both are often incontrovertible despite the lack of any evidence. Delusions have been defined as beliefs which are not shared by the person's society or culture and which are maintained despite all evidence to the contrary. However, the emphasis upon conviction (or incorrigibility) is misleading. For instance, I tend to believe that there is some good in everyone. I might be called naive or idealistic for holding this belief, but I am unlikely (I hope) to be called deluded.

Even where people hold unusual religious beliefs, they will merely be labelled 'eccentric'. The incorrigibility of the deluded person can, however, be important, where for instance he refuses to change his mind even under extreme torture. But religious or political idealists would behave in the same way, so we are no further forward. Although psychiatrists have often emphasized the highly personal nature of delusions, this seems a little unfair. Any belief, held long enough, becomes part of that person's psychological make-up. What does seem more significant is that the person may ruminate or be otherwise preoccupied with the belief, much more so than the person with strong moral convictions. Here again the key characteristic of the delusion seems to be the way it functions, rather than its content. Does it tend to dominate the person's thinking? Does it distract him from concentrating on other things? In general, does it interfere with the workings of his life?

Six kinds of delusion are commonly described:

- **Persecution**: The person believes that someone, or more often an organization, is threatening his life. The organization may be of a religious or political nature, but may also be a group of friends or neighbours. This delusion is often associated with particular experiences of taste and smell: poison in food or gas. Their unusual nature suggests that these experiences are hallucinatory. The person may also report **ideas of reference**, where he interprets hidden meanings in people's behaviour. For instance, he may believe that a cough represents a signal to begin some threatening action.
- **Jealousy**: The person may believe that his life partner has been unfaithful and identifies virtually anything as possible signs or clues to this effect. His partner's fervent denial may be interpreted as a further sign of guilt. When the partner tires of resisting, this may well be taken as an admission or confession.
- **Grandeur**: The person may believe that his abilities are wildly superior to their actual (i.e. accepted) level of competence. This idea may even extend to the belief that he is someone famous, either living or dead.
- **Poverty**: The person may believe that he and his family are poverty-stricken. It is interesting to note that this 'delusion' is less common now than it was in the days before state support.
- **Ill-health**: The person may believe that he has some life-threatening disease, which he may have passed on via infection or contagion to his children. He may identify rotting organs or decaying bones. To a large extent such 'delusions' are influenced by the person's knowledge of anatomy and medicine.
- **Guilt**: The person may experience massive self-reproach for crimes, sins or past misdeeds. He may demand punishment for these errors. This demand is often represented by sexual misdemeanours. At its most extreme he will reject his own existence: **nihilism**.

N.B. The need to take care during assessment has been emphasized throughout. When the person appears to be describing an experience that might be called 'delusional', we need to record scrupulously (exactly) what he says. We need to avoid altogether making interpretations as to the meaning or significance of 'what he has said', or premature labelling of the phenomena reported.

Many authorities have argued that there are two classes of delusion. Secondary delusions arise from some other abnormality, such as affective disorder. Here the person may believe that he has committed an unforgivable sin for which he is being punished. This delusion is secondary to the lowering of mood. A primary delusion is usually characterized by a **lack of content**. The person may note that the world is behaving strangely. He may feel eerie sensations (delusional perceptions). He may have delusional ideas or memories, remembering that the look in someone's eyes was the cause of some recent affliction. Finally, he may have a 'delusional awareness': he knows something that others do not, e.g. that the end of the world is nigh.

The assessment of delusions should attempt to capture the nature of the person's experiences, in terms of its form or content. Such a careful description may help us understand, at some later stage, the human significance of such experiences.

Perception

Hallucinations have been described as false perceptions that are in no way distortions of real perceptions. They arise as something new alongside real perception. In contrast to an illusion, a common occurrence that disturbs us sufficiently to question its reality, a hallucination is felt by the person to have an external reality. Despite any obvious objectivity, he feels that it is real. The range of possible hallucinations is virtually limitless, but commonly they are categorized according to the sensory modality involved.

- **Visual hallucinations** can range from simple lights and flashes to sightings of people, who may be named or merely classified. Such hallucinations may occur in organic disorders, where often the 'sightings' are of huge animals (the stereotypical sighting of 'pink elephants' in delirium). In general, hallucinations have real substance, using the environment, walking through doorways and casting shadows.
- **Auditory hallucinations** may range from simple noises, bangs and whistles to intelligible speech of one or more people. Where the person hears people speaking to him they may be known or unknown and may be related to some persecutory delusion, where a critical voice is common. This may be heard speaking clearly or in hushed whispers. In *echo de pensées* the person believes that he hears his own thoughts aloud and fears that others might be listening in.
- **Olfactory hallucinations** might involve gas, especially where the person feels persecuted. Or he might smell an offensive odour from his body, especially

when he also reports feelings of depression. Hallucinations of this sort are also prevalent in organic states such as the epileptic aura.

- **Tactile hallucinations** often take the form of wind blowing across the person, the sensation of vibrations or electric shocks. Often there is a strong sexual connection. The person may feel that he is being fondled or penetrated by some invisible other.
- **Gustatory hallucinations** are usually focused on food, again with the persecuted individual most evident along with the experience of epileptic aura.
- Finally, the person may experience **general somatic sensations** of a hallucinatory nature. He may feel that his body is being twisted or torn or even disembowelled. In some cases he may report invasion by animals, snakes in his stomach or frogs in his rectum; or the feeling that his flesh is decomposing.

A further four classes of 'hallucination' may also occur.

- The person may fail to perceive something that is evident to everyone else. This is commonly called a **negative hallucination**.
- The **Doppelganger phenomenon (autoscopy)** involves the person meeting an exact double who is recognized as an absolute likeness. In German folklore this is believed to be a portent of death. It is a favourite theme in literature and has been assumed to represent 'a dread of the unknown and a morbid assumption of doom'. Such a phenomenon always involves 'sinister foreboding or impending tragedy', and has often been reported by writers like Edgar Allan Poe, Franz Kafka, Fyodor Dostoyevsky, Guy de Maupassant, John Steinbeck and Oscar Wilde [9]. It has been suggested that some of these authors suffered from epilepsy, or other cerebral disorder. Reed noted, however, that Goethe claimed to have met his *Doppelganger*, despite a reputation for momentous psychological stability.
- **Pseudo-hallucinations** are the subject of much controversy, but seem to involve seeing something which even the observer recognizes to be unobservable to others. The person recognizes that that which he witnesses is a subjective phenomenon. It is very similar to the experiences of visionaries, mystics and mediums, who recognize that others are unable to see their vision.
- Finally, there is a group of **functional hallucinations** that appear to be related to the workings of the environment. Voices may be heard when taps are turned on: they stop when the taps are turned off again. Shapes and objects may appear and disappear with the turn of a light switch.

It should be readily apparent that the assessment of these experiential problems is a virtual minefield. Where the person appears to be grossly disturbed it may appear easy to detect such classic phenomena. Where the person is less disturbed, or where the person is already undergoing treatment which suppresses the phenomenon, the picture may be subtler. This may make the assessment and clarification of such phenomena more difficult.

'Problem X' and the blue banana: content-free interviewing

The description of the interview with the person with an experience of psychosis has, so far, used the consensus terminology of traditional psychiatry and psychology. I have observed such professional conventions by translating 'the hearing of voices' or 'the sight of visions' into our professional language of 'auditory' or 'visual hallucinations'. The person's 'feelings of threat when with people' become 'paranoia' and his 'strongly held beliefs' become (at best) 'over-valued ideas' and (at worst) 'delusions'.

Such labelling of experience or classification of psychic phenomena may – when accurate – be wholly appropriate. Nurses might well consider, however, what such labelling or classification adds to the person's original experience. We might bear in mind the comedian's apocryphal two-liner: 'Gee, I thought I was going crazy! Then I found out it was just schizophrenia'.

The nature of the experience of psychosis can often – to the complete outsider – appear bewildering, bizarre and beyond all reason. All nurses will have had some experience of anxiety, of low mood, of disturbed relationships, etc. People-in-care who suffer from such problems often appear to be experiencing an exaggeration of normal human experience.

The experience of psychosis is often interpreted as an alien experience: one which is unknown to all but the relative few, whom we define as 'crazy'. This is a false assumption. Everyone who dreams has the potential to appreciate the nature of psychosis. When we 'enjoy' pleasurable dreams, we awaken feeling refreshed, if not buoyant. We do so because we believed the dream to be real as we dreamt it. When we 'enjoy' a nightmare, we experience emotions at the other end of the human spectrum, for similar reasons.

There is no reason why we cannot exercise empathy when faced with a 'hallucinating' or 'delusional' person. The efforts we make to keep our distance – to avoid exploring the psychotic phenomena too closely – may describe our problems more clearly than those of the person who is the 'patient'. Nurses may fear that, by discussing the 'hallucinatory' or 'delusional' experience, they will collude with the person; somehow 'encouraging' the manifestation of psychosis. The experience of people who have experienced nurses' reluctance to address their psychotic experience contradicts this view; indeed their testimony suggests quite the reverse. By failing to offer an opportunity to review the experience, we leave the person in his original, relatively isolated, position. Alternatively, if the person is encouraged to – at least – identify the nature of his distress, this may reduce some of the isolation he experiences. He is no longer left alone with the experience.

Writers who have witnessed psychosis at close range have described this sense of isolation, few better than the New Zealand writer, Janet Frame:

I will write about the season of peril. I was put in hospital because a great gap opened up in the ice floe between myself and the other people whom I watched, with their world drifting away through violet-coloured sea where hammerhead sharks in tropical ease swam side by side with the seals and the polar bears. I was alone on the ice [10].

If nurses have a difficulty when faced by apparently bizarre behaviour or experiences, this may have something to do with the content of the person's experience: we may have become too involved with the detail of what is experienced, losing, by consequence, our appreciation of how such experiences work for – or against – the person. What are we to make of Janet Frame's account of her 'alone-ness on the ice'? For the moment, I would say we should make nothing. Rather, let us explore further this cold and isolated territory with the person and find out what the person (him or herself) makes of it.

We often assume that we need to know what, exactly, the person is experiencing if we are to address it. This is a false assumption. Indeed, the reverse might well be the case: that knowledge of what the person is experiencing or has experienced may interfere with our ability to address it objectively. The following example illustrates how knowledge of the problem may not be necessary for its successful exploration.

Nurse. So, how are you today?

Person-in-care. Not good. It's getting worse. I don't know how much more I can take.

Nurse. I see. Tell me a bit more about what is getting worse.

Person. Well, it's the blue banana, isn't it? It's back!

Nurse. Uh-huh. It's back. So it's been away?

Person. Yeah. Well, not long, but I thought that I was on top of that, y'know.

Nurse. Umm. I see. (Pause) So when did you first notice this 'blue banana'?

Person. Oh, I dunno ... maybe ... oh, years ago. It comes and goes, y'know.

Nurse. Yes. So you noticed this 'years ago'. Do you remember when exactly?

Person. Well ... yeah, when I was at college. I was studying for exams ... and ... yeah that's when it all started.

Nurse. Right! So how did it affect you then?

Person. Well ... I couldn't keep my mind on things ... anything. And ... I just couldn't shut it up.

Nurse. OK. And now it's back. How does it affect you now?

Person. Well ... I can't concentrate sometimes. It's at me all the time, y'know.

Nurse. Umm. You can't concentrate. And how else does it affect you?

Person. I got no confidence any more. I mean, I feel like nobody.

Nurse. Right. You said a moment ago that it's not there all the time. So what's it like when the blue banana's not there?

Person. Good. I mean ... great! Oh, the relief!

Nurse. Relief? From what exactly?

Person. Like I said … hassle … being made to feel like a fool. I hate it! Like I never done nothing … like I'm nobody.

Nurse. And how do you feel about that?

Person. Well … angry. Wouldn't you?

Nurse. I guess. Tell me, what would I notice about you when the blue banana is around?

Person. I find it hard to face people. Like I said, my confidence just goes. Talking to people, just being with people is real difficult. You would notice that … like I'm avoiding you or something.

Nurse. And other people. What would they notice about you?

Person. Well much the same. My family … people close … they can tell something's on my mind. They can see I'm distracted.

Nurse. Distracted? In what way?

Person. They can see that I'm struggling to contain something … it takes all of my attention …all of my energy. I got no time for anything else … for anyone else.

The example above is adapted from an interview I conducted recently with a person described as suffering from psychosis. The only change I have made is to substitute the 'blue banana' for the phenomenon the person reported. I hope that this illustration will show how we may explore the person's experience of the problem, without knowing what, exactly, is the problem. Since we do not know what the person has experienced, we are not tempted to introduce our values, or other's values, into the assessment of the problem. When people report 'hearing my dead mother calling me' or 'seeing little green men' we may be tempted to back away from exploring this on the grounds that it is absurd, threatening or simply too hot for us to handle. If the person describes the problem simply as 'X' or the ludicrous 'blue banana' our curiosity is aroused. We explore this by asking some fairly simple questions, which may provide some very interesting answers. Among the many questions that might be asked of an anonymous problem are:

'So, when did you first notice "problem X"?' (Origins in time)
'How did "problem X" affect you at first?' (History of problem function)
'And how did you feel about that?' (Past emotional context)
'In what way has that changed over time?' (Developmental history of the problem)
'How does "X" affect your relationships with others?' (Relationship history)
'And how do you feel about that?' (Current emotional context)
'And what does that mean for you?' (Holistic content)
'And what does that say about you as a person?' (Holistic context)

Through these open-ended questions we gain an appreciation of how the problem (whatever it is) affects the person, his relationships with others, his everyday life, his work, etc. We learn what other people might notice about the person which tells them that he has the problem. We find out how the person feels about having this problem and what he thinks this says about him as a person. We can also find out how 'bad' is the problem at present, how it has changed over time, what the person's life might be like without the problem and in what way this would change how he feels about himself, his relationships with others, etc. Indeed, there is virtually nothing that we cannot find out about the problem that the person is not willing to tell us. Except what the problem **is**.

This 'content-free' interviewing has a particular relevance to the assessment of psychosis. Our intention is to appreciate something of the person's experience, so that we might use this in some constructive way within the caring process. If the person reports '500 fiddlers under his bed, playing the Devil's music', we are interested to know the answers to two key questions:

- in what way this is a problem?
- what does this mean to him?

The answers to these questions are explored by the 'who, what, when, where and how' questions described in Chapter 2.

THE INTERVIEW: PICTURES IN FORM AND CONTENT

I have attempted, in this brief summary, to identify some of the categories of experiential disturbance that may be encountered during the interview of the person with an experience of psychosis. I have not listed these various phenomena to encourage 'classification' of the person's experience. Rather, this sketch is intended to introduce the nurse to the lie of the land, metaphorically speaking, in perceptual and experiential disturbance. Her responsibility, in the interview, is to collect a detailed picture of the person's description of these phenomena. I have suggested that by exploring the experience of psychosis in this way – its form and content – a picture of the person's experience may emerge; perhaps more quickly than through straightforward questioning.

The key to effective interviewing is keen and impartial observation and recording. By sharpening our pencils and our perceptions we may be able to gain a clearer appreciation of the person's experience through his own verbal account. If we need a rubber, it will be only for erasing any unnecessary interpretation of the person's report.

General observations

In addition to collecting information from the person's verbal report, the interview gives us a chance to observe his behaviour under structured conditions. As we discussed in Chapter 3, there is a need to make short notes on the person's appearance at the interview:

- how he interacted with the nurse;
- the speed of his answers;
- the use of gestures;
- any mannerisms;
- the presence of eye contact;
- signs of agitation or anxiety (e.g. getting up and pacing around the room).

A 'good' assessment of such non-verbal behaviour might be modelled on a naturalist's observation of birds: using brief, yet detailed, descriptions of behaviour to paint a verbal picture of what the interviewer witnessed. One should take care not to translate these notes into diagnostic language. For example, if the person: 'only looked up from time to time … sat turned away and was very brief with his answers', this should not be translated into: 'appeared depressed/hostile/paranoid (etc.)'.

The notes collected here may provide suggestions for further, more detailed, observations under different conditions. For example, observations may be taken of the person's behaviour in the ward, at occupational therapy or when in a group, to evaluate whether or not the presentation noted during the interview was maintained under these conditions.

The interview provides a valuable opportunity to study the person with the minimum of distraction. However, the very artificiality of the setting may produce a wholly unrepresentative picture of his behaviour. The two main values of the interview are to help the nurse decide which aspects of the person's behaviour or experience she should try to assess further, and to begin to understand something of the experience of psychosis. Both these aims are probably of equal importance.

ASSESSMENT METHODS

General presentation

A wide range of assessment scales have been developed to assess the manifest presentation of the person experiencing psychosis or to assist further in the diagnosis of specific psychotic disorders [11]. Nurses are increasingly expected to participate in both these forms of assessment, although the former – 'how' the person presents – is of greater relevance. Where the person is in residential care, especially under 'clinical' hospital conditions, it is possible to study his overall behaviour using one of the many scales available. In addition to helping clarify the nature of the person's problems, such scales also offer an opportunity to measure the extent of these problems. Such measures may prove useful in decision-making regarding necessary support and supervision and also for evaluating – in the longer term – the person's progress. The major limitation of such 'global' measures is that they rarely provide a satisfactory amount of detail for nursing care planning. They may, however, provide pointers for further – more focused – observation.

Some of the available assessment measures are summarized in Appendix B. I describe here below, briefly, three scales in popular use that are appropriate for nurses in the typical clinical situation.

The Nurse's Observation Scale for In-person Evaluation (NOSIE)

The NOSIE [12] was developed to involve nurses in the assessment of people with psychosis in hospital care. This and similar instruments recognized the crucial role played by nurses in the planning of health care. Since they spent all day with the people-in-care, they were in the best position to comment on the presence or absence of specific patterns of behaviour associated with mental disorder. A number of versions of the scale have been produced. The most commonly used version includes 30 items which make up separate subscales:

- Social competence;
- Social interest;
- Personal hygiene;
- Irritability;
- Manifest psychosis;
- Psycho-motor retardation.

The people-in-care are observed by the nursing team and rated separately on a five-point scale: 0 (Never) to 4 (Always). The scale is particularly useful when assessing people who are difficult to reach through interviewing and who may be withdrawn, mute, hostile or hyperactive. The ratings are based on continuous observation of the person-in-care, which again distinguishes it from interview-based assessment.

In studies conducted in America and the UK [13,14] the scale has been found to be a reliable, brief and unambiguous tool for the assessment of people with enduring mental disorder, requiring longer-term care. The rating is quick and simple to use and, despite requiring little training of staff, the scale is reliable. Where the person is not experiencing a psychotic disorder of a chronic nature, it has been found to be of less value.

Due to the limited number of factors covered by the scale NOSIE is ideally suited for settings where staff feel that they have limited time to complete more extensive scales. Although the scale is short, and can be completed in 5–10 minutes, comparison between people under pre- and post-treatment conditions is possible, as well as comparison between people-in-care in different areas. This latter comparison may help in deciding upon inter-ward transfers.

The Rehabilitation Evaluation of Hall and Baker (REHAB)

The REHAB was developed from a 7-year-long research study [15,16] and aims to measure 'general disability' in people with an experience of enduring psychosis. The scale may be used to identify those people-in-care with a potential for community living and identifies more general targets for treatment, serving also as an evaluative tool for measuring change across time.

The person is rated over a period of 1 week on 23 items representing two main areas of functioning. Part 1 deals with 'difficult' or 'embarrassing' behaviour and uses seven three-point ratings to produce a Deviant Behaviour Score (DB). The second part of the scale focuses on 'social and everyday' behaviour. This includes 16 items, which are summed to produce a General Behaviour Score (GB), which provides a classification of 'discharge potential', 'moderate handicap' or 'severe handicap', and also five scale scores (social activity, speech disturbance, speech skills, self-care and community skills).

The REHAB assessment package comprises record sheets, scoring manual and a guide for use of the scale, as well as individual and group profiles. Norms from their research allow meaningful comparisons to be made between any individual or group with the sample population from their various research programmes. Hall and Baker have also published details of their psychometric analysis of REHAB, which adds further support to its use as a reliable and valid instrument for the assessment of people with an enduring mental disorder.

The REHAB is perhaps most useful for surveying populations for planning purposes. Despite being technically excellent, REHAB does not provide the detail necessary to formulate individualized care programmes, especially in community settings. The assessment does, however, provide a most valuable basis for developing further the kind of detailed investigation of the person considered appropriate.

The Morningside Rehabilitation Status Scale (MRSS)

The MRSS was developed to provide a broad overview of the person 'at each stage of rehabilitation' so that their 'progress ... is accurately charted' [17]. The major advantages of this scale are that it is relatively easy to use and may be applied across the whole spectrum of rehabilitation settings.

The nurse can complete the MRSS after consulting the person-in-care, or his family where appropriate, using an *aide-mémoire* checklist of items to address. The following areas of functioning are addressed:

- **dependency scale** – the extent to which the person is reliant on others (contact with professional staff, carers, etc.);
- **inactivity scale** – the extent to which the person is involved, or shows sustained interest in 'productive activity (employment or leisure);

- **social integration/isolation scale** – the extent to which the person participates in or maintains relationships;
- **effects of current symptoms and deviant behaviour scale** – the extent to which the person's life is impaired or affects others.

The MRSS produces four scale scores and a total score, which may be used to indicate the person's overall level of functioning: high, moderate or low level.

The MRSS has limitations, in particular as a means of establishing individual care plans or for designing services. However, the scale can be completed in a few minutes by any nurse who knows the patient well, and often serves a useful function within the case-review. As its title suggests the MRSS provides an indication of the status of the individual within the rehabilitation structure. This scale offers nurses a broad 'snapshot' of the person-in-care, which may be used to monitor progress along the rehabilitation continuum and might supplement other measures of the person's overall presentation.

The use of global ratings

The scales described above were designed to increase the involvement of nursing staff in the assessment process. Traditionally, assessment was often left to the psychiatrist, or more recently, the psychologist, neither of whom spent much time within the care setting. 'Assessment' – as a result – often focused upon highly structured and artificial interview situations. Any complementary role that nurses played was, typically, highly unsystematic and usually took the form of offering advice or information from memory during a case conference.

The scales summarized above provide a general outline of the presentation of the person, at a particular point in time. These may be used as a preliminary to the selection of the more detailed methods noted briefly below. These global methods give us an indication of where we ought to begin looking in greater detail. Without the guidance of such general, or 'global' assessment methods, there is a temptation to focus attention on the first problem that grabs the attention of staff. In some cases this will turn out to be the major problem. In others, more careful consideration of the overall picture of the person might help us select more appropriate assessment targets.

THE EXPERIENCE OF PSYCHOSIS: THE WIDER PERSPECTIVE

Psychosis is clearly a highly complex phenomenon. At one level it might be viewed as a manifestation of organic dysfunction and at another as a subtype of personality disorder or depression. Although nurses may participate actively in these diagnostic considerations, arguably these do not represent the proper focus of psychiatric nursing. To fully address the needs of the person experiencing psychosis, however, nurses should be aware of the other dimensions of functioning, which might need to be addressed through one form of assessment or another. This 'wider perspective' on the experience of psychosis involves the following areas of functioning.

Change in presentation

Nursing is interested in how people grow and develop – progressing through their lives and, hopefully, overcoming or coming to terms with their life problems. In this sense nursing is interested in change: how the presentation of the person varies across time. Nurses are interested also – like their fellow health professionals – in the effect of various care and treatment processes: what difference does care or treatment make?

A range of methods has been developed for monitoring the 'natural history' of the experience of psychosis, or the differential effects of treatment. One of the most well established assessment procedures is the Brief Psychiatric Rating Scale (BPRS). The BPRS provides comprehensive rating of change across 16 'symptom constructs', each of which is rated on a seven-point scale. The scale is completed in 20–25 minutes [18]. A few minutes is spent establishing rapport, 10 minutes in non-directive interaction and 5–10 minutes in direct questioning.

The BPRS is the commonest scale used for measuring change in schizophrenia [19]. The scale is usually administered by a psychiatrist but more recently a modification has been developed for use by nurses [20]. It is recognized, however, that the successful use of the scale relies on the clinical skills of the interviewer. In the absence of a formal assessment manual, care needs to be taken when deciding who should complete the BPRS.

Positive and negative symptoms

Several authors have distinguished between **positive** (or **productive**) **symptoms** – delusions, hallucinations and thought disorder [21] – and **negative symptoms** – the relative absence of normal patterns of behaviour, involving emotional responsiveness, spontaneous speech and volition [22]. Indeed, increasingly the view is advocated that these problems represent two distinct disease processes [23], the former ascribed to increased dopamine receptor activity and the latter the result of cell loss from cerebral structural change.

The **Manchester Scale (MS)** was developed to provide a brief rating of people with more enduring experiences of psychosis [24]. The MS consists of eight items, which are rated on a 0–4 scale. Four items represent 'symptoms' reported by the person (depression, anxiety, delusions and hallucinations) and the other four derive from observation (incoherent or irrelevant speech, flat or incongruous affect, mutism or poverty of speech and motor retardation). The scale is completed within a semi-structured interview. The rater is expected to know the person, or his history, with the ratings made on the basis of observed and reported factors.

Although training to establish reliability is possible through the use of specially prepared videotapes [25] the MS is generally considered suitable for use where the raters are relatively inexperienced [26].

Depression

Some people with an experience of psychosis also show major mood disturbance. Where the person's presentation suggests a diagnosis of both schizophrenia and affective disorder, clinicians may describe the person as suffering from schizoaffective disorder. This concept has, however, a variety of definitions, which will not be addressed here. In addition to this group there are those whose presentation suggests manic depression or a psychotic depression. In all these groups there is a need to assess the affective disturbance separately from the assessment of psychosis.

Two scales already mentioned – the Brief Psychiatric Rating Scale and the Manchester Scale – include items for depression. However, both these scales offer only limited coverage of affective disturbance. In the case of the BPRS the assessor may find it difficult to distinguish between 'emotional withdrawal', 'blunted affect', 'retardation' and 'depressive mood'.

The use of self-rating scales – such as the Beck Depression Inventory [27] or the Zung Self-rating Depression Scale [28] – appears to have limited use where the person is thought to suffer from schizophrenia. Completion of such scales requires degrees of education, motivation and concentration that may be absent in such a population. Although the person may be able to recognize the experience of depression this is not the same as offering an accurate measure of the severity of the experience.

Given these considerations an observational rating scale offers the best opportunity to gain a full picture of the person's presentation and the severity of these problems. Although none of the available scales appears ideal for this purpose the **Montgomery Schizophrenia Scale (MSS)** [29] is a short scale (12 items) that measures the severity of items such as 'reported sadness', 'pessimistic thoughts' and 'inability to feel', items drawn from the Montgomery and Asberg Depression Rating Scale (Appendix B). The MSS was designed to be sensitive to change and provides an overview of the person's presentation in terms of schizophrenia and depressive symptoms.

Suicidal risk

People who are diagnosed as suffering from manic-depressive psychosis or schizophrenic disorders represent the highest suicide risk group within the psychiatric population. Although the rates of suicide are relatively comparable (15% for MDP and 10%+ for schizophrenic disorders), the former are more likely to commit suicide during a depressive phase whereas in the latter group suicide is more likely during a period of remission. In both cases a sense of hopelessness is increasingly considered to be a key factor in determining suicide risk. Where the person harbours negative expectations about the future, or feels very pessimistic about his disorder and future prospects, hopelessness is almost inevitable.

The assessment of suicide risk in people with an experience of psychosis is a very inexact science [30]. There are a number of scales that may, however, provide a helpful adjunct to other forms of assessment. Although the clinical team may not rely on these to predict suicide risk, they may provide a useful indication of likely risk.

The **Hopelessness Scale** [31] is a self-rating scale with 20 items, which takes between 3 and 10 minutes to complete. All items refer to future events, either positively or negatively, or to how things 'usually' work out for the person. If the person is manifestly depressed he may require some help to complete the scale. The nurse should be aware of the likelihood that some people may wish to conceal their suicidal intentions by falsifying their responses. The **Suicidal Intent Scale** [32] is an interview-based rating scale developed to assess the person's 'wish to die' associated with suicide attempts. Eight items address the objective circumstances of the attempt and seven items focus on the person's self-report on the attempt and its purpose. The scale takes approximately 10 minutes to complete, the interviewer using a manual to guide the questioning and scoring.

Aggression and the potential for violence

There is much evidence that violent behaviour has increased within psychiatric populations in both the UK and the USA over the past decade. This increase does, however, reflect a trend within society in general, where the homicide rate has risen by almost one-third and woundings and assaults have doubled [33]. Although the evidence of an increase in violence within hospital populations varies, there is consensus that the rise has been dramatic [34].

Why an increase should be evident within the psychiatric population remains unclear. The effect of discharging relatively 'unready' long-stay hospital clientele into the community and the subsequent instability associated with frequent re-admissions is a popular hypothesis. It is clear that nurses need to assess the potential for violence in both acute hospital wards and situations specializing in the care of people with a history of violent behaviour.

The **Modified Overt Aggression Scale** (**MOAS**) is a relatively simple daily rating scale which focuses on four types of aggressive behaviour: verbal, physical, aggression against property and abuse of self (autoaggression). Items within these categories are rated on a five-point ordinal scale [35]. This scale provides a useful outcome measure of violent behaviour but needs to be supplemented with information on the context within which such aggression occurred. To what extent was provocation present? Did the person appear to reacting to restrictions imposed either by staff or the ward environment?

The **Novaco Anger Inventory** provides a list of situations which, typically, might evoke an angry response. This includes provocation, threats to self-esteem and frustration. The scale measures the degree of anger evoked using a five-point scale [36]. The distinctive value of the scale is its focus on covert hostility in relation to specific situations, rather than displays of overt aggression. Although the scale has limitations in terms of its predictive validity it does provide the nursing team with more information on the situations that might form the basis of therapeutic intervention. Novaco's recent research suggests that the anger rating is predictive of subsequent aggression in Californian state hospitals [37].

SIGNS AND SYMPTOMS OF ILLNESS: THE FUNDAMENTAL NEGATIVE BIAS

Within this chapter – and in the bibliography in Appendix B – the reader's attention is drawn to the relative utility of different assessment instruments and the problems they purport to address. Given my introductory remarks on the nature – if not also the possible meaning – of the experience of psychosis, we cannot leave this chapter without considering some of the limitations of assessment approaches that begin with an assumption about the nature of the problem which is the focus of the assessment.

Many of the scales described here and in other chapters assume that the problems shown by the person signify or are symptomatic of some illness, disorder or dysfunction. I am interested neither in disputing nor advocating this viewpoint. This view does, however, produce some specific problems for nursing, given its philosophical premise that the 'unique individual' or 'person' is the subject of our attentions. To what extent do symptom checklists and scales elucidate further the disorder or illness assumed to lie 'behind' the patterns of behaviour or verbal reports of the person?

In Wright's view the award of a diagnosis (or label of any kind) leads to a 'muting of differences within the labelled group' [38]. She acknowledges that although diagnostic manuals (in this case the DSM-IIIR) remind the diagnostician that, although 'people described as having the same mental disorder ... have at least the defining features of the disorder, they may well differ in other important respects that may affect clinical management and outcome' [39].

Despite such warnings the process of 'within-group deindividuation' is so insidious that it may reach the point of dehumanization. Wright expressed the concern that the resultant diagnosis might involve a classification of people, rather than a classification of the disorders that people have.

As long as the primary focus of diagnosis is the 'disorders' then, by implication, little attention will be focused on personal assets or environmental resources, which might result in the 'remedy' for such disorders. Wright's solution is to develop a 'four-front approach':

- deficiencies and undermining characteristics of the person;
- strengths and assets of the person;
- lacks and destructive factors in the environment;
- resources and opportunities in the environment [40].

This approach is relevant to any of the human problems (or disorders) addressed in this book. It may have a specific relevance, however, to assessment of psychosis, often assumed to be an alien entity which inhabits the person and which is largely isolated from other 'worlds' within the person or his environment.

Unravelling the problem: revealing the meaning

Many of the popular assessment scales, including those acknowledged in this chapter, aim to quantify the experience of psychosis. This aim is wholly laudable. Discrete measures are invaluable for determining service provision, or monitoring the person's progress. We should take care, however, not to neglect the clarification of the problem: what exactly appears to be 'going on' within this unique experience? What is this experience 'all about'?

There are few acknowledged assessment scales which adopt a more qualitative approach to the assessment of psychosis. As nurses are expected to re-focus their attention on the 'unique individual', I presume that more interest will be shown in the descriptive exploration of the experience of psychosis through semi-structured interview methods. One such method has emerged recently, which holds much promise both for professionals understanding the nature of one aspect of the experience of psychosis and also as a means of preparing for the therapeutic work necessary to address it.

My Dutch colleagues Marius Romme and Sandra Escher [41] have developed an interview schedule that provides a means of gaining a perspective on the experience of 'hearing voices'. The mere fact that they talk about 'hearing voices' rather than 'auditory hallucinations' attests to the inherent humanity of their approach: they believe that the experience is inherently meaningful, not a 'hallucination'.

Romme and Escher's interview schedule covers 12 areas and aims to develop a rich picture of the experience itself and the effect of the voice-hearing experience within the person's life. The interviewer explores:

- aspects of the voice-hearing experience;
- characteristics of the voice;
- organization of the voice in relation to the person;
- triggers that appear to provoke or diminish the voice;
- antecedents of the voice-hearing experience;
- effect of the experience on the person's well-being;

- identification of the voice;
- interpretation of 'meaning';
- coping strategies;
- youth history and trauma;
- social network;
- healthcare history.

Romme and Escher's approach is an 'empowering' approach to what is often a highly threatening experience [42]. They observe that as they encourage the person to talk about the experience: 'this reduces the anxiety associated with the voices and often the frequency. ... [By] analysing [the voices'] way of communicating with the person [this] might provide clues about whom they represent in the daily life of the person [43]'.

I hope that psychiatric nurses will follow Romme and Escher's lead by developing such 'exploratory' forms of assessment in their own work. Although such exploration is important for all areas of mental distress, it may have the greatest application in the psychoses, traditionally viewed as the 'underworld' of human experience.

NOTES

1. The uncertain status of the term 'psychotic' will be acknowledged throughout the chapter.
2. Laing, R. D. (1967) The schizophrenic experience, in *The Politics of Experience*, Penguin, Harmondsworth, p. 85.
3. Peplau, H. E. (1990) in *Psychiatric Nursing: Theory and Practice*, (eds W. Reynolds and D. Cormack), Chapman & Hall, London, p. 107.
4. Parse, R. R. (ed.) (1995) *Illuminations: The Human Becoming Theory in Research and Practice*, National League for Nursing, New York.
5. Podvoll, E. (1991) *The Seduction of Madness*, Century, London.
6. In Laing's view 'Freud descended to the Underworld' – the ultimate metaphor for madness. Here he met stark terrors. He [Freud] 'carried with him his theory as a Medusa's head which turned these terrors to stone'. Laing, R. D. (1965) *The Divided Self*, Penguin Books, Harmondsworth, ch. 1.
7. The following discussion is heavily influenced by the writings of Reed, G. (1972) *The Psychology of Anomalous Experience*, Hutchinson, London.
8. In this context we might seriously consider the position of all religious cultures, but especially the 'born-again Christians', many of whom claim to have had a personal communication with God.
9. For a concise description of the *Doppelganger* phenomenon, see Reed, G. (1987) in *The Oxford Companion to the Mind*, (ed. R. L. Gregory), Oxford University Press, Oxford.
10. Frame, J. (1980) *Faces in the Water*, Women's Press, London.
11. For a detailed overview of assessment instruments, see Barnes, T. R. E. and Nelson, H. E. (eds) (1994) *The Assessment of Psychoses: A Practical Handbook*, Chapman & Hall, London.

12. Honigfeld, G., Gillis, R. O. and Klett, C. J. (1966) NOSIE-30: a treatment sensitive ward behaviour scale. *Psychological Reports*, **19**, 180–2.
13. Phillip, A. E. (1979) Prediction of successful rehabilitation by nurse rating scale. *British Journal of Psychiatry*, **134**, 422–6.
14. Honigfeld, G. (1974) NOSIE-30: history and current status of its use in pharmaco-psychiatric research, in *Psychological Measurement in Psychopharmacology*, vol. 7, (ed. P. Pichot), S. Karger, Basel, pp. 238–63.
15. Baker, R. and Hall, J. N. (1983) *Rehabilitation Evaluation of Hall and Baker (REHAB)*, Vine Publishing, Aberdeen. (Available from the publishers, 2a Eden Place, Aberdeen.)
16. Baker, R. and Hall, J. N. (1988) REHAB: a new assessment for chronic psychiatric patients. *Schizophrenia Bulletin*, **14**(1), 97–111.
17. Affleck, J. W. and McGuire, R. J. (1984) The measurement of psychiatric reha-bilitation status: a review of the needs and a new scale. *British Journal of Psychia-try*, **145**, 517–25.
18. Overall, J. E. and Gorham, D. R. (1962) The brief psychiatric rating scale. *Psychological Reports*, **10**, 799–812.
19. Machanda, R., Hirsch, S. R. and Barnes, T. R. E. (1989) A review of rating scales for measuring symptom changes in schizophrenia research, in *The Instruments of Psychiatric Research*, (ed. C. Thomson), John Wiley, Chichester.
20. McGorry, P. D., Goodwin, R. J. and Stuart, G. W. (1988) The development of the Brief Psychiatric Rating Scale (Nursing modification) – an assessment proce-dure for the nursing team in clinical and research settings. *Comprehensive Psychia-try*, **29**, 575–87.
21. This distinction was first introduced by Hughlings Jackson in the 19th century. See Berrios, G. (1984) Positive and negative symptoms and Jackson: a conceptual history. *Archives of General Psychiatry*, **42**, 95–7.
22. Strauss, J., Carpenter, W. T. and Bartko, J. (1974) The diagnosis and under-standing of schizophrenia: Part III. Speculations on the processes that underlie schizophrenic symptoms and signs. *Schizophrenia Bulletin*, **1**, 61–9.
23. Crow, T. (1980) Molecular pathology of schizophrenia: more than one dimension of pathology? *British Medical Journal*, **280**, 66–8.
24. Kraweicka, M., Goldberg, D. and Vaughan, M. (1977) A standardised psychiatric assessment scale for rating chronic psychotic patients. *Acta Psychiatrica Scandi-navica*, **55**, 299–308.
25. Hyde, C. (1989) The Manchester Scale: a standardised psychiatric assessment for rating chronic psychotic patients. *British Journal of Psychiatry*, **155**(Suppl. 7), 45–7.
26. Machanda, R., Saupe, R. and Hirsch, S. R. (1986) Comparison between the Brief Psychiatric Rating Scale and the Manchester Scale for the rating of schizophrenic symptoms. *Acta Psychiatrica Scandinavica*, **74**, 563–8.
27. Beck, A. T., Ward, C. H. and Mendelson, M. (1961) An inventory for measuring depression. *Archives of General Psychiatry*, **4**, 561–71.
28. Zung, W. W. K. (1965) A self-rating depression scale. *Archives of General Psychia-try*, **12**, 63–70.
29. Montgomery, S. A., Taylor, P. and Montgomery, D. (1978) Development of a schizophrenia scale sensitive to change. *Neuropharmacology*, **17**, 1053–71.
30. In Hawton's view available assessment instruments are only of limited value,

possessing a very low predictive power. Hawton, K. (1994) The assessment of suicidal risk, in *The Assessment of Psychoses: A Practical Handbook*, (eds T. R. E. Barnes and H. E. Nelson), Chapman & Hall, London.

31. Beck, A. T., Weissman, A., Lester, D. and Trexler, L. (1974) The measurement of pessimism: the Hopelessness Scale. *Journal of Consulting and Clinical Psychology*, **42**, 861–5.

32. Beck, A. T., Schuyler, D. and Herman, J. (1974) Development of suicidal intent scales, in Beck, A. T., Resnick, H. L. P. and Lettieri, D. J. (eds) *The Prediction of Suicide*, Charles Press, Maryland.

33. Walmsley, R. (1986) *Personal Violence*, Home Office Research and Policy Unit Research Study No. 89, HMSO, London.

34. The report on the Bethlem Royal and Maudsley Hospital's register of violent incidents showed that the number of violent incidents had trebled between 1976 and 1987. Noble, P. and Rodgers, S. (1989) Violence by psychiatric inpatients. *British Journal of Psychiatry*, **155**, 384–90.

35. Kay, S., Wolkenfield, F. and Murrill, L. (1988) Profiles of aggression among psychiatric patients. I: Nature and prevalence. *Journal of Nervous and Mental Disease*, **176**, 539–46.

36. Novaco, R. (1975) *Anger Control: The Development and Evaluation of an Experimental Treatment*, Lexington Books, Lexington, LA.

37. Novaco, R. (1991) Anger and violence among state hospital patients. *Aggressive Behaviour*, **17**, 88.

38. Wright, B. A. (1991) Labelling: the need for greater person-environment individuation, in *Handbook of Social and Clinical Psychology: The Health Perspective*, (eds C. R. Snyder and D. R. Forsyth), Pergamon Press, Oxford.

39. American Psychiatric Association (1987) *Diagnostic and Statistical Manual of Mental Disorders*, 3rd edn, rev., American Psychiatric Association, Washington, DC, p. xxiii.

40. Wright, B. A. (1991) Labelling: the need for greater person-environment individuation, in *Handbook of Social and Clinical Psychology: The Health Perspective*, (eds C. R. Snyder and D. R. Forsyth), Pergamon Press, Oxford, p. 480.

41. Romme, M. and Escher, S. (1993) *Accepting Voices*, MIND Publications, London.

42. Romme, M. and Escher, S. (1996) Empowering people who hear voices, in *Cognitive-Behavioural Interventions with Psychotic Disorders*, (eds G. Haddock and P. Slade), Routledge, London.

43. Romme, M. and Escher, S. (1996) Personal communication.

<table>
<tr><td>

9

</td><td>

The person and the environment: boundaries of the self

</td></tr>
</table>

Not in Utopia ... but in the very world ... the place where in the end
We find our happiness, or not at all!

Wordsworth

We do not have solitary beings. Every creature is, in some sense, connected to and dependent on the rest.

Lewis Thomas

THE ENVIRONMENT: AN INTRODUCTION

Throughout much of this book we have emphasized the assessment of the person and his functioning. This narrow view may well be a characteristic of the psychiatric method: we know that people are (to some extent) a function of their environments, but we act (often) as if they occupy a vacuum. We act as if pathology always lies within the person, rather than within the person's relationships with his world.

If my concern is in any way grounded, the cause may lie in our scientific approach to understanding the world and the people within it. In our efforts to understand human distress we have developed experimental studies within which the researcher manipulates a hypothesized cause and randomly assigns subjects (people) to different levels of exposure to this cause. Leaving aside all other considerations, the philosophical limitation of such an 'experimental' approach is that it treats subjects (people) as objects [1]. What can such an approach to human enquiry ever tell us about people – how they live their lives and how they manage 'the slings and arrows of outrageous fortune'?

It seems self-evident that people do not suddenly become mentally ill. Human distress – whatever form it might take – does not well up within the person and, without warning, manifest itself as a psychiatric disorder. Equally, where the disorder is thought to be 'enduring', it does not lie dormant – except in that metaphorical sense – only to 'catch light' as if igniting itself from within. At the time of writing, science does not appear to believe in the phenomenon of spontaneous combustion. We might care to remember that mental distress is not self-ignited, however metaphorically we might care to use the expression. Mental illness is more complex than this.

We have acknowledged throughout the text nursing's growing interest in holism and the concept of the unique individual. If we accept these concepts, then we must accept that mental distress may be **of** the person, but is not necessarily **in** the person. Our sorrows – as well as our joys – lie somewhere between us and the world that defines us.

Throughout the preceding chapters I have referred repeatedly to behaviour – how we act in our lives and how we act upon our lives. Much of our behaviour involves reactions to our environment. We react to traffic lights, bicycle bells, fire alarms or the sight of someone important entering the room. We react to major disasters and trivial incidents. We may even be indiscriminate in such reactions: becoming more upset over trivia than apparent trauma.

We also act upon the environment: pressing this and pulling that to gain access to everything from money at our bank cash dispensers, to fresh air and more or less sunlight. Increasingly, we talk of people who appear to manipulate their relationships with others as 'pressing the right buttons'.

We are linked inextricably with our environment: the world we inhabit. Our 'selves' – who we are – lie within our skins. Our 'world' – that which helps define who we are – lies immediately beyond our skins. The interface – between our 'selves' and our 'world' – is literally no more than skin deep.

We are in constant touch with our world. Such contact – the skin—world interface – is the inescapable fact of existence. This fact applies as much to the person described as a psychiatric 'patient' as it does to ourselves, the onlookers from the insecure peninsula of normality. Where the person is considered to be severely disturbed, it is all too easy to forget that his environment has played a part in the creation of that disturbance. How much a part remains unclear. This is not about laying blame. If we do not accept that everything we do is in some way related to our world, then we conjure with notions of spontaneous combustion.

In the groove

It is axiomatic that the 'problems of living' [2] which we label abnormal, and which we define as 'mental illness', involve the particular circumstances under which the person lives. This is especially the case when such problems are defined within a hospital or clinic setting. The rules and regulations of the institution are the metaphorical bells and buzzers that control the person-in-care's functioning to a greater or lesser extent. This 'institution' might be a rehabilitation hostel in the community, a residential home for old people, a day hospital, a 'drop-in' mental health centre or an acute admission ward in a district general hospital where the person is a newcomer, if not a 'new patient'. I shall refer to all of these settings as 'institutions'. All 'provide procedures through which human conduct is patterned, or compelled to go, in grooves deemed desirable by society' [3].

Institutions or environments?

Some readers might resent the use of the term 'institution'. This has become a dirty word in this politically-correct age of enlightenment in psychiatric care. However, as our discussion develops, it may become apparent that the term has no real 'value' connotations other than those we award. It may represent the humanitarian just as easily as it represents the restrictive organization of a life in care. I intend to say little about individual people here. In this chapter I am more interested in the sea of existence within which the person swims. To what extent will this 'sea' wash him ashore on some idyllic desert island or merely drown him in more troubles? What is the nature of the person—world relationship?

One of our considerations must be the way the environment is organized, in an architectural sense. However, most of our interest should lie in the abstract organization – the schedule of rules and regulations, both explicit and implicit. Some of these will be pinned to noticeboards, others will be simply a part of the verbal culture, if not the 'mind set', of staff. All such rules and regulations are potent influences on the behaviour of the people-in-care as well as those who care for them. These are the boundaries that contribute to the definition of the self. These boundaries may be just as evident within families, which are institutions in their own right.

In one sense we are looking, indirectly, at staff behaviour (or behaviour of others who might be deemed to 'care' for the person) and its effects upon the person. Architects and planners may provide the environmental shell but nurses (and to a lesser extent other professionals) are responsible for constructing and manipulating the 'living environment'. This is especially so in the **total institution**: those environments that represent the totality of the person's experience, such as the 'secure environment' of the forensic ward. I hope that I do not patronize my colleagues too much when I say that many staff are oblivious of these processes. They may be largely unaware of their surroundings, content to work through a shift thinking, perhaps, about having a drink or meal after work or next week's cup tie. For the staff team the environment is a temporary, if not invisible, thing. For those who will still be there after the staff have left for the pub or are on the terraces – the clientele – the 'environment' has a quite different meaning. It may serve as either a reassuring cocoon or a suffocating constraint.

The function of the environment

To understand something of the effects of the environment we need first to establish its general function.

- What happens to people within this particular setting?
- Does it promote the growth of the individual, or does it function as a shelter: a genuine asylum in a storm-tossed world?
- Does it retard growth or encourage dependence?
- In addition to these general questions, we need also to consider how we might measure – or, to use the popular parlance, **audit** – the workings of the environment.

I shall try to refrain from adopting either of the stereotypical views of the institution. I do not believe that they explain the plight of the person with an experience of mental illness. Neither do I see the institution as necessarily virtuous. My own position can best be summarized by quoting the words of Thomas à Kempis: 'occasions do not make a man either strong or weak, but merely show what he is'.

Institutional environments have the capacity to bring out the best or the worst in people. This assumption seems to hold true even when the institution concerned is the family. In previous chapters I have alluded to the views of R. D. Laing on the putative influences of the 'world' – including the family – on the person's experience of mental health or ill-health [4]. Now, 30 years later, Laing's perspective is in danger of being dismissed as an aberration. It is now assumed that there are no 'schizophrenogenic' families (or mothers). Instead there are families characterized by 'high expressed emotion (HEE)' [5]. My colleague Ben Davidson described the EE hypothesis (or theory) as a sanitized (or de-politicized) version of the world-according-to-Laing. Davidson recognized that it is easier to attribute 'relapse' to some abstract, unwitting interpersonal process than to acknowledge that – given the way they live – some families drive one or more of their members crazy. Whether they do so intentionally or unwittingly seems to miss the point.

When we consider how we might assess the environment, we should be interested in discovering ways of determining how different environments work so that we can ensure the maximum opportunity for growth and the least likelihood of deterioration. Our interest should be not only in clinical or institutional environments, but should include some consideration of the family environment, however problematic such an assessment might be.

THE PERSON AND THE ENVIRONMENT

The relationship between the individual and his environment may be compared to the relationship between a record and a record-player. The kind of music played, whether classical or popular, is determined by the recording. The quality of the music played depends, however, on the record-player. The same record can sound harsh and squeaky, or smooth and full of tone, depending on the kind of record-player used. The same is true of people. The language they speak, the behaviour they show and the beliefs they hold may all be influenced by their culture: the world they inhabit. However, the quality of their performance depends upon inherited talents and potentials or upon functional abilities developed during their lives [6].

The debate still rages over which is the more important influence on a person's behaviour: environment or heredity. To employ another metaphor, the question is rather like asking which is more important to the running of a car – the petrol or the engine?

In our consideration of the role of the environment I accept that the person's behaviour may have its origins in (for example) some dysfunctional biochemical state. I accept also that the person's environment plays a part in his 'presentation of self' [7]. Our institutions provide us with grooves similar to those of a record, and we follow these grooves to satisfy societal standards of appropriate behaviour. The psychiatric environment – even when it is no more than abstract notions of sanity or madness – provides similar grooves. Those in power (staff) determine the constituents of 'appropriate behaviour'. The person-in-care either conforms to or resists this pattern.

'Appropriate behaviour' within a psychiatric institution is, invariably, unacceptable behaviour in the natural world of the outside. Dependency is valued and assertiveness is problematic. As soon as people-in-care begin to show 'inappropriate' institutional behaviour, they are 'showing' that it is time for them to leave the institution. They either move on to some less restrictive environment, or move further in to the restraining arms of the institutional system.

When we come to consider the role of the environment, the key question is: 'To what extent does the environment assist the person to show "inappropriate" behaviour?' We need also to ask to what extent this influence is in the best interests of the person.

Stigma and the myth of normality

These consideration about 'appropriate' and 'inappropriate' behaviour imply further considerations about normal behaviour. The layperson might be excused for thinking that the people in the care of the psychiatric services are in some way 'not normal' [8]. They might also believe that the staff who care for or treat them on behalf of society **are** normal. These considerations are only relevant here since they are the part of the social construction of stigma.

The experience of mental illness (or the imposition of such a diagnosis) is the second of three forms of stigma described by Goffman [9], the others being forms of physical deformity and those associated with race, creed, etc. Stigma is 'an undesired differentness', which turns those whom the stigmatized person meets away from him, 'breaking the claim that his other attributes have on us' [10]. The world in Goffman's view is collapsed, therefore, into 'those who do not depart negatively from the particular expectations at issue' (who might be called 'the normals') and those with one of the three forms of stigma [11].

Increasingly, people with an experience of mental illness have sought to act as advocates for themselves or others with similar life experiences [12]. We cannot discuss the role of the environment without considering the effect the rise of the user-advocacy movement in mental health (if not disability in general) has had on the provision of services for such people. In one sense the user-advocacy movement seeks to validate the experience of mental illness, often challenging the medicalization of such experiences [13] and generally calling into question the content and processes of care and treatment for 'the mentally ill'. Today's user-advocacy movement is a descendant of a well-established tradition of 'user-voices' [14]. It seems clear, however, that late-20th century psychiatry is now on the horns of a major dilemma in trying to acknowledge the validity of the experience of mental illness on the one hand and trying to maintain, on the other hand, the tradition of psychiatry, which is based, fundamentally, on divisive notions of normality and abnormality.

Goffman anticipated the rise of user-advocacy when he noted that stigmatized people are not as impressed by the stigma as 'normals' are. Indeed they may emphasize these distinguishing characteristics and are 'unrepentant about doing so' [15]. Goffman noted also that the stigmatized person:

> tends to hold the same beliefs about [his] identity that we [normals] do; this is a pivotal fact. His deepest feelings about what he is may be his sense of being a 'normal person', a human being like everyone else, a person, therefore, who deserves a fair chance and a fair break. ... Yet he may perceive, correctly, that whatever others profess, they do not really 'accept' him and are not ready to make contact with him on 'equal grounds' [16].

Goffman also makes the important observation that: 'the notion of the "normal human being" may have its source in the medical approach to humanity ... [seeming] to provide the basic imagery through which laymen [sic] conceive of themselves [17].'

These considerations are critical factors in our assessment of the environment of care of contemporary psychiatric nursing services. I have noted in previous chapters nurses' assumption that they (and perhaps only they) address the 'whole' of the person's experience, through holistic nursing. Increasingly, nurses talk of 'working in partnership', embracing collaborative forms of care and models of caring. The assessment of the person's care environment needs to ask the following questions.

- To what extent are nurses and people-in-care equal?

- To what extent is the form of care and the process of caring based on true collaboration?
- To what extent are nurses (or indeed any other member of the team) free to dispense with the concept of stigma?
- To what extent are nurses required to address the person-in-care as someone characterized by 'undesired differentness'? [19].

The total institution

Our concept of the total institution is derived mainly from the classic text by Erving Goffman, the American sociologist. Goffman described how it was normal practice for people to move from one environment to another, to engage in different activities or patterns of behaviour [20]. We sleep, eat, work and play with different people, usually in quite different situations. In the 'total institution' such natural barriers are conspicuously absent. Goffman observed that in many cases all such social, recreational, occupational and self-care activities might take place under the one roof, often with little movement of the residents. In this sense the setting for top-security prisoners and people-who-are-patients differs little. Neither have much of a 'life' outside the confines of the institution.

Of course not all psychiatric settings are total institutions in the sense defined by Goffman. It is more appropriate, perhaps, to distinguish the extent to which any environment approximates a total institution.

- To what extent does the environment of care restrict the person?
- To what extent does the environment of care promote normal living?

Why should we ask such questions? We have known that care environments can be damaging to their residents. Barton's classic text on institutional neurosis showed how care could lead to a deterioration in the functioning of individuals [21]. This was more likely to happen where people wore the same clothes, ate from the same bowls, shared the same public toilet and bathing facilities and were regimented by the same set of restrictive institutional practices. The 'patient', as described by Barton, was stripped of his personality in much the same way that prisoners and refugees are stripped of their individuality. With this loss of their intrinsic self comes a deterioration in physical habits, an increase in apathy and a general loss of interest in life itself.

Clearly, we now know what kind of environment would be best for people-in-care. How often do we put this into practice? In evaluating the quality of institutional care we have to accept that there are limitations on how 'natural' or therapeutic these environments can become. This acknowledgement should not deter us from asking how far can we push back the boundaries of the restrictive environment. To what extent can we normalize an abnormal situation?

The half-way house

With the advent of more progressive policies for people in mental illness has come the development of a range of alternative institutional settings. This began with rehabilitation units within the hospital grounds, gradually being extended to hostels and group homes in the community and, in more and more cases, more ordinary forms of housing provision. These have led people from the 'abnormality' of the old-style locked 'back ward' to the uncertain reality of life in the natural community.

All such settings function as stepping stones. They are not closed environments, like the total institution described above. However, we still need to question the extent to which the life enjoyed by the person is anything like as normal as is often assumed.

- To what extent is the person free to come and go?
- To what extent is he restricted?
- To what extent does the environment exert a significant influence?
- To what extent might the environment be modified to facilitate his human growth and development?

Although 'drop-in' centres and day hospitals are much more transitory environments, they should not escape a similar kind of analysis. The person may spend only a small proportion of his day there, but the content may be more significant than the time of the exposure. Consequently, the issues addressed in this chapter apply equally to day hospitals for people with acute or enduring forms of mental distress, as well as older people with psychiatric disturbance.

The therapeutic environment

We cannot leave this discussion of 'institutions' without discussing the concept of the therapeutic milieu as it pertains to the small-scale living or therapeutic community on a larger scale. Most of us like to think that the clinical environment is arranged to suit the person's needs, and to reduce his distress. The term 'therapeutic milieu', however, has a special meaning, and the notion of the 'therapeutic community' is even more specific in terms of its philosophical base and practical function. Both are pertinent to our discussion here.

After the Second World War a number of experimental projects began to offer a different kind of care and treatment to people with a range of mental health problems. The rehabilitative process used shunned the use of the disciplinarian, custodial practices that were the legacy of the early asylum days or a distortion of the 'moral treatment' tradition. Instead, emphasis was given to sharing decision-making between staff and people-in-care. Staff no longer had a monopoly over the direction of the environment. Where antisocial behaviour was evident, efforts were made to tolerate, rather than punish, to encourage the person to assume more responsibility for his actions.

The roles of staff within such settings differed greatly from the 'custodial' context: less attention was paid to rank and status, and an atmosphere of informality was cultivated. The environment concentrated almost exclusively on confronting people with the reality of their own behaviour, usually through individual or (more often) group psychotherapy [22]. In one sense such environments achieved an atmosphere of normality through the appearance of informality and lack of structure. In another sense, however, it was heavily organized and – therefore – institutionalized; through its detailed programme of daily meetings, discussion groups, debate and decision-making (often) over even the most trivial of matters. Such intensity is hardly to be found in the sitting-room of the typical semi-detached house. In many ways it was sufficiently intense to make even the most custodial staff member wince.

The development of the therapeutic community did, however, exemplify a major effort to recognize and address the environment as a major influence on the people cared for within its walls.

ASSESSING THE ENVIRONMENT – AN OVERVIEW

Organizing the assessing of the environment

Much of the assessment methodology discussed so far can be used, with discretion, by nurses at any level in the rankings of the hierarchy. The same cannot be said of the decision to study the environment. The decision needs to be taken by someone in authority, although all members of the team may provide an input to the process of assessment. Although all assessment needs to be undertaken with care, special problems may emerge when the environment is brought under review. Some of the observational practices recommended for analysing environments resemble 'time-and-motion' methods. Staff who have not been involved fully in the assessment process might be forgiven for assuming that their 'working', rather than the workings of the environment, is under scrutiny. Such a misconception could sabotage the whole exercise.

Any assessment of the environment is usually undertaken for one of the following reasons.

- **To assess the 'quality of care' in a particular setting**. This often involves an analysis of one or more of the following factors:
  — the amount of therapeutic interaction;
  — levels of disturbed behaviour;
  — levels of appropriate activity for the setting;
  — expressed levels of satisfaction among the people-in-care.
- **To identify the effects of specific changes in the environment**. This might involve the effect of one or more of the following:
  — rearrangement of the furniture;

— revision of staff rotas or routines;

— people joining or leaving the environment.

- **To evaluate the changes in any of the factors mentioned above over a discrete timescale.** Rarely is it sufficient to identify problems and propose solutions. In any environment it is important to monitor these interventions across time: do these solutions last in the medium or long term? Although such an assessment may be undertaken to resolve some major problem, or following some external criticism of the environment, this kind of assessment should be routine in all care settings.

The assessment of the environment is a kind of 'quality-control' measure. It begs the question: 'Does the environment achieve what it sets out to achieve?' Such a question has as much relevance to the care setting as it does to the production setting, where the ideas of quality control and goal achievement were born [24].

Assessing the design of the environment

The first issue we should consider is the fabric of the environment. This constitutes the skeleton, or framework, of the ward, unit, centre, etc. Around this framework is draped the social world which staff and the people-in-care inhabit. I shall not address this in any detail, for clearly this is a subject in itself. However, in assessing any environment it is clear that we must look at how it is built, as well as its function.

- Does it have small rooms or large, echoing chambers?
- Are the ceilings 20 feet from the ground, resembling St Pancras Station?
- Does the 'day room' resemble a large living-room in a modern semi-detached?
- Is the colour scheme stimulating, drab or dazzling?
- Are there pictures and *objets d'art* appropriate to the age, cultural background and interests of the client group?
- Does the lounge have a pool table in one corner and a Space Invaders machine in the other?

Such questions are not simply aesthetic. Many attempts to improve institutional environments have involved trying to turn the 'back ward' into a page from a designer's catalogue. Hessian wall coverings and hi-tech furniture may, however, be just as alien and uninspiring to the residents as the gloss-painted walls and tubular steel armchairs they replaced. The design of an environment is not concerned solely with comfort. Its primary aim is to facilitate a certain kind of social behaviour. The assessment needs to ask: 'What kind of social behaviour needs to be promoted here?' and 'To what extent does this environment achieve that?' The staff team should consider these questions with respect to any part of the environment of care: sitting areas, bedrooms, bathrooms, toilets, kitchens. To what extent do these environments, in their present form, encourage the kind of behaviour appropriate for these situations?

Some people assess the quality of the person's environment by comparing it with similar staff facilities. Are the toilet paper, cutlery, menu, levels of privacy (etc.) the same for staff and the people-in-care? If not, why not? This is hardly a foolproof system, for someone is bound to comment that the needs of the people-in-care are different. However, many of the improvements in clinical environments have come about through staff sharing facilities with the people-in-care in the manner of the therapeutic communities mentioned earlier. In assessing the quality of the person's environment it may be worth while considering how long the nurse could tolerate the level of privacy, comfort, stimulation and freedom afforded by different aspects of the environment.

Assessing the staff team

The members of staff are as much a part of the environment as the television set and the wallpaper. The assessment needs to consider how they appear to the person. This 'appearance' may play a significant part in the construction of their behaviour. I have mentioned already the air of informality cherished by the therapeutic communities. Some aspects of that philosophy have been accommodated by contemporary services. Uniforms for nurses have all but disappeared. In some situations they are replaced by conspicuous ID tags or massive key-ring attachments to belts. Uniforms function to locate the staff: the age-old complaint over visitors being 'unable to tell the staff from the patients' is apposite. Many managers like to be able to distinguish clearly between 'patients' and 'staff', and uniforms, conspicuous IDs, etc. prove useful in this respect. From the person-in-care's perspective they also provide a barrier between one person and another. For those who wish to be 'looked after' this may be viewed as helpful. For others who wish to be 'worked with' this may prove a major source of conflict. Again, we need to ask the question: What is the environment for?

The various grades of uniform, and the ranks that accompany them, function as further barriers between those wearing uniforms. The uniform, therefore, encourages social distance. To what extent is the staff team 'distanced' from the people-in-care? To what extent might this distance be construed as a 'good' or 'bad' thing?

Power, authority and interpersonal processes

Formal titles and forms of address create social distance. First-name terms, on the other hand, signify collegiality, friendship, trust and a degree of intimacy. The use of such forms of address can be classed as 'overfamiliarity'. In such contexts it would be necessary, perhaps, to assess why a member of staff felt threatened by this invasion of her professional identity?

The use of nicknames involves a similar concern. Calling James 'Jacko' may be a form of endearment. It might also be patronizing. In many cases the nickname is highly inappropriate: calling an older unmarried woman 'Gran' or any older man 'Dad' might cause offence.

When assessing the function of staff within the environment we must begin with their raw status as staff. To what extent do the uniforms, titles, insignia, pet names (etc.) function as mechanisms of control? Such information may tell us much about the social psychology of the institution. Since I have stressed the 'interpersonal context' of psychiatric nursing throughout this book, it is important that we gauge the extent to which staff are able to relate to the people in their care and *vice versa*. We also need to know the extent to which the encumbrances of authority and professionalism may obstruct them from doing so.

The organization of the environment

The operation of the environment is determined by two classes of instruction. The first involves 'abstract' rules and regulations. These are often enforced as though they were written on tablets of stone. When these rules are questioned, often no record can be found: they represent the verbal culture of the ward. The second is the formal organization of the interaction of staff and persons: the 'routine'. This is usually well documented, on a noticeboard if not on a tablet of stone. When we consider the role of rules and regulations, we need to evaluate their effect.

Does the environment dictate the same rule for everyone:

- when to rise for the day;
- when to go to bed;
- when to have a bath or wash his hair;
- where he can smoke;
- whether or not he can drink alcohol;
- whether or not he can have a friend in his room;
- whether or not he may change the decor of his room?

Some kind of order is necessary where a large number of people live under one roof. The assessment needs to consider, however, the extent to which the environment is restrictive. Some people would say, 'Of course the person can't decide when to have a bath, or paint his wall ... he's in hospital after all' [25]! Again we are back to our original dilemma. What is the hospital for? Can its traditional face and function be adapted and modified to suit 'new needs'?

I make no recommendations one way or the other. I am simply acknowledging that the way our environment is organized has an effect: sometimes it encourages us to conform, and we follow the grooves in the record. In other instances we rebel, either publicly or deviously. In those settings where people appear to be 'bucking the system', we need to consider whether the environment rather than the person needs changing.

I have drawn a thread of person-centred care throughout this book. This might be wholly impractical in many settings, especially where staff are required to provide a shepherding function. Yet even in situations where staffing levels are low, or the organization of staffing is less than efficient, it is all too easy to blame the environmental disorder on the 'mental state' of the people-in-care. In looking at the organization of activities throughout the day we need to evaluate whether the organization encourages or discourages the performance of the desired behaviour.

- Does the care system include specifications about the arrangement of privacy at bathtimes?
- Do the staff and the people-in-care eat at the same tables?
- Do people spend a lot of time 'waiting': for food, drugs, appointments with staff or other forms of staff attention?
- Do the staff spend much time engaged in 'observations' of people deemed to be at risk?
- Do such patterns of 'observation' preclude human interaction?

In many closed institutions the person's day is ordered beyond the level necessary for avoiding cold dinners or congestion in the living area. Our assessment needs to ask: Is such a level of organization and control therapeutic or restrictive?

The orientation of the institution

Richard Lovelace, the English poet, was the first to remark that 'stone walls do not a prison make, nor iron bars a cage'. The quotation is particularly apposite when we consider the function of institutions, as distinct from their appearance. Many a care setting may appear comfortable, airy and potentially therapeutic. We need to analyse its function to decide whether such a promise is realized. Most analyses of the function of environments, from Goffman in the 1950s to the present day, have involved asking the question: 'For whose benefit is the institution run?' Numerous studies have suggested that the answer is not always 'the people-in-care'.

In the early 1970s Raynes and King studied the 'quality of care' of children in residential settings. Local authority homes, voluntary homes and hospitals were studied in order to detect any significant differences [26]. Although they focused on the care of children with intellectual impairment and physical disabilities their findings continue to have relevance for anyone requiring continuing care in residential situations.

Raynes and King developed a scale to measure the quality of care which indirectly influenced today's generation of social-change agents. Their scale measured:

- **Rigidity of routine**: the degree to which management practices were flexible – i.e. to what extent did staff accommodate 'individual differences' among residents, varying routines according to the day of the week, time of year, occasion, etc.?;
- **Block treatment**: the degree to which the residents were treated as individuals or merely as members of a group – i.e. did the residents bathe, use the toilet, have meals, etc. according to individual need, or was this determined by a care practice policy?;
- **Depersonalization**: the degree to which the residents had the opportunity to acquire and maintain personal possessions, enjoy privacy, use their initiative, make decisions, etc.;
- **Social distance**: the degree to which the residents engaged in 'normal' interaction with staff – i.e. did the residents dine with the staff team or interact with staff on an individual basis? Did the residents receive individualized care from one identified member of the team, or were they 'processed' by several?

Raynes and King found that, although there were major differences between the different residential units studied, these differences were not explained by the overall size of the institution, the actual size of the care units or differences in staff—person ratios. Instead the differences in role orientation served to distinguish one setting from another. Raynes and King argued that there was a direct relationship between the orientation of staff and the pattern of care they ultimately offered. In short, they found that those staff who had been trained in large institutions were more task-oriented and spent little time engaging in close interaction with the residents. Those who had been trained outside large institutions were more orientated towards the individual, displaying this orientation through higher levels of individual contact.

Similar studies have shown that, even where the fabric and structure of the environment are changed to allow increased individualization of care, the negative features of the total institution highlighted by Raynes and King will survive if the person running the unit retains a custodial philosophy [27].

The features highlighted above are echoes of some of the considerations already mentioned. Barton highlighted the 'inflexibility' of routines in his study, and this was one of the key elements in Goffman's research. Many other researchers have pointed out that institutions deprive people of an opportunity to engage in complete cycles of activity, e.g. shopping, preparing and cooking food, eating the meal and then doing the washing up. Instead they are consistently catered for, often like guests in a second-rate hotel. Staff attitudes play a large part in influencing 'block treatment' or the process of 'personality stripping'. Traditionally we have distinguished between 'custodial' and 'therapeutic' staff. Such distinctions are not always clear-cut. It is clear, however, that any analysis of the person's environment must take account of the prevailing attitudes of the staff. Nurses who tend to view those in their care as 'people', similar to themselves, will tend to be more person-oriented, whereas those who are task-oriented tend to be dominated by the use of diagnostic categories or subtypes in their experience of the person [28]. The authoritarian tradition of nursing is of obvious relevance here. It relates strongly also to the issue of social distance, as we have already discussed.

In theory, psychiatric nursing is based upon the establishment of open, trusting, therapeutic relationships between staff and person. In assessing the person for treatment or help-giving, we must consider whether or not it will be possible to offer help. The question can only be answered by an analysis of the climate of care, as expressed through the attitudes of staff and the patterns of care they project. The research of Barton, Goffman and Raynes and King is between a quarter-century and 50 years old. It is interesting to note that we are still struggling, in many situations, to provide care consistently through one identified nurse; or we continue to be faced by criticisms from the user-advocacy movement that contemporary psychiatric care is dehumanizing.

I have emphasized these historical accounts of 'context of psychiatric care' to show how knowledge does not necessarily lead to change. Where nurses embark on an assessment of the care environment we assume that they do so with the 'process of change' firmly in mind. They are not undertaking a piece of objective research. They are studying what goes on under their very noses, what issues from their policies, protocols and conventions. They are studying how those abstract ideas interact with the physical environment, producing the 'atmosphere' which characterizes the care setting.

Assessment of the living environment

The considerations listed above are a disparate grouping. How can one possibly evaluate the quality of a ward or a day-care environment, covering everything from the architecture and decor of the building to the caring orientation of the staff? Such a wide-ranging assessment will be very difficult, if not impossible. I include these merely as considerations. One level of 'assessment' might look only at the fabric of the ward, problems people meet in moving from A to B and the ease with which they can turn taps on and off or unravel the toilet tissue. Another level might deal exclusively with the daily timetable: does it accommodate the celebration of birthdays, having a lie-in on Sundays or having a sandwich in front of the television instead of the regulation 'high tea'? Other assessments might try to evaluate the function of staff attitudes – towards specific people-in-care, towards routines, individual-ized care or staff dress. Our assessment of the environment might focus on specific facets such as those mentioned, but may in some situations attempt to take the complete 'environment' as the canvas of care.

Jubilee Mews – case illustration of an extraordinary community

Increasingly, people with more serious or enduring forms of mental illness are receiving structured support to live within the natural community, rather than within the artificial community of the hospital. Jubilee Mews is a three-house development built on an 'ordinary street' within a suburb of Newcastle-upon-Tyne, UK. Each house is home to four 'residents', all of whom have suffered from serious mental illness for many years. Bus stops, local shops, pubs, churches, post offices and all the other amenities of a 'local community' are within walking distance. Although Jubilee Mews comprises a group of specially built properties, the houses are indistinguishable from the neighbouring homes of other 'ordinary people'.

The interior decoration of each house was chosen to reflect the personal tastes and choices of the residents, in an effort to promote a sense of belonging and ownership. Each resident has their own room and front door key and access is gained in the event of an emergency only with the resident's prior consent. The residents' right to privacy is respected at all times. Above all, residents are encouraged to participate in all aspects of daily living and play an active part in the day-to-day decision-making. The residents participate in community meetings, which are held regularly and which provide them with a 'voice' to express their views on all aspects of their care and life within Jubilee Mews.

The provision of this kind of care aims to 'approximate' the world of the natural community. It seems evident that projects like Jubilee Mews are in some senses set apart from the ordinary world: they are extraordinary environments for people who have led lives which are, by and large, out of the ordinary. The extraordinary support offered by a home like Jubilee Mews may be the necessary step that has to be taken for people wishing to resettle in the world of 'ordinary people'.

Value standards in a caring environment

Many developing mental health services, like Jubilee Mews, are giving greater emphasis to assessing the abstract environment, characterized by the values upon which the whole care process rests. These kind of services have taken the concerns expressed first by Goffman, later by Raynes and King and Wolfensberger, and provided living examples of 'valued' and 'valuing' environments for people with special needs. Jubilee Mews has identified seven specific principles that govern the delivery of care. Each of these principles can be viewed as a function of the environment and can be assessed by examination (specifically) of the care policies and (more generally) of the organization of the environment.

- **Rights**: It is assumed that all people have a right to be respected and empowered to make decisions regarding their own lives. They also have a right to expect that they will be supported and safe to make such decisions.

- **Citizenship**: It is assumed that all residents should be supported to allow them to become involved as valued members of the local community and society in general. This reflects their equal status as citizens.
- **Independence**: It is assumed that residents have a right to support and education to enable them to make informed choices as individuals. Through such choices they may increase their level of independence and sense of self-determination.
- **Choice**: It is assumed that residents have a right to support to make informed choices based on the resources available to them.
- **Privacy**: It is assumed that residents have a right to expect that they have a right to privacy. Their wish to spend time alone either in private or in a relaxing and comfortable environment over which they feel a sense of ownership should be respected.
- **Fulfilment**: It is assumed that residents have a right to expect support in fulfilling their full potential. This might involve education or other means leading to the realization of their needs, desires and ambitions.
- **Dignity**: It is assumed that residents should be valued as unique individuals. They should be supported in the expression of their personal beliefs and actions within a non-discriminatory environment [29].

The traditional forms of 'care' offered to people with a mental illness have been characterized by discriminatory or restrictive practices. These values, which underpin the policies and practices that are the environment of Jubilee Mews, reflect an effort to reverse these practices, which devalue and therefore harm further people who require mental health care [30]. Assessing the environment from this abstract perspective is rarely easy. It involves analysing care plans, and checking policies and philosophies. More importantly, it involves observing the activities within the environment to gauge the extent to which these values are or are not translated into action.

ASSESSMENT OF THE ENVIRONMENT: SPECIFIC CONSIDERATIONS

In the second part of this chapter I shall consider more specific ways of assessing the person's environment. The two methods I shall discuss are standardized measures, developed through research to provide a highly specific picture of what is happening within the environment. In view of their specific nature, they tell a very incomplete story. However, these methods may be further examples of the kind of 'thermometers' mentioned earlier: they may help us to take the temperature of the environment from a variety of angles.

The Ward Atmosphere Scale (WAS)

When we talk about the atmosphere in a ward or unit we do not mean the air pressure or the various gases circulating around us. Instead we are referring to another 'invisible' feature of the environment that is equally influential – the various attitudes, relationships, rules and regulations and other organizational factors that go to make up the 'social environment'. We have considered many of these items already. But how do we assess the 'social environment', especially when we cannot see it?

In the early 1970s the Ward Atmosphere Scale (WAS) was developed for use with staff and the people in their care. It tried to assess their respective perceptions of the ward atmosphere [31]. The format has been revised several times, with perhaps the best-known version being the 100-item questionnaire, which requires the staff member or person to circle 'True' or 'False' against each item. Examples are:

11. Patients (*sic*) never know when a doctor will ask to see them.
30. The patients are proud of this ward.
82. Patients are encouraged to show their feelings.

The various items on the scale represent ten discrete dimensions, which can be grouped under the following three headings:

- relationships (1–4);
- treatment programme (5–7);
- administrative structure (8–10).

The ten dimensions analyse the atmosphere as follows.

- **Involvement** assesses the extent to which the people-in-care take an active part in the routine running of the ward.
- **Support** assesses the amount of help and understanding available from members of the staff and from fellow people-in-care.
- **Spontaneity** assesses the extent to which people are encouraged to express their feelings openly towards staff or other people-in-care.
- **Anger and aggression** assesses the extent to which these emotions are tolerated or encouraged by way of therapeutic expression.
- **Autonomy and self-direction** assesses the extent to which people-in-care are encouraged to take responsibility for their own affairs or relationships with others.
- **Practical orientation** measures how much preparation the person is given for his discharge back into the community.
- **Personal problems** assesses the amount of help given to people-in-care to identify and understand their problems and emotions.
- **Activity planning and organization** assesses the importance of routine and order, and their relationship to the planning of schedules and activities.
- **Programme clarity** assesses the extent to which the person understands the

rules and regulations of the ward and the various procedures involved.
- **Staff control** assesses the amount of restriction imposed upon people-in-care through rules and regulations and other controlling measures.

This scale is the outcome of considerable research [32]. The WAS was revised for use in community treatment programmes: half-way houses, hostels, rehabilitation centres and day hospitals. The revised scale – the Community Oriented Program Environment Scale (COPES)— has 102 items, which are scored 'True' or 'False' [33]. These are summarized using the same ten dimensions on the original WAS.

Both the WAS and COPES have shown marked differences between environments that are manifestly 'therapeutic' or 'custodial'. In an early ward-based study people who were involved in a therapeutic programme reported greater levels of involvement and general 'satisfaction' than people receiving more standard forms of care [34]. Similar findings have been reported for the COPES format [35].

Although the WAS and the COPES are simple to use, the value of the information they produce should not be underestimated. The picture of the environment offered by both scales is relevant to any 'institutional' setting. This is obviously most true of the relationships and administrative dimensions, which are part and parcel of any institution: school, hospital or prison. The scores on the treatment programme dimensions, which involve personal development, would be expected to differ across different environments.

Moos found that this scale tells us a great deal about the people-in-care's perception of their environment. On some parts of the scale staff and people-in-care are in complete agreement, for example regarding the levels of organization. However, people-in-care may rate 'staff control' higher than staff. Moos's research has also shown that, where there are large numbers of people-in-care and few staff, the levels of 'support' and 'spontaneity' are low and the amount of 'staff control' is high. Finally, where the environment is more 'open', with fewer restrictions on people-in-care and less of an 'institutional' atmosphere, this is reflected in high scores for 'spontaneity', 'autonomy and self-direction', 'personal problems' and 'anger and aggression'.

The cynic might well argue, 'Well, we knew that already', and in some settings they could be right. Some environments are obviously open, supportive and therapeutic. Others are obviously confining, restrictive and custodial. Between these two extremes there exists a vast grey area where we are uncertain of the extent to which the environment is a positive or a negative force. The WAS and its community-oriented derivative may help resolve some of our doubts. However, even where we are certain of the status of the environment, surely there is no harm in confirming the therapeutic 'temperature' of the ward or day unit. This may help us also identify in which areas (or dimensions) the setting is rich or deficient. By using such a scale, we can evaluate how the environment changes – or remains the same – across time.

The Family Crisis Oriented Personal Evaluation Scales (F-COPES)

So far we have discussed only people living in 'extraordinary' environments typical of the traditional 'therapeutic' setting, whether this be in hospital or some other clinical context. The environment that exerts the most influence on people – whether they are people-in-care or 'ordinary' people – is, however, the family. Many people attribute their success (or failure) as people to values or other 'gifts' or 'insults' bestowed during the crucial developmental stages of their childhood and adolescence. Metaphorically speaking, children learn to become adults within the bosom of the family.

A family also has the capacity to restrict the development of its members, if not to inflict significant psychological damage. Mention has been made already of the hypothetical effects of 'high expressed emotion' on people described as suffering from schizophrenia [36]. Much evidence exists to suggest that negative marital and family relationships are implicated in a wide range of mental health problems [37].

The WAS and the COPES assessed how the environment 'worked' in terms of the relationship between the person-in-care and the clinical team and its supportive structure. Such environments might be seen as artificial families. Certainly, what goes on within the institutional environment is no more or less than an exaggeration of the relationships and rules that represent family life.

The F-COPES [38] is an assessment that measures how families respond to, and possibly resolve, problems. It assesses the problem-solving behaviours and attitudes of the family. These are represented on five subscales:

- acquiring social support;
- reframing;
- seeking spiritual support;
- mobilizing family to acquire and accept help;
- passive appraisal.

The scales comprise 30 items, each of which is rated on a five-point Likert scale, from 'Strongly agree' to 'Strongly disagree'. The scales are scored individually, and a total score is derived from summing the 30 responses.

The family members are asked to rate how they would face or respond to problems.

When we face problems or difficulties in our family, we respond by:

- seeking encouragement and support from friends;
- watching television;
- believing we can handle our own problems;
- having faith in God.

The scale provides a discrete measure of the family members' perceptions of their responses to family difficulties or crises. The family members' scores may be compared to available norms for adults or adolescents of both sexes.

Examples of other family-oriented measures are included in Appendix B [39,40,41]. The common feature of these measures is the emphasis on the 'function' of the family: how members relate to one another and how they address the life-problems which may have been precipitated by one of the family. They are not measures of 'pathology' or 'symptoms'. Such measures may prove more 'real' than assessments that focus attention on one family member – the pathologized 'scapegoat' so vividly described in the psychiatric literature.

CONCLUSION

The assessment of the environment of care may present nurses with the greatest challenge of all. To some extent this challenge is heightened by the lack of control which nurses often feel they possess over the conditions of care, if not the very fabric of the environment itself. In traditional 'medical' facilities – such as hospital wards – the nursing team is held accountable for the care of the 'patients', but may have only limited responsibilities for determining the kind of 'therapeutic' conditions that might result in meeting the needs of the people-in-care.

We should not forget either that some environments are expected to 'control' the people-in-care. This is true of special care settings – such as forensic settings – but is also increasingly true of wards attached to general hospitals, where significant proportions of the people-in-care may be at risk from self-harm or personal neglect. In such settings the kind of environment necessary to meet their 'needs' may differ greatly from that required for people who wish to reclaim their autonomy through therapeutic engagement with the nursing team.

The reader will be aware that the comparisons which are often made by managers between clinical environments and other situations that 'house' people – such as hotels or leisure facilities – are naive in the extreme. Although the principles that govern the assessment of 'quality' in all human environments are the same in principle, in practice an acute psychiatric ward cannot be compared to a hotel, and *vice versa*. Where nurses are caring for people with highly divergent needs, finding a standard for the quality of the overall environment may be problematic. Despite these challenges, the kinds of principle that have been outlined here, as guiding human assumptions about the rights, dignity and autonomy of people, carry the highest recommendation. Various assessment scales will provide useful indications of the 'support' that is available within the social and physical environment. Ultimately, nurses may need to develop their own methods to quantify and describe the important dimensions of their special environment and the policies and protocols that help to define all the people who live within it.

NOTES

1. Ericson, K. T. (1967) Person role and social uncertainty: a dilemma of the mentally ill. *Psychiatry*, **20**, 263–74.
2. Berger, P. L. (1966) *Invitation to Sociology: A Humanistic Perspective*, Penguin, Harmondsworth.
3. Bierstedt, R. (1963) *The Social Order: An Introduction to Sociology*, McGraw-Hill, New York.
4. Laing, R. D. and Esterson, A. (1964) *Sanity, Madness and the Family. Vol. 1: Families of Schizophrenics*, Tavistock, London.
5. Leff, J. and Vaughan, C. (1976) *Expressed Emotion in Families: Its Significance for Mental Illness*, Guilford Press, New York.
6. Barker, P. (1993) Understanding people – normal human development: cognitive aspects, in *Mental Health Nursing: From First Principles to Professional Practice*, (eds H. Wright and M. Giddey), Chapman & Hall, London.
7. Goffman, E. (1969) *The Presentation of Self in Everyday Life*, Allen Lane, London.
8. This is of course wholly reasonable, given that psychiatry means 'the study and treatment of mental **disease**'. Allen, R. E. (ed.) (1990) *The Concise Oxford Dictionary of Current English*, 8th edn, Clarendon Press, Oxford.
9. Goffman, E. (1963) *Stigma: Notes on the Management of Spoiled Identity*, Penguin, Harmondsworth, p. 14.
10. *Ibid.*, p. 15
11. *Ibid.*, p. 15
12. Read, J. and Wallcraft, J. (1992) *Guidelines for Empowering Users of Mental Health Services*, MIND Publications, London.
13. Chamberlin, J. (1988) *On Our Own*, MIND Publications, London.
14. Porter, R. (1987) *A Social History of Madness: Stories of the Insane*, Weidenfeld & Nicholson, London.
15. Goffman, E. (1963) *Stigma: Notes on the Management of Spoiled Identity*, Penguin, Harmondsworth, p. 17.
16. *Ibid.*, pp. 17–18.
17. *Ibid.*, p. 17.
18. Department of Health (1994) *Working in Partnership: The Report of the Mental Health Nursing Working Party*, HMSO, London.
19. The emphasis on Goffman's notion of 'undesired differentness' finds further reinforcement in the increased emphasis given to biological models of mental disorder. See Gournay, J. (1995) New facts on schizophrenia. *Nursing Times*, **91**(25), 32–3.
20. Goffman, E. (1961) *Asylums: Essays on the Social Situations of Mental Persons and Other Inmates*, Doubleday, New York.
21. Barton, R. (1966) *Institutional Neurosis*, 2nd edn, John Wright, Bristol.
22. Jones, M. (1976) *Maturation of the Therapeutic Community: an Organic Approach to Mental Health*, Human Sciences Press, New York.
23. Baron, L. (1987) *Asylum to Anarchy*, Free Association Books, London.
24. The concern for the 'quality' of health care, however, is not new: see Maxwell, R. J. (1984) Quality assurance in health. *British Medical Journal*, **288**, 1470–2.
25. It is notable that Mary Barnes painted the walls and doors of her room ... and later described this as a vital part of the therapeutic odyssey that led her 'back'

from psychosis to sanity: Barnes, M. and Berke, J. (1971) *Mary Barnes – Two Accounts of a Journey Through Madness*, MacGibbon & Kee, London.

26. Raynes, N. V. and King, R. D. (1974) Residential care for the mentally retarded, in *The Handicapped Person in the Community*, (eds D. M. Boswell and J. M. Wingrove), Tavistock, London.

27. Tizard, J., Sinclair, I. and Clarke, G. (1975) *Varieties of Residential Experience*, Routledge & Kegan Paul, London.

28. Turner, V. (1977) How the nurse can help preserve the person's individuality. *Nursing Mirror*, **20, 27 January**.

29. Details of the structure and value base of Jubilee Mews are presented courtesy of Brendan Hill.

30. Emerson, E. (1992) What is normalisation?, in *Normalisation: A Reader for the Nineties*, (eds H. Brown and H. Smith), Routledge, London.

31. Moos, R. (1968) The assessment of the social atmosphere of psychiatric wards. *Journal of Abnormal Psychology*, **73**, 595–604.

32. Moos, R. (1974) *Evaluating Treatment Environments: A Social Ecological Approach*, John Wiley, New York.

33. Moos, R. (1972) The assessment of the psychosocial environment of community oriented psychiatric treatment programs. *Journal of Abnormal Psychology*, **79**, 9–18.

34. Gripp, R. F. and Magaro, P. A. (1971) A token economy program evaluation with untreated ward comparisons. *Behaviour Research and Therapy*, **9**, 137–49.

35. Milby, J. B., Pendergrass, P. E. and Clarke, C. J. (1975) Token economy versus control ward: a comparison of staff and person attitudes towards ward environment. *Behaviour Therapy*, **6**, 22–30.

36. Leff, J. and Vaughan, C. (1976) *Expressed Emotion in Families*, Guilford Press, New York.

37. Barker, P. (1992) *Severe Depression: A Practitioner's Guide*, Chapman & Hall, London.

38. McCubbin, H. I., Olsen, D. H. and Larsen, A. S. (1981) Family crisis oriented personal evaluation scales (F-COPES), in *Family Assessment Inventories for Research and Practice*, (eds H. I. McCubbin and A. Thompson), University of Wisconsin, Madison, WI.

39. McCubbin, H. I., Patterson, J. M., Bauman, E. and Harris, L. H. (1981) Adolescent-family inventory of life events and changes (A-FILE), in *Family Assessment Inventories for Research and Practice*, (eds H. I. McCubbin and A. Thompson), University of Wisconsin, Madison, WI.

40. Moos, R. H. and Moos, B. H. (1983) Clinical applications of the family environment scale, in *Marriage and Family Assessment: A Source Book for Family Therapy*, (ed. E. E. Filsinger), Sage Publications, Beverly Hills, CA.

41. Olson, D. H. (1991) Commentary: three-dimensional (3-D) circumplex model and revised scoring of FACES-III. *Family Process*, **30**, 74–9.

PART THREE

The further shores of nursing assessment

We devoted much time in the previous chapters to discussing ways of collecting information about the person-in-care. Our objective has been to come to some kind of understanding of who he is and what is the nature of his problems of living. Even at the simplest level such an enquiry involves the formation of judgements, about the person, his problems and life in general.

The everyday activity of 'collecting information' and 'making judgements' is – by definition – an ethical pursuit. The British philosopher G. E. Moore proposed that questions such as 'What ought we to do?' were tied up inextricably with questions about the 'things' to which such questions are directed.

In contemplation, if a man begins with certainties he shall end in doubts; but if he be content to begin with doubts, he shall end in certainties.

Francis Bacon

10

Moral and ethical issues in assessment

All colours when placed in the shade appear of an equal degree of darkness among themselves. Placed in the light they never vary from their true and essential hue.

Leonardo da Vinci

Nothing can be more unphilosophical than to be positive or dogmatical on any subject.

David Hume

Modest doubt is called the beacon of the wise

Shakespeare

INTRODUCTION: KNOW LITTLE – KNOW MUCH

Assessment is about ways of looking at people-in-care; and ways of helping people to look at themselves. I have discussed some of the problems of making observations on the nature of people's lives and the difficulties involved in making judgements or pronouncements based upon these observations. The reader is probably well aware by now of my doubts about 'how easy' or 'how meaningful' might be the business of assessment.

Increasingly, we talk about nursing being a holistic (or wholistic?) activity, within which the whole person – from the biochemical to the spiritual – is somehow addressed. I shall address this topic specifically in the final chapter. If true holism is our *raison d'être* as a profession, then I fear that we might be doomed to failure. The idea that I might come to know who (in totality) are the people in my care beggars belief, especially when there exists so little time for such a grand endeavour. I have long since settled for the idea that (certainly) I and (probably) most of the people in my care are a mystery. The process of nursing assessment may aim to throw some light on the great human mystery. However nursing assessment remains, for me, a means to reduce my ignorance about the people in my care. If they become a little less ignorant about who they are and what it means for them to be alive and in distress, then the whole assessment process can rightly be called a success.

Whatever our aspirations, nursing assessment remains a fairly limited means of getting to know people. In time, as we develop new methods, it may get better. In addition to methodological weaknesses there are other problems, which might be classified as philosophical, moral or ethical in nature. In this penultimate chapter I shall share with the reader further some of my doubts about assessment and my ability to do 'it' successfully, far less reach the wholeness of the person-who-is-the-patient. Here we shall consider our attitudes towards the 'patient body' in general, bringing into sharper focus our philosophical and ideological bases. By the time readers have finished this chapter they will appreciate that I am not alone. They too may feel ready to join the mass of doubters who seek to know much by knowing little.

WHO DO YOU SEE WHEN YOU SEE ME?

It is an inescapable fact that we are obliged to judge people in our care. Increasingly our society expects nurses as well as physicians to predict the course of some illness or to predict the likelihood that someone will harm themselves or others. In the mid-1990s the UK has witnessed public atrocities, where men have slaughtered – apparently at random – children in their schools or people in general in their streets. Society believes these people are either 'mad' or 'evil' or both. Quite rightly, our society – needing to re-establish a sense of security – wants someone (anyone) to tell them why these people committed such atrocities and who might be at risk of repeating such acts in the future. Many have come forward to offer their 'explanations' and their 'solutions'. Real answers to these enigmatic questions may be a long time coming, if they ever do.

I have no idea whether people who commit such atrocities – whether in Waco, Hungerford or Dunblane – are suffering from some special form of madness, or whether they are a sign of a society slowly but steadily going mad. The wisest – and easiest – answer may be that they are a bit of both. These *causes célèbres* suggest one of the major problems that nurses face when coming to assess the people in their care. Mental illness, by its very definition, occupies a special territory. The clear-cut 'signs and symptoms' that are evident in many physical disorders are not so evident in mental illness. We have to make subjective judgements about what we see, or even what we think we see, and what it all might mean. Much of the emphasis of this book has been upon methods of trying to ensure that we have indeed seen (or heard) or otherwise witnessed something.

In the first part of this chapter I want to extend our efforts to gain a more objective picture of the person by considering the problem of seeing things that may not be there at all. In some situations we may be so blinded by stereotyped perceptions that we may fail to see the 'real' person. Such stereotyped images are not peculiar to the clinical setting. Our family and friends become so used to seeing us and being with us that often we feel that they do not really notice us. This kind of un-compliment is something that we repay them as we too relate only to their stereotype.

The classification of patients

Standard medical diagnosis is concerned with evaluating some deviation of physical or physiological functioning. This may be one of **degree** – when a person has high blood pressure; or of **nature** – when someone has a gastric ulcer. The diagnosis is based upon an appreciation of normal physiological functioning. The doctor does not diagnose a condition within a person. Rather she identifies a disorder within one of the person's physiological systems. As a result the person is described as having a certain condition: he has emphysema or congestive cardiac failure. We do not refer to these people as though they were synonymous with their condition. The person with emphysema is not called an 'emphysemic'. We adopt this convention (of classifying the totality of the person) only when we view the problem as chronic, or perhaps incurable. For instance we used to refer to 'diabetics', 'spastics' or 'asthmatics'. The long-standing nature of the person's condition encourages others to see the person and his condition as inseparable [1].

It is common practice for nurses to want to know what is wrong with a person before they begin to work with him. Student nurses, especially, are often anxious to establish the person's diagnosis so that they will know how to treat him. In one sense this is something to be encouraged. This way we might assume that the person will receive the correct care and attention. In another sense the diagnostic label may merely stereotype the person: squeezing him into a diagnostic pigeonhole, which only crudely summarizes the nature of his problems and says even less about 'him'. The person might well be excused for thinking: 'I am not a real person, I'm a schizophrenic (or whatever)'. Often the labels we apply to people are assumed to represent their total identity, but one which is very much a spoiled identity [2]. Goffman took the view that stigma did not involve so much 'a set of concrete individuals who can be separated into two piles, the stigmatized and the normal, as a pervasive two-role social process in which every individual participates in both roles ... at least in some phases of life' [3].

I shall consider stigma more specifically in a moment. The importance of this point is that in medical diagnosis (such as diabetes) we do not assume that disorders in one area of functioning always bring about disorder or dysfunction in other areas. Indeed a person may have several disorders at the same time, but this does not mean that they all originate from the same cause. Moreover, the individual can retain his personal identity throughout his various trials and tribulations. He has a number of complaints or ailments. He has not been taken over by them. It seems clear that the distinction made between 'the mad' and 'the sane' or between 'normal' and 'abnormal' people is a function of the systems and structures erected to deal with madness: structures which, as Porter acknowledged, 'turned people into rigidly dichotomized patients (aliens) and psychiatrists (alienists)' [4].

The all-embracing disorder

Although psychiatric medicine uses the same kind of labelling process and the same kind of descriptive terminology, the principles of classification have a wholly different rationale and effect. As I shall discuss later, in many cases our assertion that the person suffers from a certain mental disorder is more of an assumption than a proven fact. Although unequivocal proof of the existence of mental disorder is rarely given, most of us accept (as an article of faith) that such disorders exist. However, we should not pretend that the disorders we are talking about are in any way similar to epilepsy, gastroenteritis or colonic cancer.

Not only is there disagreement as to the constitution of many psychiatric disorders but even where such conditions are clearly defined difficulties are met in establishing a reliable diagnosis. When we say that a diagnostic criterion exists, we mean that any suitably-trained person should be able to identify the presence or absence of the condition providing that they use the same assessment process. More than 30 years ago studies began to show that many categories of psychiatric disorder used 'overlapping criteria' or were poorly defined [5]. People showing much the same symptoms may be assigned to quite different diagnostic categories. The key feature here is that the diagnostic label reveals so little about the person and the way he functions. Often the person's behaviour (or symptoms) are not greatly related to his diagnosis. It has long been recognized that, despite the assertion that schizophrenia has a common global incidence, the diagnosis was made more commonly in the USA and Soviet Russia than in many other Western countries. In the USA, the chances of being labelled schizophrenic vary, however, from one state to another and even from one ward to another. Despite the revisions made to the various diagnostic manuals (now DSM-IV and ICD-10) the view continues to be expressed that the best predictor of how a person will be diagnosed is where the psychiatrist was trained and the therapeutic model that guides his practice [6].

The same concern might be expressed about nurses. It was once shown that not only did they tend to look at the people in their care in the same way as their medical colleagues [7], but their application of labels like 'hostile' or 'hyperactive' often depended more on their background training than any obvious pattern of behaviour shown by the person-in-care. In a study involving the use of the term 'confused', massive discrepancies were found among nurses and doctors. Some used the term to refer to simple disorientation, whereas others meant the kind of disturbed state characteristic of severe dementia or hallucinosis [8].

In the mid-1990s some psychiatric nurses are being 'trained' specifically in the use of diagnostic methods to identify the presence of positive and negative symptoms of schizophrenia [9]. The use of diagnostic labelling is a convention with obvious positive qualities. It serves as a means of communicating simply about the person among professionals, and may also help identify treatment goals and methods. It is apparent, however, that the label may at times be not only irrelevant, but highly inaccurate. A label conveying so little information about the person merely 'typecasts' him. More importantly, it may be very difficult for the person to escape from such a stereotype [10]. The key question for nursing here is: 'Is the diagnosis of symptoms part of the "proper function of nursing" [11]?'

The self-fulfilling prophecy

Diagnostic classifications should distinguish people with psychiatric disorders from so-called 'normal' people. If they fail to fulfil this criterion their value is called into question. In a classic, and still controversial, experiment, Rosenhahn showed that it can be difficult to distinguish 'normal' people from the psychiatrically disturbed. He arranged for eight research assistants to gain admission to 12 different mental hospitals in the USA by simply telling the admitting doctor that they heard the sounds 'thud' and 'crunch' [12]. They showed no other problems.

Once they were admitted to hospital (with a diagnosis of schizophrenia) they stopped reporting these sounds and behaved 'normally'. It took an average of 2 weeks before they were discharged as 'schizophrenia in remission'. Rosenhahn noted that nowhere in the vast literature on schizophrenia were hearing the sounds 'thud' and 'crunch' listed as a symptom of the disorder. He concluded that the diagnostic criteria (which have since been amended twice), failed to differentiate the 'sane' from the 'insane'. This was reinforced by the observations of other 'patients' who became suspicious of the 'pseudopatients' about two or three days after their admission. Once people are labelled as schizophrenic, staff attitudes towards the 'person' change. Their normal behaviour may be overlooked or profoundly misinterpreted. The psychiatric label can have a life and influence all of its own.

Rosenhahn's paper caused a storm of outrage in the American psychiatric establishment, since it challenged the value of the classification system (of the time) and the competence of psychiatrists to use it appropriately. My aim in recalling this experiment is quite different. As I have noted repeatedly, nurses are not (yet) required to diagnose people. Rosenhahn's concerns are, therefore, of largely academic interest. However, once a person has been classified, nurses must beware of stereotyping him. We must guard against assuming that the person is no more than the diagnostic label suggests. Once diagnosed we may expect the person to behave in a particular way, to fulfil our expectations. If he behaves differently we may interpret this as further signs of his problems or 'disease state'. We may begin to create, albeit unwittingly, an environment which may be intent upon ensuring that he fulfils the criteria of the label that has been applied. This is the self-fulfilling prophecy in action.

GENDER AND ASSESSMENT

Gender influences our lives from the moment we are born. In the early days there are no differences between the sexes, except for the genitalia. However, they are treated differently. Traditionally, females are seen as being more fragile and are encouraged to be dependent and passive. Males are seen as hardy and are encouraged to pursue a path of aggressive self-reliance. As children, the sexes are prompted to think, act and even feel differently. Even in the case of hermaphrodites the child reared as a female will become a woman, while an identical child reared as a male will become imbued with male interests and acquire male privileges. In most cultures women are reared to be passive, accepting, unquestioning, beautiful, supportive and cooperative. Girls are restricted from an early age from enjoying the freedom and adventure that boys enjoy. They are restrained most specifically in their cumbersome dresses, which restrict their movement. They carry this symbolic restraint throughout their lives until as adult women they teeter precipitately on stiletto heels, or are partially handicapped by elongated painted talons, which serve no functional purpose. These erotic 'enhancers' are designed, transparently, to meet the needs of the voyeuristic male. *Homo sapiens* may have left his primate family behind but we remain animals at heart.

Where women stray from this path they may be conveniently labelled as 'tomboys' or, in the best Hollywood tradition, characterized as 'dowdy'. The social training of women is designed to meet their limited roles as mothers, housemaids, male assistants or sex objects.

Sexist psychology

These comments betray a gross generalization. They are, however, no more of a generalization than if I implied that men are strong, self-reliant leaders and hunters. Here I am merely acknowledging that it is little wonder that the sexes grow up differently. Traditional reasons given to explain such differences – biology and personality – are now largely discredited. The reality is that in a male-dominated society women are judged by male standards. Joanna Rohrbaugh commented wryly upon the 'female Catch-22'. She notes that women can never win when they are defined and evaluated by male standards. In aptitude tests where men score higher on mathematical or spatial ability, these tasks are assumed to be of supreme importance. Where women display an advantage, as in verbal ability, they are classed as different, rather than better [13].

Psychology has been a male-dominated science throughout its long history. When Freud tried to translate it into even more scientific terms he set the seal on its sexist status with his idiosyncratic view that women were creatures who were mourning the loss of the penis. Many of his followers tried to perpetuate this particular myth about sex differences. The clue to all of this, as Rohrbaugh pointed out, is power: penis envy may be a curious translation of power envy.

What is the relevance of all this to psychiatric nursing assessment? Without wishing to project a closet feminist line, it is apparent that women have been the victims of massive prejudice in the mental health field, as well as within wider society. Many women's problems reflect male prejudice. This is true even where women perpetuate the myth. Any woman who refuses to toe the feminine line is seen as competing with men and may be classed as 'aggressive' or 'butch' or with some other complex or chip on her shoulder. Where she acts out the feminine role to the full she may be described as neurotic, frigid or hysterical. Some of my nursing colleagues remain uncomfortable about 'women behaving badly'. Their capacity to 'see' the person who lies behind the stereotype may be impeded as a result.

Mental disorders in women

The prevalence of certain mental disorders in women has often been explained by reference to their unique biological system. Hysteria was first proposed by Hippocrates, who thought that female psychological disorders were hidden signs that the woman's body was pining for a child: thus we gain the concept of the 'wandering womb', from the Greek *husterikos*. Although we now recognize the foolishness of this idea, we retain the notion that hysteria is peculiar to women.

Depression in its various forms appears to affect women more consistently and seriously than men. Some have argued that this is because women are in a continual state of mourning – mourning the freedom and privilege they have never had, or have sampled all too briefly [14]. Arieti believed that women are depressed more often than men because we still live in a patriarchal society, in which women are raised to be dependent upon another person [15]. Returning to the notion of penis envy, it may be more accurate to suggest that depressed women are mourning not for the castration of their penis, which would be pure fantasy on their part, but because they really have been castrated – in a metaphorical sense. The symbolic penis of which they have been deprived is the male role in the world, including all the opportunities and privileges connected with that role [16]. Arieti and Bemporad also noted how women in operas are depicted typically as (for example) sick, frail, exploited, loose and promiscuous, mechanical, beautiful when young, but with a youth of short duration. 'We can conclude that either a woman's life is made miserable by men and therefore she has a right to be depressed; or she is regarded by men in such a negative way as to justify being in a state of despondency' [17].

Anorexia nervosa – the so-called 'slimmer's disease' – and bulimarexia – where starving, gorging and purging routines are intermingled – are strongly associated with women. Traditionally these have been depicted as sexual disorders. The analyst might argue that these women refuse to eat because they fear impregnation: they gorge themselves from time to time as unconscious desires to become pregnant break through. This sounds curiously like a latter-day Hippocrates at work. Feminist analyses of eating disorders take a different view with both feet planted on empirical soil. An early study of bulimarexic women noted that nearly all reported a perceived or actual male rejection incident. Their discontinuation of relationships with men was not concerned with pregnancy fears, but a fear of performing inadequately and being rejected again [18]. Not surprisingly, the women in this study reported an extreme concern with their weight and appearance, and concerns that they were unattractive to men. This feminist analysis is not entirely at odds with the analytic tradition. It is accepted that such eating disorders are an expression of sexual conflict. However, whereas the Freudians emphasize the fear of impregnation and the underlying rejection of femininity, the feminists emphasize the fear of rejection and the underlying eagerness to be feminine. Controlling their physical selves might be the one power that such rejected women possess.

Disorders of living

It is not my intention here to present a feminist critique of traditional psychiatric attitudes towards women. I merely acknowledge that in some areas women have greater and more persistent problems than men: certain anxiety states, depression, some habit disorders and aspects of social relationships figure strongly in this respect. In many cases this appears to be more a function of their social upbringing and position within society than a function of any biological or personality sex differences. As Rohrbaugh has pointedly commented: in a frantic attempt to please others, some of these women become conventional, martyred caretakers, who are then vulnerable to the depression that accompanies the empty-nest syndrome. Some become depressed trying to conform to the expectations of the Dominant Other. Some women starve themselves in demands for autonomy or in a vain attempt to attain a distorted image of physical beauty, which they see as the path to happiness and fulfilment through male attentions. Still other women rely upon superficial social charm and emotional appeals to manipulate the men in their lives [19]. In the beauty context Judith Bat-Ada commented caustically: 'All the special glitter that this male society produces for women – the makeup, the high heeled shoes, the tight little dresses – single us out as women as effectively as did the yellow stars on the coats of the Jews,' and, more specifically, on the influence of soft pornography: 'Women hate themselves for not being like the magazine models they see men panting after. We don't measure up to the measurements touted by the magazines, and we know it. We despair, but because there is nowhere to go with that despair, it turns inward and becomes self-hatred [20].'

More than a decade on from that observation I would hope that women might have taken more of their own power, but the news from the clinical front continues to be bad. The issue is, of course, still more about power than disease. Why should women need to 'manipulate' men? How could women ever begin to challenge the 'feminine (or the beauty) myth'?

How to begin? Let's be shameless. Be greedy. Pursue pleasure. Avoid pain. Wear and touch and eat and drink what we feel like. Tolerate other women's choices. Seek out the sex we want and fight fiercely against the sex we do not want. Choose our own causes. And once we break through and change the rules so our sense of our own beauty cannot be shaken, sing it and dress it up and flaunt it and revel in it: in a sensual politics, female is beautiful [21].

In our attempts to assess the nature of any problem of a psychological nature in women we should be aware that some, if not many, of these problems may be bound up in the experience of being a woman. Although, as Rohrbaugh noted, millions of women are already re-evaluating their assumptions, attitudes and value systems, the questioning of established values should not be exclusive to women. As a man, it is important that I come to grips with some of my own prejudices, dysfunctional attitudes and distorted value-systems. I have made a point of emphasizing the role of women throughout this book as the 'therapeutic agency', where the person-in-care is mostly referred to in the male gender. I have done so in an attempt to reverse the traditional procedure of depicting the weak and dependent person as a woman and the person who invariably comes to her rescue as a dashing 'father-figure'.

Female consciousness made a remarkable flourish over the 1970s and 1980s. I fear that it is being distorted again by powerful market forces, if not also the political rearguard in many countries which desires a return to some of the older values. In our own society hoardings, newspapers, television and the cinema continue to pressure women to conform to the male fantasy of the sexual object or the male reality of the homemaker and child-rearer. Certainly many more women are able to assert a more honest kind of sexuality, which is equal and different to men's.

Stereo-terrorism

Many signs suggest that the pressures upon women to project a 'female stereotype' are being subtly reinforced by the pressures on males to project the male – or macho – stereotype. Perhaps both sexes are terrorized by gender stereotypes. American cinema is most notable in this particular campaign, as it resurrects over and over the idea of the screen hero (from the relative reality of Indiana Jones and Rocky to the fantasy of Judge Dredd). The former American president Ronald Reagan, who had been a screen hero of sorts, often shored up his leadership status by being filmed for television chopping wood or arm-wrestling other presidential candidates into submission [22]. In his later years in the presidency Reagan was ridiculed for his apparent foolishness, which may only have been a harbinger of the dementia that was later formally acknowledged. Sadly, President Reagan was not allowed to age gracefully. He will go down in history as the 'Grecian 2000 President' who fought the signs of physical age but lost the fight with mental ageing. And age is, of course, yet another spectre of terrorism by stereotype.

More and more energy and money is poured into the fight against ageing, pulling in its wake an enhancement of the ageism that we have tried – at least through political correctness – to challenge. We adopt a prejudiced view of old people [23] because our society is founded on the following assumptions.

- Youth is more important than age (or perhaps even experience).
- Work, activity and efficiency are important ("just being' is a waste of time).
- Death and suffering must be resisted (or denied).
- God is dead (hence human life is everything).
- Mental health is possible (when it is no more than a romantic fiction) [24].

There is no room here to discuss the implications of these 'world views', which seem inherently foolish to me. This may, however, be no more than a sign of advancing years. I may already be the 'old fogey' so many are trying to avoid. The reader will consider the implications of these and other forms of stereo-terrorism for themselves and their work. They seem unlikely to go away. They are not 'out there'. They are within us! Whenever we judge others we do not define them – we define ourselves.

The assessment of men

The tragic situation of many women is also a tragedy for men. It is well known that many psychological and physical disorders in men are a function of the massive restraint they exercise over their emotions and their desperate efforts to attain the physical or status ideals which may be wholly beyond them. For every 'body-builder' who dies as a result of steroid abuse, there must be ten men who drown their failure to realize the macho ideal in drink or drugs or who become the archetypal family abuser.

When assessing people who either are in the process of becoming 'patients' or who are well established in their psychiatric 'careers', we need to penetrate the veneer of the sexual stereotype that most, if not all, of us erect around ourselves. Our assessment should attempt to understand the effects that sexual stereotyping may have upon the person as well as the effects it may have upon our perception of the person. Although psychiatry has a major task in hand in attempting to repair the disservice done to women, it has hardly even begun to consider the psychological damage that men endure. That they endure their distress covertly is one of the reasons why we have been able to keep the book on men closed for so long. Now as traditional societies implode, as women begin to assert themselves, as unemployment robs men of their hunter-protector mission and more 'enlightened' attitudes to sexuality prevail, male mental distress is no longer able to keep its own dark secret. This fact is betrayed by the suicide statistics for younger men, if by nothing else. Given the social and economic climate this seems unlikely to improve.

There are signs, however, that some kind of a 'man's movement' is emerging which might take as part of its brief the way men have – down the ages – been restricted by the social construction of maleness. Some of the proponents of the 'new man' ideal have challenged some of the 'male myths' which have developed as a consequence of the (quite appropriate) challenge to patriarchy from the women's movement. They recognize, however, that men can be a victim of their maleness, at the same time as they make women victims of their problems with their maleness [25]. If the 'men's movement' has a single objective it appears to be to build (literally) a new paradigm of masculinity, one established on cooperation. Men need to: 'show the way out of the sickness competition has created in the hearts and souls of men for thousands of years. These "leaders" must answer the challenge and move over and stand shoulder to shoulder as brothers in a new era, rather than as bosses, captains, generals, and masters or gurus [26].'

This is not the place to discuss the position of men within psychiatry, since it appears to be, at best, an emergent one. In time we may gain a fuller appreciation of what it 'means' to be male in a world where the male role has all but disappeared. In time we may come to appreciate the special significance that mental distress has for men, what its influences are and what might be its special form of resolution. For now we need to be content with knowing less than a little.

THE ASSESSMENT OF OTHER PEOPLE WITH DISABILITIES

Within any psychiatric population we may find people who are physically as well as psychiatrically disabled. This may be wholly physical, as in cerebral palsy or choreoathetosis, or mental, where a range of levels of intellectual impairment may prevail. In recent years we have popularized the notion that the physically disabled person may be normal in all other respects. This new philosophy is very slowly extending itself to the person with a mental 'handi-cap' (now referred to in the UK euphemistically as a 'learning disability'). At present society discriminates to varying extents against disabled people; but discriminate against all of them it does, with impressive consistency. In the assessment of people with psychiatric disorder who may also be suffering from some accompanying physical or mental impairment we need to consider the extent to which our views of the person are coloured by other labels that are applied.

Disable-ism: what's in a name?

In an early but valuable and readable contribution to our understanding of the effects of disablement, Miller and Gwynne made the important observation that, although the word 'cripple' is seen as offensive, the synonyms are hardly an advancement in humanitarian terms. Popular alternatives such as the infirm, the disabled, the invalid or the deformed all carry negative prefixes, expressing the absence of socially desirable attributes [27]. As noted above, the re-titling of people with a 'mental handicap' as people with a 'learning disability' (suggesting that they cannot learn) has been hailed as a great advance. Society's biggest handicap seems to be a compulsion to label!

In more primitive societies, or I should say less bureaucratic and competitive societies, the crippled person is better accepted. Although he may be denied the privilege of high office, he is usually given a role that is commensurate with his abilities. In such societies the disability is seen more as a natural phenomenon that might happen to anyone. As a result cripples suffer less discrimination. In the West our tradition of discrimination has a long history. The Bible, Greek myths, drama and literature since the Renaissance, and contemporary comics and children's fairy stories are filled with crippled villains or 'bogeymen'. The Bible gives clear guidelines for excluding cripples, or virtually anyone with a physical affliction or blemish, from entering the priesthood [28]. This tradition has stood the test of time. In some religions it is common for such crippling afflictions to be seen as a punishment for misdeeds in previous lives. It is hardly surprising that the cripple is poorly catered for in such a climate of retribution. In short, our labelling of the 'crippled' person is not merely descriptive; it serves a function. It is designed to locate him somewhere at a distance from the rest of us.

This symbolic distancing was, of course, fulfilled geographically in the establishment of colonies and institutions for the disabled. The classic discriminatory statement made against the disabled person can still be heard in any restaurant when the waiter or waitress turns to his obviously 'normal' carer and asks: 'Does he take sugar?' This form of person-blindness is not exclusive to the layperson. I recall an eminent psychiatrist in my youth proclaiming that people with intellectual impairments never suffered from proper psychiatric disorders, because they were not bright enough. On a more disturbingly ignorant level, a parent told me how she had asked her general practitioner why her mentally handicapped son seemed to follow his father's instructions but paid little attention to her. 'They're like dogs, you see. They only obey one master,' was the authoritative reply. I fear that the doctor knew as little about the canine fraternity as he did about his human 'patient'.

In such examples we have clear illustrations of people who are 'blinded' by the signal of disability. Or rather, they show how people have a vivid impression of a stereotype that blinkers them. A person with a disability commented on D. H. Lawrence's depiction of Lady Chatterley's enfeebled husband:

> However one rates the human species, a man must be considered as a whole. His body is an incredibly wonderful piece of fully automated engineering, but in itself it is not a man. His mind, soul, spirit, is an even more wonderful and complex thing, but in itself it still does not constitute a man .... He is much more than the sum of these parts, but a deficiency in one means a deficiency in the whole. Lawrence's view that after Sir Clifford became a cripple he was no longer a man is extreme, but it contains more truth than we like to admit. A cripple is still a man, but, as it were, on a smaller scale. His totality is diminished, his image distorted. He is not a whole [29].

The writer affirms with impressive candour that, although people with disabilities may be accepted to a limited extent, their sexuality presents major problems for the lay public and often more so for those caring for them. Surprisingly, the blind, who are deficient in a crucial sense, are not discriminated against in the same way. Some kind of Jungian complex may be at play here. Blindness does not have the same sinister connotations that a physical abnormality has in the collective unconscious. Instead, as history demonstrates, blindness is often seen as an asset: e.g. in poetry or the exercise of philosophical wisdom.

The latent power of discrimination

The stereotyped disabled person in the psychiatric services can take various forms. In those settings where people with physical and/or mental disabilities are integrated with people with mental illness, the intellectually impaired person may be seen as less complex and more one-dimensional, the key dimension being intelligence. Where staff are anxious to exercise their skills on the stronger meat of ego-defence mechanisms or ephemeral group processes, the intellectually impaired person may be viewed as 'retarded', 'subnormal' or 'a bit simple'. In a conversation with staff on a long-stay hospital ward some years ago a man was described to me as a mentally subnormal. I asked what this meant. 'Well, he's got very simple needs ... a very simple guy.' How did he know? I enquired. 'Because he doesn't appreciate things.' So why didn't he help him to appreciate things? 'Because he wouldn't understand. He's too simple.' As I noted earlier, I fear that, when we make such judgements, we say more about ourselves than about the object of our judgement.

Such judgements operate as highly focused self-fulfilling prophecies, uttered with the conviction that used to be the prerogative of the American white discussing American 'people of color', or the British describing Indians at the height of the Raj: 'Why is the Negro inferior?' 'Because he is ignorant.' 'Then why don't you educate him?' 'Because he can't learn. He's inferior.' George Bernard Shaw once remarked that in America 'they force the Negro to shine their shoes for them, and then look down upon him because he is a bootblack'.

Now, having learned the new language of political correctness, we realize that it was 'white folks' who were deficient all along. Professor Leonard Jeffries of the City College of New York coined the term 'melanin impoverished' to refer to 'white people'. Given that 'white folks are deficient in melanin', this shows that they are 'less biologically proficient than blacks' [30]. If political correctness has done nothing else it has obliged us to confront the foolish belief that our received language is not imbued with all manner of powers, most of which are beyond our control. The readers will consider to what extent their language disadvantages those to whom it refers.

In all institutions set up to deal with dependent people there is a danger that the residents will become an equivalent of the victim of racial prejudice. Because some of the people are highly dependent, requiring total care and attention, everyone is perceived in this way. In many settings for older people the residents are reduced to the lowest common denominator, that of physical incapacity. As a result, other needs may be discounted or rarely considered. Where they are acknowledged, they may be seen as secondary or subsidiary concerns. The person may be viewed as more sick, frail, helpless, or incapacitated than he really is. This perception is maintained by the fact that the philosophy of care is orientated towards physical care. As Goffman has shown, this is another example of the self-fulfilling prophecy [31]. The person's needs are seen as largely physical in nature. Consequently, this is the only kind of care on offer. As a result, the persons' demands are largely of a physical nature. (They can only request what is on the 'menu'.) These demands in turn reinforce the staff view that the person's needs are purely physical in nature.

THE CREATION OF THE STEREOTYPE

Why do staff develop a stereotype of the disabled person as dependent, helpless and childlike? This idea may be fuelled by the amount of time the staff spend working closely with people who may indeed fulfil this stereotype. Highly dependent people may consume much staff time. This tends to colour their attitude towards 'working in a disabled area'. There is a tendency to over-generalize, suggesting that all disabled people behave in the same way as the high-dependency group. Any residential setting for the care of people with dementia is an obvious example. Here there may be several people who are very frail, disoriented and perhaps reduced to a basic level of functioning. However, every person – by the law of averages – cannot be similarly disabled. If we are willing to remove our blinkers we will find varying levels of cognitive functioning, healthy emotions and differing levels of motor and social behaviour. Indeed, these 'functions' may fluctuate within individuals from one day to the next. However, people with any kind of disability who refuse to fit the stereotype are branded as trouble-makers or disruptive elements. The 'crazy anti-hero' who takes on the system finds an empathic chord with audiences the world over – from *One Flew Over the Cuckoo's Nest* to the '*Dream Team*'. How many of us know that, when we struggle to manage and contain the 'difficult' people in our care, we are only struggling with ourselves?

Where the care system is routine and rigid – especially where independence or the expression of individuality is not catered for – disruption is almost bound to occur. Where such people are viewed or treated like difficult children, their reaction will naturally be one of resentment or anger. Often this merely adds fuel to the fire and provides further evidence that the person must be 'mad'. Conformity to the stereotype of the passive, pathetic and everlastingly grateful person is the criterion by which we often judge the 'good patient'.

Stereo-awareness

These few comments about some of the problems with stereotypes that we might meet during the course of assessment are in no way exhaustive. I offer these comments merely as stimulus for further deliberations. Although I have talked exclusively about people-who-are-patients, it is clear that we tend to stereotype ourselves – the carers – in the same way. Where interpersonal conflicts crop up within a team, these may be attributed to the 'emotionality' of the female staff; the old age or youth of various members; or the fact that someone's stupidity is causing frustrations or tension. Sexism, ageism and intellectualism are three of the commonest stereotyping devices used by staff on each other. They correlate highly with the common use of similar strategies with people-who-are-patients. As I noted earlier, we now know that 'black folks' and 'white folks' are equal-but-different. When we began to acknowledge this over 30 years ago it was the oldest possible news for 'black folks' and the worst possible news for some 'white folks'. If our colour is all that we have, then we may not have much.

Getting an education

Increasingly nursing education recognizes that true education involves the development of knowledge about ourselves, for surely we all are students till the day we die. The proper root of the English word 'education' lies in the Latin *educere*, meaning 'to draw forth' or 'bring out', or 'develop from a latent condition' [32]. When we 'get an education' we inevitably learn the obvious, which we have long struggled to avoid. People who aim to become psychiatric nurses need to develop a proper sense of themselves: their attitudes, beliefs, prejudices, etc. Only once this period of learning is over will they be ready to look realistically at people-in-care. In this sense my comments in the past few pages may already be unnecessary. Where nurses are being prepared to appreciate their own prejudiced perceptual set, they will require less prompting to un-blinker their vision of the person in their care. Such self-awareness will clear the air: clearing a way to a truly objective, impartial assessment of the person. If the reader has persevered with me over the past few pages, she will at least know something of the nature of my own prejudices and my efforts to let them go.

People not patients

One of the questions I have refrained from asking during the preceding chapters is: 'Does the person really have a problem?' We should not take it for granted that, simply because a person carries a certain label or has been referred for assessment with a certain complaint, this is any proof of the existence of real problems. We would do well to remember the moral of Rosenhahn's story in this respect. I am not saying that we should be in perpetual doubt. I merely advise against taking too much for granted. Many nurses believe that it is not their job to challenge the authority of the psychiatrist with whom they work. I would agree. Reporting information that suggests a different interpretation of the person's status is not a challenge to diagnosis, or anyone's authority; it is simply 'good nursing'. The nurse has a responsibility to remain as impartial as possible, while offering the person support and advocacy [33]. Many, if not all, psychiatrists in a hospital setting rely upon the reports of nurses to arrive at their final diagnosis. The nurse cannot afford to hide her opinions or judgements without risking endangering the person in the process.

It is a truism that many people suffer psychiatric treatment because of the problems within families or even society itself. Our most famous psychiatric 'commentator' questioned our responsibility to make people 'fit into' a mad society. Perhaps it is our responsibility to reshape society to make it less distressing for its inhabitants [34]. On a more domestic note it is clear that our perceptions of mental disorder can be grossly misleading. James Thurber's apocryphal tale of the man who saw a unicorn in his garden [35] is a wry reminder that sloppy labelling can not only be offensive but might also work against us.

A man told his wife that he had seen a unicorn in the garden one morning. 'You are a booby, and I'm going to have you put in the booby hatch,' she replied. The man, who had never liked the words 'booby' or 'booby hatch', thought for a moment and then said, 'We'll see about that.' His wife telephoned the police and a psychiatrist. When they arrived she proceeded to tell them about her husband's sighting of the unicorn. They began to believe that she was the insane one. When her husband arrived on the scene he failed to confirm her story, so off **she** went to the 'booby hatch'.

We might do well to remember that sometimes, when we are studying 'crazy behaviour', we might be better employed in looking at the conditions that give rise to these apparently crazy phenomena. Especially, though not only, when we are working with families, we might ask ourselves: What exactly do we think we mean when we say that someone is mentally ill? The concept of mental illness is little more than a comfortable convention. Like an old overcoat, we dare not investigate it too closely in case it starts to fall apart.

MENTAL ILLNESS AND MENTAL HEALTH

Throughout this book I have mixed the use of technical terms like 'psychosis' or 'anxiety' with the concept of 'problems of living'. I have tried to avoid talking about psychiatric nursing as a mere subsidiary of the diagnosis of mental disorder. From this viewpoint nurses are, at least in theory, involved in collecting a much wider body of information about the person's functioning than is necessary for the formation of a diagnosis. I have repeatedly suggested that nursing – if it has a 'proper focus' – is concerned with the human responses to psychosis or anxiety, rather than with these phenomena themselves. We cannot leave the discussion of nursing assessment, however, without considering some of the dilemmas inherent in psychiatric diagnosis, since these dilemmas might represent further reasons why we should be attempting to extend our own assessment expertise and technology.

We have noted already the observation that diagnosis is influenced by the ideological orientation of the diagnostician: her 'school of thought'. In considering nursing assessment we need to ask what sorts of things nurses believe about the people who are their patients. I find the answer an elusive one. Despite our adoption of the title of 'mental health nurse' there appears to be no central theoretical model of mental (ill) health that might help unite nurses in the way they look at people. McKenna's research suggested that nurses were more comfortable with 'models of nursing' which gave them a structure for their relationship, as in the Roper—Logan—Tierney model, which employs 'activities of daily living'. Models which require them to 'get close' to the person and 'develop' a relationship were the least popular, such as Peplau's theory of interpersonal relations [36].

In the UK, at least, nurses used to follow their leader, adopting the theoretical model of the consultant-in-charge, accepting his notions of mental illness in the best-behaved tradition of the handmaiden [37]. It might be a romantic fiction to assume that, because nurses now have access to a wide range of nursing models, they are any less influenced by the psychiatric theory of their medical colleagues.

Models of mental disorder range from traditional psychoanalysis to anti-psychiatry. In between there are various convictions about what is wrong with the person. These are influenced by medical viewpoints (the biophysical school); psychodynamic or intrapsychic beliefs; and sociological viewpoints (social psychiatry). In some countries (e.g. Italy) the school of thought may be heavily influenced by political standpoints.

The horns of the dilemma: health not disorder

Nurses have been encouraged from their first introduction to their discipline to accept the idea that mental illness is similar in form and function to any physical illness. By implication it is assumed that mental health can be similarly defined. Over the past 30 years – my lifetime in psychiatry – the disruptive effects of psychiatrists like Szasz and Laing, sociologists like Goffman and more recently the philosopher-historian Foucault [38] have led us to question our rather concrete view of mental illness. Here I want to comment upon only some of the more notable problems involved in trying to understand what is wrong with the person. I proffer no solutions. I am merely sharing some of my doubts and anxieties. We are in a position analogous to riding the horns of a rather hyperactive dilemma. We need to learn how to position ourselves on this dilemma to afford ourselves as much comfort as we can. I see no sign of the dilemma disappearing or of us having an opportunity to dismount.

There has been a growing trend among a number of health care workers to acknowledge that the traditional distinctions between one disease category and another hinder us from understanding fully the meaning of health and its numerous irregularities. The medical tradition has encouraged us all – professional and laypersons – to think of illness in terms of **pathology**: the functional or structural changes caused by disease. However, it is clear that not all human disease follows the rules laid down in the textbooks. Selye's seminal research into the role of stress in health and disease concluded that people react to stress in a variety of ways [39]. It may be more important to try to understand how people become 'sick' than simply to catalogue the variety of disorders that they might suffer from.

The 'holistic' model of health care that is accepted implicitly by nursing favours an ecological view of humanity where everything is interconnected. This is in stark contrast to the medical model, which explodes the person in order to study disease in one part of his functioning. We are now beginning to experience a change of heart. Once we viewed people from the limited perspective of Newtonian physics: like a special class of billiard ball responding passively to the forces exerted upon and through them. Now, we are beginning to see illness and health as more dynamic features of the person's total functioning and interaction with his world.

The non-specificity of mental illness

I have observed repeatedly that identifying mental disorder says little about the people to whom the label is applied. In an incisive analysis of the diagnostic approach Mathew Dumont highlights what he calls the 'non-specificity of mental illness' [40]. Taking schizophrenia as an example, he reminds us that Bleuler, who first coined the term, described a number of 'primary symptoms': associative looseness, affective disturbance, autism and ambivalence. These were all prefixed with the letter 'A' to make them easier for medical students to learn. Delusions and hallucinations were classed as 'secondary symptoms'. Bleuler did not suggest how often the four As occurred together, nor did he indicate how often these 'symptoms' occurred in the non-schizophrenic population. However, the idea of the disease of schizophrenia was born (created) thus in 1911.

The picture has cleared little today. Despite the massive body of evidence from research, the meaning or origins of 'schizophrenia' seem no clearer [41]. We are aware of something being amiss but are uncertain as what exactly that might be. The illusion that there are natural boundaries to the thing we call schizophrenia has been maintained for generations. This assumption has allowed various researchers to draw meaningful inferences from statistical trends which, like the edges of a moving cloud, tend to fulfil the fantasies of the beholders. If we remove the labelling process, with all its classist, racist, sexist underpinnings, what we are left with is a diffuse population of disturbed people who are in no specific or characteristic way neurologically damaged [42]. It may be that a major reason for the clustering of major mental illnesses among the lower socio-economic classes is the whirlpool of teratogenic influences to which the poor are subjected [43]. This seems as likely an explanation as genetic influence.

How are people whole?

In Chapter 1, I suggested that we function on a range of levels. One of the major problems in trying to understand mental illness is that we have tended to split people up into compartments. As we noted earlier in this chapter, a mental disorder is often seen as taking over the person. Much of the debate of the last hundred years has focused upon the dualism between mind and body: are they separate or are they the same?

Dumont tried to solve the problem by comparing the way we function to the formation of ice on a lake. In order for the drop in temperature to lead to the formation of ice, a complex chain of actions and interactions must take place. These involve, mainly, the electromagnetic forces around individual molecules of water. This leads to the formation of crystals, which congregate to form what we call ice. Dumont compared the formation of patterns of behaviour to this complex process of action and interaction. When we reach out to save a child from falling (a single behaviour) this action is derived from a template which connects memory, intelligence, imagination, emotion, perception and numerous other individual functions, by a network of (metaphorical) gossamer threads. The net result is a template that resembles a hologram. Like a hologram it may appear in one form but function in another, quite different, dimension.

This model of behaviour seems to reflect contemporary science and technology in much the same way that Freud was influenced by ideas about the internal combustion engine, which led to his concepts of drives, energy and catharsis. Dumont argued that if one accepted the hologram analogy the idea that a gene – coding for a very small cluster of amino acids – could cause the structure of a huge, amorphous mass of behaviour like schizophrenia was like assuming that the structure of water can explain the outline of a cloud. It is an error of scale of such magnitude as to be something of a thought disorder itself [44]. Whatever mental illness is, it seems unlikely that a process of classification will help us determine the best treatment interventions. If holism is a valid health-care model then we must view people in ecological terms, connected to and continuous with other functions of their biological, cultural and social existence.

Dumont's ideas might seem a little radical to many nurses reared upon a simple diet of diseases and syndromes. Perhaps they might be forgiven for thinking that he is denying the very existence of mental illness. Nothing could be further from the truth. He acknowledges that people suffer disturbance and distress. However, these must be seen as problems that are a function of their total experience as persons: projecting through their own biological space to interact with their social and cultural world, and ultimately with the influences of the environment, whether, natural or man-made. Dumont's view recalls Peplau's view – which I have used several times already – that we need to let go of such simple disease models in favour of treating 'patients as persons' [45].

Is health possible?

Most of us accept the notion of health and sickness as concrete things, if only for simplicity's sake. When we come to analyse what we mean by such terms we start to feel the horns of the dilemma even more sharply. Yet we might do well to question exactly what we mean by illness, to appreciate better the meaning of health.

More than a decade ago Sedgwick made the highly provocative assertion that there are no illnesses or diseases in nature [46]. Illness is something humans define. We select certain states, which we choose to call illness. These are the natural causes that lead to the death or loss of function of a limited range of species: people, pets, domestic livestock and the plants we cultivate for gain or pleasure. All of these may be classed as disease-ridden or illness-prone. We do not normally talk about spiders, lizards or desert grass as sick or diseased. These are of little importance to us. Sedgwick argues that the labelling of disease or illness is a social value system. Illness simply does not exist: it is a social construction.

We have grown to believe that illness is defined by our biomedical wizardry. This also is mythical. Concepts of illness were in use centuries before man even understood the circulation of the blood. Even today different cultures interpret sickness or disease differently, as a disturbance either of the body or the spirit, and occasionally both.

Illness as deviancy

So what does all this mean? Is Sedgwick saying that we simply believe in illness and make it happen? No. Merely that our perceptions of illness are heavily influenced by concerns that have little to do with pathology. In the introduction I suggested that illness might be seen as deviancy: the ill person is different from other people; he differs from the established norm of biological or psychological functioning. However, when we are talking about 'the norm', do we mean healthy? Massive variations regarding the meaning of 'healthy' occur within as well as across cultures. Sedgwick noted that in 1911 it was found that hookworm was seen as part of normal health in parts of North Africa. In one South American tribe the disease of dyschronic spirochetosis (which is marked by coloured spots on the skin) is so common (normal) that anyone without the condition is disqualified from marriage.

Social and cultural norms clearly influence our perceptions of normality and pathology. In Western society the doctor has traditionally held the exalted status equivalent to the witch doctor or priest in more primitive societies. Doctors are, as a result, called upon to comment upon not only obvious physical problems but also matters such as contraception, sexual relationships, child-rearing practices and emotional management. In *The Psychopathology of Everyday Life*, Freud popularized the notion that no one was free of neurosis. A psychotherapeutic growth industry has developed, despite any firm evidence of its value, which encourages people to seek solace or repair for what may well be 'natural emotions'. In the wake of an upsurge of iatrogenic disorders, doctors are now urging people to recognize that problems of living cannot be remedied by taking tranquillizers or antidepressants *ad nauseam*. These are some of the problems of living that are the responsibility of the world, its politicians and ultimately its individuals. It seems axiomatic that we need to solve such problems by our own moral actions.

We have done many a human being a disservice by medicalizing his natural suffering: by applying a label to something that should be seen as a function of that person's distress as a result of his interaction with his own world [47]. Readers might be forgiven for thinking that I have been attempting to confuse them over the past few pages. I have questioned the logic by which we arrive at definitions of psychiatric disorder. I have questioned the philosophical and sociological bases upon which we construct our models of health or sickness.

These questions merely reflect a recognition that the understanding of health, illness or what is assumed to be wrong with the person can never be a simple business.

ASSESSMENT AND ETHICS

Ethics is the discipline that governs our actions towards others under any condition. In the health care arena this must begin with assessment. If nurses are not ethical – right and just – at this stage, how can they ever redeem themselves at any later stage of care delivery?

The nurse as an agent of treatment

Nurses might be excused for thinking that they fulfil only a minor role in the successful treatment of people with a psychiatric disorder. Largely, this is a function of the confusion between the terms 'care' and 'treatment'.

> [T]he hospital family consists of mothers (nurses); fathers (physicians) and children (patients) and is based upon the patriarchal family system of western society ... the subordinate position of nursing is reinforced by the care/cure myth that values caring, the traditional female nursing role, less than curing, the male medical role ... [this is] further emphasized by the fact that doctors are well paid for curing, but not so nurses for caring [48].

The gentle irony of this situation is that, although curing and caring are different, both are essential. Healing in its fullest sense involves both care and cure. It has been observed repeatedly that nurses often do both in practice. For this reason nurses can never afford to take their relationships with the person-in-care lightly. Society, and indeed the person, may assume that other staff are more important, for whatever reason. This does not absolve nurses from their responsibility to be aware of their own importance. Nursing assessment should never be assumed to be inferior to medical diagnosis: it is merely different.

The ethics of asking questions

'Asking questions' is the most consistent thread woven through this book. What right do we have to ask the person questions about any aspect of his life? The simple answer is that we have no such rights. The person need not answer any questions, or participate in any part of the assessment process, if he does not wish to. In a legal setting the person has a right to 'remain silent'. This should extend to psychiatric assessment. However, the person may simply choose not to answer, so the question is academic.

We need to be aware that the person might feel threatened by an interview or some other form of assessment. In some situations the content of the assessment questions may be more threatening than the form they take. We should respect the person's concern on this issue and should try to make life easier by modifying the questions, or trying to put him more at ease. However, if the person is unwilling to answer certain, or any, questions, what right have we to coerce him further? Apart from the absence of any such right, such an action will merely prejudice further relations with the individual.

The role of prejudice

It is commonly assumed that nurses are angels in disguise. Although I am a great believer in the humanitarian potential of everyone, by the law of averages, nursing – like any other professional group, must have its quota of bigots. I doubt very much whether even a library full of ethical essays would change their attitudes. Even if we see ourselves as liberal and free-thinking, we should not forget our potential for prejudice. I have already covered three areas where our stereotyped notions of people may obscure our ability to see them clearly. In other areas we may be blinkered by moral or religious standards. Wife- or child-battering, sexual deviations and even the use of foul language are areas where our own moral philosophy might bring us into conflict with the person. Even political prejudice might be involved if we are confronted by someone with radically opposing views to our own. These problems are not such a problem with the seriously disturbed person where, if we choose, we can attribute his behaviour to 'the ravings of a madman'. In less severe cases conflicts might be experienced if the nurse interprets his behaviour as meaningful. She must guard against such conflicts influencing her judgement.

Once when facilitating a workshop one of the nurses participating said that she had felt very uncomfortable with the role play. I was intrigued: 'In what way was it uncomfortable?' The nurse said that she could not find anything to use as a life-problem in the role play. 'You don't have any problems?' I inquired. 'Oh no,' came the reply, 'I have plenty of problems, just none that I was willing to share here.' This was really interesting, I thought: 'Well, you will have learned something from this, then?' The nurse seemed bemused. 'Learned what?' 'Well, if nothing else, you will have learned something of what it is like to be a patient.'

Sadly, this is not altogether a rare occurrence. We assume that because people are patients they will open out their lives for us gladly. When they do not, we often accuse them of 'denial' or 'resistance'. When we begin the assessment encounter we need to be sensitive to what that encounter might mean for the person. Sensing what it might mean for us could be a useful yardstick.

The ethical use of the assessment

The assessor cannot separate herself from the use to which her information will be put. Unlike diagnostic data, assessment in nursing is rarely used for statistical purposes. I have already emphasized the need to identify problems that are problems for the person-in-care rather than any other person. Nurses have a limited role as the person's advocate, acting on his behalf when necessary, even to the extent of helping ensure that the assessment goals are in his best interests. In this context it is important that the nurse does not let herself be used to 'trick' the person into confiding material he might previously have been unwilling to disclose. If the nurse has established a good relationship with a person, he may make such disclosures because he trusts her. If the nurse wishes to pass on such information, she should seek his approval. Otherwise she will risk breaking a confidence and prejudicing the relationship. She may even risk damaging the person further. We would do well to recall Florence Nightingale's dictum that above all else nursing 'should do the patient no harm'.

It is worth while for the nurse to advise the person at the very outset exactly why she wants to ask certain questions and what she intends to do with the information. By stating the aims and objectives of the assessment the nurse is keeping an open agenda: there are no hidden motives or uses to which the information will be put. This openness will do much to strengthen the relationship.

Ethical records and ethical notes

I have stated a number of times already my conviction that we should try wherever possible to confine ourselves to stating 'the facts' rather than interpretations of the facts. When we comment upon a person we should strive to report verbatim what he said and did; what he thought and felt about what he did. We should leave it at that. There is no need for interpretation.

Some years ago I worked with a young man who spent most of our first meeting discussing the records I was keeping, which were lying closed in their folder on the desk. He also talked a lot about the sorts of thing he knew other people to have said about him. He had asked a number of people (GP, social worker and psychiatrist) whether he could see the records they were keeping, asking whether they could be destroyed after he had ended his contact with the service. He reported that he had lost a number of jobs 'on account of my health record'. Later I was intrigued to find a reference in his notes to this young man's 'pathologically suspicious and paranoid behaviour'.

On the surface, this man did appear to be making unreasonable demands. Logically, he had a valid point. The records that were kept by the psychiatric service were concrete documents. At that time they could not be handed over to the person. He could not even view them. And there was no question of their contents being destroyed once he ended his contact with the service.

Coleman suggested, over a decade ago, that if people were able to keep their own health records this would rule out much of the danger of breaches of confidentiality [49]. Today in the UK people are free to ask to read their medical records. This development would, however, be only a partial solution for the young man I mentioned. He was concerned more about what was being put into the records. Such fears can be well grounded and certainly need not be paranoid.

Each time we meet a new 'patient' the diagnostic sketch already in his record will colour our perceptions. I tend to avoid reading case notes before meeting a person for the first time to reduce the likelihood that I shall only 'see' the person who is described in the notes or referral letter. This is not always possible. I raise the issue here merely as provocation for the reader. To what extent does your assessment begin with a 'clean slate', or are you merely adding to an already prejudged opinion? At worst, to what extent is the nursing assessment a convoluted system of 'Chinese whispers'?

Ethics and confidentiality

There are undoubtedly many pressures put upon nurses to report the content of confidential discussions held with people-in-care. It is important that we are aware of the limitations of the relationship and the conditions under which this confidence may be breached. It is a good idea to tell the person what the aim of the assessment is. Then he is in no doubt about the purpose to which his comments might be put. If the nurse tells the person that she wants to find out how he feels so that she can plan his care with the rest of the team, then it is implicit that anything she says may be reported back to the rest of the team. If he asks for clarification on this point, honesty must prevail.

If the nurse takes rough notes, which may later be transcribed into a case file, the nurse can read these notes back to check that her observations were correct. If the person asks to see what she is going to write about him, she may let him see the rough notes. Once the notes are written up, formally, they become a legal record and access becomes a more complex affair. The situation might be resolved by encouraging the person to hold the care plan: this approach, which is gaining in popularity, is however restricted to certain kinds of 'notes', usually for certain kinds of people-in-care. I offer no easy solutions here. I expect that readers will consider the ethical challenges for themselves, on the basis of these few points.

The ethics of breaking a confidence

Are there any situations in which a confidence shared within the assessment may be broken? Muyskens [50] listed three situations in which the nurse might feel obliged to breach confidentiality with the person.

The first is where the person is in a temporary fit of depression or anger and discloses his intention to harm or kill himself, which would clearly prejudice or destroy his prospects for leading a full, autonomous life. The nurse's decision here is clearly a paternalistic one. She makes a judgement over the head of the person, in much the same way as parents do over children. Although the information may have been imparted in confidence, the nurse believes that the person's best interests will be served by breaking this confidence.

In the second example the rights of some third party might be threatened. Muyskens quoted the example of a mother who threw her child down a flight of steps, afterwards claiming that it was an accident. Later, in a state of depression, she confessed to a nurse, imploring her to remain silent. What is the nurse's moral duty? Muyskens noted that in most states in the USA a **legal** responsibility would exist to report the incident. Is the moral requirement any different? He acknowledged that, since the risk of further damage to the child cannot be predicted, the decision is a difficult one. He decides, however, that the protection of confidentiality does not extend to situations where the rights of a third party are at risk, no matter how small.

In the third example he argued that confidentiality may be breached where there is some danger to the general public. A person who talks about his resentment against society, and his ambition to 'get even', may simply be talking. However, he may be a threat to the lives of innocent people. His ambitions must be publicly acknowledged.

It has not been my intention here to review all the possible ethical dilemmas that might confront the nurse in her assessment of the person-in-care. I have selected only those that appear most common concerns or are fairly regular obstacles to the development of ethical assessment. The requirement to protect the freedom and dignity of the person does not begin and end in treatment: it is sketched in the assessment and often becomes the blueprint for ethical practice thereafter.

CONCLUSION

In this chapter I have shared some of my concerns about assessment. I have expressed concern that even when we try to be 'person-centred' one stereotype or another may hinder us from ever becoming truly person-centred. I have discussed some of the doubts that have been expressed about the value of the concept of 'mental illness'. Traditional practice tends to guide all of us – whether professionals or laypersons – towards thinking that the complex mish-mash of human misery can be reduced to identifiable organic or psychological states, with identifiable causes and outcomes. This seems by all accounts to be an over-simplistic view of people and their worlds. The more we know about mental illness, the less we appear to understand. I have offered no ready solutions: just encouragement to avoid being simple-minded.

Finally, I discussed a few of the key issues involved in the practice of ethical assessment. The issues I have addressed are of a fairly concrete consistency and should pose no problems for the nurse who is uneasy with philosophical debate. I have made a few suggestions as to how the planning of ethical assessment can provide the framework for the subsequent ethical care of the person. Taken together, these three facets represent my sole contribution to the philosophy of assessment.

I am conscious that this chapter, on the 'philosophy' and 'ethics' of nursing assessment, is longer than the exposure given to assessment in total in many nursing textbooks. I have long cherished the belief that assessment will tell us 'what needs to be done' in the name of care. If the reader takes the full meaning of my expression 'learning from the person' then they may appreciate that, at least, assessment is much more important than any intervention which might follow. I hope that in time nurses will become more comfortable with, and knowledgeable about, the philosophical issues I have sketched out here. Perhaps by then we will feel more comfortable too with the mechanics of the practice.

NOTES

1. Adams, H. E., Doster, J. A. and Calhoun, K. S. (1977) A psychologically based system of response classification, in *Handbook of Behavioural Assessment*, (eds A. R. Ciminero, K. S. Calhoun and H. E. Adams), John Wiley, New York.
2. Goffman, E. (1963) *Stigma: Notes on the Management of Spoiled Identity*, Penguin, Harmondsworth.
3. *Ibid.*, p. 163.
4. Porter, R. (1987) *A Social History of Madness: Stories of the Insane*, Weidenfeld & Nicholson, London.
5. Zigler, E. and Phillips, L. (1961) Psychiatric diagnosis: a critique. *Journal of Abnormal and Social Psychology*, **63**, 607–18.
6. National Institute of Mental Health (1974) *Schizophrenia Bulletin, Issue 11*, Government Printing Office, Washington, DC.
7. Cormack, D. F. S. (1976) *Psychiatric Nursing Observed. A Descriptive Study of the Work of the Charge Nurse in Acute Admission Wards of Psychiatric Hospitals*, Royal College of Nursing, London.
8. Simpson, C. J. (1984) Doctors and nurses' use of the word confused. *British Journal of Psychiatry*, **145**, 441–3.
9. Barker, P. and Reynolds, W. (1996) The proper focus of psychiatric nursing: a critique of Gournay. *Journal of Psychiatric and Mental Health Nursing*, **3**(1), 75–80.
10. It is notable that so many of the members of the user movement choose to define themselves as 'survivors' of the psychiatric system. In the UK the best example is *Survivors Speak Out*.
11. Barker, P. and Reynolds, W. (1996) The proper focus of psychiatric nursing: a critique of Gournay. *Journal of Psychiatric and Mental Health Nursing*, **3**(1), 75–80.

12. Rosenhahn, T. (1973) On being sane in insane places. *Science*, **179**, 250–8.
13. Rohrbaugh, J. B. (1980) *Women: Psychology's Puzzle*, Harvester Press, Hassocks, Sussex.
14. Chessler, P. (1971) Person and patriarch: women in the psychotherapeutic relationship, in *Women in Sexist Society*, (eds V. Gornick and B. K. Moran), Basic Books, New York.
15. Arieti, S. (1979) Roots of depression: the power of the dominant other. *Psychology Today*, **12**, 54–92.
16. Arieti, S. and Bemporad, J. (1978) *Severe and Mild Depression: The Psychotherapeutic Approach*, Basic Books, New York.
17. *Ibid.*
18. Boskind-Lodahl, M. and Sirlin, J. (1977) The gorging–purging syndrome. *Psychology Today*, **10**(2), 50–5, 82–5.
19. My view, expressed here, is influenced greatly by Beck, C (1979) Mental health and the aged: a values analysis. *Advances in Nursing Science*, **1**(3), 79–87.
20. I am indebted to my daughter, Charlie Barker, for extending my understanding of the state of 'wimmin' and for drawing this work to my attention: Bat-Ada, J. (1982) cited in *Take Back the Night: Women on Pornography*, (ed. L. Lederer), Bantam Books, New York.
21. Wolf, N. (1990) *The Beauty Myth*, Chatto & Windus, London, p 241.
22. This quotation is taken from Rohrbaugh, J. B. (1980) *Women: Psychology's Puzzle*, Harvester Press, Hassocks, Sussex.
23. I use the term 'old' since the convention 'older' seems ridiculously relative. If age is an important index we might as well discriminate clearly. If we can have 'young people' there must, by implication be 'old people'. The problem is deciding who lies between.
24. Beck, C (1979) Mental health and the aged: a values analysis. *Advances in Nursing Science*, **1**(3), 79–87.
25. Thomas, D. (1993) *Not Guilty – Men: The Case for the Defence*, Weidenfeld & Nicholson, London.
26. Lee J (1991) *At My Father's Wedding: Reclaiming Our True Masculinity*, Piatkus, London, p. 167.
27. Miller, E. J. and Gwynne, G. V. (1972) *A Life Apart*, Tavistock, London.
28. Leviticus 21: 17–23, quoted by Miller, E. J. and Gwynne, G. V. (1972) *A Life Apart*, Tavistock, London.
29. Cited in Hunt, P. (ed.) (1966) *Stigma: The Experience of Disability*, Geoffrey Chapman, London.
30. Cited in Beard, H. and Cerf, C. (1992) *The Official Politically Correct Dictionary and Handbook*, Grafton/Harper Collins, London.
31. Goffman, E. (1961) *Asylums*, Doubleday, New York.
32. Hoad, T. F. (1986) *The Concise Oxford Dictionary of English Etymology*, Oxford University Press, Oxford.
33. Schrock has suggested that nurses need to fulfil such a role in order to coordinate the activities of the various groups of professionals involved in the delivery of care. Schrock, R. A. (1980) Planning nursing care for the mentally ill. *Nursing Times*, **17 April**.
34. Laing commented: 'Psychiatry could be, and some psychiatrists are, on the side of transcendence, of genuine freedom, and of true human growth. But psychiatry can

so easily be a technique of brainwashing, of inducing behaviour that is adjusted, by (preferably) non-injurious torture .... I would wish to emphasize that our "normal" adjusted state is too often the abdication of ecstasy, the betrayal of our true potentialities, that many of us are only too successful in acquiring a false self to adapt to false realities.' Laing, R. D. (1965) *The Divided Self*, Penguin, Harmondsworth, p. 12.

35. Taken from Thurber, J. (1953) *The Thurber Carnival*, Penguin, Harmondsworth.
36. McKenna, H. (1994) *Nursing Theories and Quality of Care*, Avebury, Aldershot.
37. Cormack, D. F. S. (1976) *Psychiatric Nursing Observed. A Descriptive Study of the Work of the Charge Nurse in Acute Admission Wards of Psychiatric Hospitals*, Royal College of Nursing, London.
38. Eribon, D. (1991) *Michel Foucault*, (trans. B. Wing), Harvard University Press, Cambridge, MA.
39. Selye, H. (1976) *Stress in Health and Disease*, Butterworth, Boston, MA.
40. Dumont, M. P. (1984) The nonspecificity of mental illness. *American Journal of Orthopsychiatry*, **54**(2), 326–34.
41. Boyle, M. (1990) *Schizophrenia: A Scientific Delusion*, Routledge, London.
42. Gournay, K. (1994) Redirecting the emphasis to serious mental illness. *Nursing Times*, **90**(25), 40–1.
43. Dumont, M. P. (1984) The nonspecificity of mental illness. *American Journal of Orthopsychiatry*, **54**(2), 326–34.
44. *Ibid.*
45. Peplau, H. E. (1995) Another look at schizophrenia from a nursing standpoint, in *Psychiatric Nursing 1974–94: A Report on the State of the Art*, (ed. C. A. Anderson), Mosby/Year Book, St Louis, MO.
46. Sedgwick, P. (1982) *Psycho Politics*, Harper & Row, New York pp. 28–42.
47. Taken from Illich, I (1976) More wealth, less health – an interview with Ivan Illich. *Psychology Today*, **2**(6).
48. Passau-Buck, S. (1982) Caring versus curing: the politics of health care, in *Socialisation, Sexism and Stereotyping*, (ed. J. Muff), C. V. Mosby, St Louis, MO.
49. Coleman, V. (1984) Why patients should keep their own records. *Journal of Medical Ethics*, **1**, 27–8.
50. Muyskens, J. L. (1982) *Moral Problems in Nursing*, Rowman Littlefield, Tottowa, NJ.

<table>
<tr><td>

11

</td><td>

Assessing the whole person: healing our lives and mending our minds

</td></tr>
</table>

Advice is like snow; the softer it falls, the longer it dwells upon, and the deeper it sinks into the mind.

Samuel Taylor Coleridge

I love the man ... who can gather strength from distress, and grow by reaction. 'Tis the business of little minds to shrink, but he whose heart is firm, and whose conscience approves his conduct, will pursue his principles unto death.

Thomas Paine

INTRODUCTION

I noted in the introductory chapter our fascination with holism and the belief that nursing is now, at last, a holistic activity [1]. We might assume, therefore, that all people-in-care will be addressed as 'whole people' rather than patient entities. Were this the case, then we might assume that the 'whole' needs of such 'whole' people would have been identified through some process of holistic or perhaps 'wholistic' assessment. But what exactly do we mean by the whole person; and how do we go about establishing who is this whole-person (apart from any other kind of person) and what are these whole-needs?

I step into this chapter with some trepidation. I once was fond of saying that I was not sure who I was, far less who were any of the people in my care. After spending more than half of my life in psychiatric nursing I remain uncertain of the identity of those in my care. I would like to say that, at long last, I know who I am. At the time of writing, I remain unsure. By the end of this chapter, I may be a little clearer as to who I am and who are the people in my care.

METAPHORS OF MIND

Gregory Bateson is reputed to have told the story of a man who wanted to know about the mind, what it was and whether computers would ever be as intelligent as humans. The man asked only one question, which he typed into the most powerful computer he could find: 'Do you compute that you will ever think like a human being?' The computer rumbled and stuttered as it analysed its own computational habits. Eventually it printed out a single reply, which the man grabbed excitedly. On it he found six words which responded without answering the question. The computer had replied: 'That reminds me of a story ...'.

Most of our libraries boast whole walls of books and papers which purport to explain the concept of mind. The contents of those books and papers – the theories or research studies upon which they are based – are no more than stories themselves. These reflect the efforts we have made to get to grips with the mind by talking about it.

Mind: the positive space

The mind itself may be no more than a meta-story that explores, but fails to explain, the business of being and living. The mind and the body appear interdependent: looping back upon one another, leaving us uncertain of where we began the search. Oriental philosophy and psychology appears to 'toy' with the mind—body split, but may – long ago – have grasped its essential paradoxical nature of such dualism.

> We shape clay into a pot,
> but it is the emptiness inside
> that holds whatever we want.

This 'eternal truth' from the *Tao Te Ching* may well be the best metaphor for our unflinching efforts to discover the location of the mind [2]. As we begin to be seduced more and more by the dazzling explanations of 'mental functioning' offered by neuroscience [3] we may care to consider that, although the 'mind' may be **held** by the brain, this does not mean this it **is** the brain.

The story of caring for the mind

It was once taken for granted that mental illness involved an affliction of the mind. Nowadays we are a lot smarter: now we're not so sure. Whatever the nature of mental illness it is clear that many people so afflicted have needed, and have been given, some kind of care down the ages. The concept of 'caring' and nursing may not figure prominently in the 'story' of psychiatry and mental health, but no story about the institutionalized care of people with mental distress would be complete without a consideration of psychiatric nurses.

Throughout history, all societies have sought to identify, contain and treat mental disorder. Psychiatric nurses in Britain are, in this sense, descendants of an ancient order. They can trace their lineage back to 9th Century Celtic monks, who first developed the process of 'human caring' [4]. If a patron saint were needed it might well be John of God who, as the lowly João Cuidad, was imprisoned in 16th-century Portugal following what we might now call a manic episode. Cuidad was so shocked by his experience that, following his release, he committed his life to the care of the mentally ill and destitute [5]. There is evidence that many psychiatric nurses who have made significant contributions to the field have at one time or another suffered from mental illness [6]. Although not a psychiatric nurse, Florence Nightingale would rank among them, having experienced prolonged bouts of despair and suicidal thoughts. The experiences of such nurses (or carers), like those of John of God, may even have enhanced their capacity to care. A more complex challenge faces those nurses – and the reader may be among them – who have been blessed so far with relative 'mental health'. I say relative, for it would be a bold person who would claim mental health, either as a right or as a constant feature of their being. I have expressed some of my reservations about the definition of mental health and 'normality' throughout the preceding chapters. I remain uncertain of my own right to such a description.

The challenge which so-called 'normal' nurses face is: How do we become aware of what it means to experience significant mental distress? How do we find, within our own experience, the 'wound' that might help us heal those in our care [7], if not ourselves? In what way are we and the people in our care more alike than different [8]?

The proper focus of psychiatric nursing

In making my own small contribution to the validation of psychiatric nursing as a core aspect of mental health care, I challenge the idea that psychiatric nursing ever was an appendage of general nursing. Psychiatric nurses do, of course, complement the care offered by doctors, other nurses and the whole panoply of health professionals. Arguably, their unique role has always been to facilitate the psychosocial, if not spiritual, 'healing' of the person with mental illness. How they exercise this 'psychic healing' function may distinguish them not only from other professionals in mental health care but also from all other nurses.

I have noted how it has become fashionable to assert that all forms of nursing are 'holistic', in some way addressing the totality of the person. Given the nature of mental illness, involving in every case some damage or insult to the 'self', care must be focused on the personal, the psychosocial and the spiritual identities of the patient. This latter emphasis should not be mistaken for religious ideology, although for some nurses that might be important.

My view of the history of psychiatric nursing is uncontroversial, and has been confirmed by archival research [9]. What may be controversial is my belief that psychiatric nursing is a spiritual activity; that nurses participate in the 'psychic healing' of the person with mental illness. By employing this provocative belief as the anchor for this concluding chapter I imply that the exploration of the spiritual dimension(s) of the experience of mental illness must, perforce, be part of the assessment process.

Somewhere within the body of this chapter, if not this book, lies the enduring question: What do psychiatric nurses do? It probably is the question uppermost in the mind of the 'reflective practitioner' who is the reader. It may well be the question I am least confident about answering. Whatever nurses do it must involve a complex of interpersonal relations. Given the form of care – human meeting human – and the content of those meetings – interaction, exchange and mutual influence – we could not discuss caring without inter-personal relations. If 'psychic healing' is one of the goals of nursing, interper-sonal relations must be the process by which it is realized. Perhaps the less-frequently asked – and arguably more important – question is: What do people-in-care need nurses for [10]?

Re-authoring life

Something significant takes place within those relationships. Their ordinary nature often disguises their significance: people telling stories about their lives. Often these stories make grim and harrowing telling, as well as hearing. They remain, however, no more than stories. The significance of true [11] psychiatric nursing may well lie in recognizing how such relationships heal everyday lives, and that by 'healing our lives' we all might make a contribution to 'mending our minds'. In this sense the assessment process may not only help us appre-ciate 'what is going on' within the world of the person, but may also fulfil some kind of therapeutic function: by relating the stories of his life the person may begin the re-authoring of his life [12]. By being party to this process, I believe that nurses might also heal their own lives.

I had intended to soften the impact of any provocative statements by offering an advance warning. Perhaps that statement – that the 'healers' might also be 'healed' by the act of 'healing' – may well have been the first of my provocative statements. It seems so obvious to me that I tend to take it for granted.

Before I fumble further with my definition of what is psychiatric nursing – and by implication what it is not – I need to say what psychiatric nursing is **about**. And, before I discuss the relationship between 'healing lives' and 'mending minds' perhaps I should illustrate what I mean by life and the mind.

PEOPLE: THE NATURAL PHILOSOPHERS

Two and a half thousand years ago Socrates warned that 'the unexamined life is not worth living' [13]. Bateson's computer story may be only a witty update on that age-old moral. People are natural philosophers, devoting much of their lives to establishing the meaning and value of their experience and to constructing explanatory models of the world and their place within it. Each reader of this chapter will close the book having constructed in their own mind their personal meaning of what they have read. They would need to be anaesthetized, or seriously drunk, to avoid doing so. What we find – when we take a look at ourselves – may, however, not always be what we expected.

The search for meaning

People with mental illness may well spend more time than most reflecting on their experience of self. Mental illness is an alien experience and most 'sufferers' are only too aware either that they are not the people they once were or that they are, in some way, different from the rest of humanity. This awareness of disturbance or alienation connotes the illness of the mind, a human problem which may be translated into social, psychological and medical relations. These add up to a spiritual – or whole-life – crisis where the person is trapped in the search for meaning, which we all undertake as we journey from the cradle to the grave.

There is a view that some people with mental illness are unaware that anything is amiss. Such a proposition is often made in the case of people with psychosis or dementia. I shall return to this issue later. For the moment I ask you to consider what you understand by the term 'sentient beings'. For me, being human, being here with you – even within the pages of this book – depends on my status as a 'sentient being', knowing what it is to be happy or sad; united with others or alienated from society; secure in a loving relationship or disoriented to the point of panic. These experiences are common-or-garden varieties of mental health or mental distress.

Such a concept of mind suggests the coming together of perceptions, judgements, actions, interactions and emotions. We often say that the mind is greater than the sum of these parts, but that is no more helpful than saying that I am more than a body with a history. I would rather say that our perceptions, judgements, actions and emotions have relationships with one another, albeit at a conceptual level – producing the spiritual me.

I believe – but cannot justify my belief – that our 'humanness' is located in the mind: the abstract mirror that reflects the thinking, behaving and emoting which represents the bodily business of our lives. The mind – who we are – is in turn reflected back through our thoughts, feelings and actions.

It is there – in that two-way mirror – that our knowledge of ourselves lies. Often we can only 'see' ourselves reflected vaguely, as if 'through a glass, darkly'. Many people with mental illness may, like Alice in Wonderland, have stepped through the mirror, to experience the confusion of not knowing what is real or imaginary, which side they are on and whether they are in or out of step.

We remind ourselves of the metaphorical nature of mental illness to emphasize that mental illness often has no location: it is everywhere and nowhere, apparently at the same time. Mental illness often reflects the whole of a person's lived experience, without emphasizing any particular part. It is this 'lived experience', rather than mental illness itself, that nurses manage in the name of care [14].

The awefulness of care

On meeting a person with severe mental distress it is difficult not to be struck by the awefulness of their experience. Indeed, it is necessary to preserve a sense of awe in their presence. Since I am not aware of having suffered, to date, from any obvious mental illness, I have no direct experience of the territories charted by those who have been in my care. I consider myself fortunate to have had a chance to look over their shoulder, to espy something of those territories. Just such a territory was described vividly by the New Zealand writer Janet Frame:

> I will write about the season of peril. I was put in hospital because a great gap opened up in the ice floe between myself and the other people whom I watched, with their world, drifting away through a violet-coloured sea where hammer-head sharks in tropical ease swam side by side with the seals and polar bears. I was alone on the ice [15].

Since I have experienced these territories – vicariously – I have no great fear of mental illness. I hope, however, that I invest such experiences with great respect. Perhaps an analogy with the lifeboatman's relationship with the sea is apposite: holding no fear but much healthy respect.

We have only a limited understanding of how exactly psychiatric nurses help people with mental illness. Some of that understanding comes from nurses reflecting on the experience of caring. Some comes from the teachings of patients. Much of it comes from the mutual examination that goes on within the nurse's relationship with the person-in-care. It is popular today to talk about the 'empowerment' of people with mental illness, and here I make my next provocative statement. We do not empower our patients; the person with mental illness empowers us. The only way we can be of real service is to learn from the person. Having learned what to do for the patient, from the patient; nurses often gain some understanding or insight, which changes them – however imperceptibly. This small change in their professional demeanour influences the next interaction, and so on *ad infinitum*. The nature of the interaction that goes on within that relationship results in a blurring of the distinction between who is the nurse and who is the person-in-care. I become like a dance. This reminds us of the question, posed long ago by W. B. Yeats:

> O chestnut tree, great-rooted blossomer
> Are you the leaf, the blossom or the bole?
> O body swayed to music, O brightening glance
> How can we know the dancer from the dance?

Caring: the hopeline

If nurses do anything of note within those interactions, it is to offer hope. They hold out a 'hopeline' to people who are often devoid of hope. One of the key tenets of nursing must be that people are not the problem – **the problem is the problem**. Adopting this view allows people to distance themselves from their problems. San Blise described how, rather than chastizing or otherwise trying to 'control' a 'hostile' woman, she advised her: 'You must be a really strong person. You have one of the worst cases of schizophrenia I have seen.' The woman responded: 'Are you saying that I have schizophrenia? ... That's what's causing all that stuff. Thank God! I thought I was losing my mind! [16]'

This woman was not 'a schizophrenic'. She was a woman who had a problem with something the nurse called schizophrenia. I am confident that – especially from the woman's perspective – this was not simply semantics. Like the people described in the previous chapters, this woman was neither morally responsible for the problem nor possessed of some fundamental flaw. The people we have discussed here have **had problems with** 'psychosis', 'mood disturbance', 'anxiety' and so on. Effective nurses recognize that people can have relationships even with things that might be seen as parts of themselves; they assume that people and their problems are not one and the same thing. By adopting this view, nurses facilitate the hope that such problems can be overcome or otherwise left behind on the life-path. To facilitate hope one must first believe that people can change and grow. This is more than a philosophy. This is the map of the territory of care. Where people-in-care do not make progress some of this might be a function of the carer's pessimism. We need to foster a fierce belief in people's possibilities for change.

Looking after – standing still

When I became a nurse 25 years ago I was taught much about what was wrong with 'patients' – and entertained with a litany of theories as to how such phenomena might have developed. I learned how to recognize deterioration or exacerbation, but paid little attention to how positive change might be facilitated. I spent much time observing patients (*sic*), but spent little time with them, sharing their lifespace, sharing their life stories. That was what psychotherapists did. Nurses looked after people, which often meant helping them remain stationary.

When I reflect on the changes that occur in my own beliefs and behaviour, many of these seem to occur as a consequence of conversations with people I hold in high esteem. I may only be reading their words in a book, or they may only be talking to me on a telephone line, but my sense of change derives from the stories we tell one another. The reader will have considered the importance of similar stories in their own life. What part have such relationships – whether fleeting or sustained – played in your growth and development; your forward movement down the life path? Your answer to that question will determine the importance you attach to the stories you hear as part of the assessment process.

Effective nurses help patients develop their natural reflective processes. Psychiatric nurses help people to 're-author' their lives, through the story-telling process [17]. In that sense psychiatric nursing is a most ordinary pursuit. Although a few nurses are beginning to work with people (usually called clients) out of consulting rooms at community clinics, much psychiatric nursing takes place in the most mundane of settings: from the day rooms of hospital wards to the living rooms of the person's own home. What nurses do there can all too easily be mistaken for mundane interaction and mundane conversation.

ASSESSMENT AND SELF-EXAMINATION

Psychiatric nursing is one semi-public context within which people re-affirm their need for self-examination as a core element in the life process. I began 15 years ago to work with women with severe depression who had been hospitalized over many years, many of whom had made repeated attempts on their lives. As I began to explore their experiences – individually, sometimes with their husbands and families, and in groups – I began to feel like an intruder; as I listened in to these stories from the edges of life. Viktor Frankl suggested that the anxiety that people with melancholia experience is what Kierkegaard called 'the giddiness which overcomes us on the peaks of freedom' [18]. For those women that giddiness involved a perception of the gap between what life was and what they thought it ought to be. That gap was experienced as an abyss – over the edge of which they felt themselves falling, along with the rest of the world and its meaning. It was within those experiences that I began to appreciate the edge of my own professional abyss, the gap between what I felt able to do and what I thought I ought to be able to do. In time I realized that the women and I shared the same problem. We both needed to act within our lives now, with all our perceived limitations, in the face of all our living nightmares. As Harry Stack Sullivan observed, we were more alike than different [19].

Nightingale said that nurses should do the patient no harm. I would add that nurses should do as little as necessary to ease distress and to influence the person's growth and development. How nurses facilitate this development, through their relations with patients, has been recognized as a research topic for over 40 years. In this sense interpersonal relations represents the proper focus of nursing: it is the royal road to care.

Personal realities

When asked what exactly they do, how they do it and why do they do this, rather than anything else, nurses' answers are often vaguely specific or vaguely general: 'I give out medication' or 'I work in the community'. An even vaguer but arguably more accurate answer is that nurses respond to the person's own response to illness, disorder, dysfunction or whatever [20]. People signal their felt-sense of distress. We might say that they 'intuit' their illness. They use their emotional intelligence to recognize what is happening at the 'whole' level. A friend and colleague – who has had many experiences of manic depressive psychosis – told me that she has very specific sensations when 'going high' (manic), which soon manifest themselves in a kind of 'video-screen' in front of her forehead, where her thoughts and feelings (perhaps her 'self') are displayed [21]. Despite having worked with many people with a diagnosis of manic depression over 15 years, I had never heard the 'story' of impending mania described in exactly that way. Without hesitation I can say that I have no idea what such an experience really means, far less what causes it. I have come to the realization, however, that – given time and support – the people who own such experiences can reach their own understanding. This personal reality is the only reality worth getting excited over. The biggest handicap professionals face is the need to know something that the person-in-care does not know. This is the curse of the 'certainty principle' [22]. I am repeating the obvious, which most of us know intuitively: people-in-care teach us. Effective caring begins (and ends) by getting an education.

If you accept that proposition, then you might agree that nurses do not address – in any way directly – the basis of mental or physical illness. Indeed, you might even agree with me that mental illness (*per se*) is not the focus of psychiatric nursing. Rather, nurses respond to the person's experience of illness. The focus of psychiatric nursing – which provides us with our reason for being there – is to engage with the person's experience of distress.

Nursing meaning – nursing function

The 'caring' function of nursing is often misrepresented as doing something 'active'. Some years ago I studied what nurses did when faced with a person with distress related to severe depression [23]. The most commonly reported nursing response was to try to ease the person's distress through 'reassurance'. Increasingly nurses are recognizing the value of what might be called 'gentler' approaches to caring: emphasising the way in which they might influence the conditions that allow change to occur in a way appropriate to the individual.

In this context, an unusual definition of nursing is to be found in table billiards [24]. The term 'to nurse the balls' means the stroke 'used to keep the balls in the best position for the scoring of cannons'. By nursing the balls, rather than employing more vigorous strokes, the billiard player increases the likelihood of achieving a high score; of realizing optimum performance. In forestry the action of planting a sapling in the shadow of an established tree is also called 'nursing': providing the 'sheltering' conditions under which growth and development are most likely to occur. When the **nurs**eryman attends to the sapling he does not 'make' the small tree grow. Instead, he aerates the soil, prunes the branches **care**fully and ensures that toxins are avoided and that the soil is enriched with nutrients if necessary. The **nursing** that the tree receives reflects the conditions under which growth and development might occur.

NURSING – THE EDUCATIVE INSTRUMENT

Hildegard Peplau said that, among other things, nursing was a maturing force and an educative instrument. By means of effective nursing individuals and communities can be aided to use their capacities to bring about changes that influence living in desirable ways [25].

Nursing, in Peplau's terms, is very much about such a firm, controlled yet gentle facilitation of optimum performance. Nurses do not change people. Nurses help people use their own capacities to bring about their own desirable changes in living.

When people are helped to appraise their life, its problems, the meanings they attach to these events and the myriad possible actions open to them, they gain a new perspective. That awareness of 'something different' is one of the critical signposts on the human life path.

Personal science: finding words for true knowledge

The development of such alternative perspectives might be seen as part of a 'personal science of human problems'. Although people may make discoveries which are similar to those of others, in the final analysis such discoveries always possess a unique meaning. Take the example of depression. Irrespective of the putative causes of the depression, most people share a fear of what is ailing them. They will feel powerless to respond constructively to the depressive event and, with the passage of time, may descend into the 'Slough of Despond' which Bunyan described in *The Pilgrim's Progress* — where hopelessness and desolation become one [26]. These 'sensations' are common to severe depressive states and are reported by most sufferers, although the language and the metaphors may differ. We are indeed more alike than different. And yet people draw their own meaning out of the experience of illness; a meaning which is, by definition, beyond my ken.

TREPHOTAXIS

When I reflect upon the people I have worked with over the past 25 years I have no idea what they experienced; but I have shared – by mutual agreement – my experience of their reflections on their personal science and they, presumably, have had a reciprocal sharing of my experience of their experience. The complexity of those interactions is difficult to get one's tongue around. Wittgenstein's view that language is the only reality may well be appropriate, of which more later.

My knowledge of myself and others is bounded by the language that defines my experience. As Peplau wisely remarked 'language influences thought; thought then influences action; thought and action together evoke feelings in relation to a situation or context' [27]. Indeed, how language operates and how we might help the person reframe his emotions and behaviour remain highly fertile research territories.

Language is used also to redefine nursing, by the creation of models of nursing practice. I have lost track of how many such models are now in existence, each claiming to be the evocation or distillation of the 'art and science' of care. Believing that we were getting lost in the many definitions of what is or is not nursing, I decided – some years ago – to proffer a solution called **trephotaxis**. Trephotaxis is a neologism cobbled together from the Greek, meaning 'the provision of the necessary conditions for the promotion of growth and development' [28]. We deploy 'trephotaxis', or we become 'trephotarcs', when we facilitate the conditions under which people discover the experience of growth and development [29].

What these 'necessary conditions' might be varies from one person to another. Indeed, these conditions may vary from one moment in a person's life to another. Nothing lasts. Why should we expect the conditions within which our experiences are embedded to last? Given that people are more alike than different we can expect some commonly occurring conditions. The nurse has a responsibility to know, through assessment, what 'needs to be done' to provide the conditions necessary for growth and development from the cradle to the grave. Midwives provide the original conditions, when they help us over the hurdles and through the hoops into the world. Nurses in the hospice setting help people through different hoops and over different hurdles as they leave the world. Psychiatric nursing may well be about following people as they journey the road less travelled in between [30].

Healing lives

Growth is a possibility for all patients, even for those facing death. I have written elsewhere of my experience in caring for my father, who lived with cancer for 5 years and who, when he had had enough of the struggle, asked me to help him prepare for his death [31]. He did this very explicitly by asking me to bury him: to 'say a few words', since he was not in any sense religious. This was a brave request since, within his culture, everyone was buried by a priest or minister, whether believers or not. His choice was doubly difficult since my mother was, and remains, a strong believer. That invitation began a change in my relationship with my father, which indirectly changed my life. My father had always been a background figure – quiet, supportive, but largely unknown to me. In the last few months of his life he talked for the first time of the joys and the suffering of his life: his barefoot days in the slums of Sunderland which was the beginning of joy, and his part in the Allied forces' relief of Belsen, which was part of the suffering. These were not the stories of which soap operas are made, far less film scripts. Simple yet profound story-telling on the last stages of his life path. Stories that healed his life and began the healing of my own.

When people fail to realize such growth they may well be suffering more from professional pessimism than psychopathology. Whatever the presumed 'condition' from which the person suffers, true nursing addresses the potential for growth; how the person can grow in human terms, with the result that the disorder – whatever it might be – either presents less of a problem or may even appear no longer to be manifest. I repeat, nursing addresses the person's relationship with the disorder. We have a responsibility to help the person nurture the hope that he might leave the disorder behind him. A half hour spent with a depressed person – discussing the awefulness of their life and the depths of their despair – is likely to end with the person feeling more desperate and with you having assimilated at least some of that despair. If, having acknowledged the human significance of the despairing view, the same time is spent discussing how the person manages to live with their difficulties, where they draw their strength from, where they might renew old supports or discover new ones, the person will change physically; becoming more active, lively and perhaps even more optimistic. This experience – which I have witnessed countless times – illustrates Hilda Peplau's dictum that 'people make themselves up as they talk'. This is, however, no ordinary talk, although to the outsider it might appear so [32]. Nursing, which has always dealt in the currency of language, is illustrating how the careful use of language can aid and abet the growth process. I say 'aid and abet', for clearly we facilitate rather than make this happen.

Assessment and curiosity

The history of psychiatric nursing is replete with examples of 'trephotaxis', the most significant being within the territory of interpersonal relationships.

Consider the following proposal: 'The nurse has to become an acute observer, who maintains an active curiosity and a habit of asking questions about her own and the patient's feelings and behaviour and an interest in developing insight into her own and other person's stereotyped ways of thinking about and behaving with patients' [33]. The same authors suggested that 'the careful observation of small changes in a patient that could be built upon and expanded is a significant part of this process' [34]. That quotation illustrates the value of curiosity: through inquiring into the nature of relationships, both nurse and patient (*sic*) may grow more knowledgeable about what exactly is going on between them. With knowledge might come the understanding which both seek. The authors, Morris Schwartz and Emmy Lanning Shockley, published those American views 40 years ago. It is sobering to have to acknowledge that nurses were so 'intimately' involved with psychiatric patients (*sic*) before the phenothiazine revolution. How much progress – in nursing – has been made in the intervening 40 years?

That emphasis upon nurses helping people grapple with their everyday life problems continued in Britain in the mid 1960s when Elizabeth Barnes, the former Matron at the Henderson Hospital, edited the first significant British text on the therapeutic community and the therapeutic role of the nurse [35]. This was developed further by Annie Altschul's research, in the late 1970s, into nurse—patient relationships [36], which remains to this day the most valued (and valuable) British contribution to the clarification of the form and function of interpersonal relationships in nursing. I am reassured that Professor Altschul maintains her belief in the central importance of 'nursing *in vivo*', using the milieu of the everyday social and interpersonal world to productive ends.

ASSESSMENT AND THE WHOLE SYSTEM

A common misconception about psychiatric nursing is that nurses simply encourage patients to talk about how they feel, thereby 'working through' their difficulties. Some 30 years ago Hilda Peplau said: 'I am not at all convinced that mere catharsis is useful' [37]. Rather, she went on to say, nurses should 'allow patients to express negative feelings; whilst encouraging discussion, allowing the nurse an opportunity to observe the behaviour, catalogue it as a pattern, and perhaps get some data to help her understand the pattern'. Peplau was illustrating the importance of formulating hypotheses: in order, in my words, 'to begin to find out, more exactly, what is going on here' with a view to 'finding out what needs to be done' to facilitate growth and development.

Rosemary Parse said that nurses address the whole 'lived-experience' of the person. What is meant by that? [38]. Figure 11.1 illustrates the intimidating complexity of the human situation.

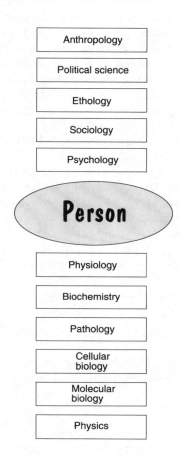

Figure 11.1 The levels of the human condition.

At the organic level we need physics, molecular biology, cellular biology, pathology, biochemistry and physiology – in ascending order – to appreciate how the body of this person works. When we move beyond the individual, we need – again in ascending order – psychology, sociology, ecology, political science and finally anthropology to appreciate the psychosocial boundaries of the individual. The person is, metaphorically, the pivot for this human see-saw, at the opposite ends of which lie the atomic self and membership of the human race. The person has various relationships up and down these hierarchies – although without reflection most of us are unaware of these relationships. How the person-who-is-patient relates to these various organic and psychosocial selves is the content of the nursing enquiry.

Let me offer an everyday example. Many people with mental illness take medication as part of their treatment. Some are fearful of taking drugs, which they assume might be toxic or addictive. Such beliefs are located within the psychological or sociocultural selves. While having such fears, they experience distress and disturbance somewhere within their organic selves. The nurse's responsibility is to address these fears; to help patients become informed about these drugs; to weigh up their advantages and disadvantages; and finally to help them decide whether or not they will take them. The person is helped also to clarify and make sense of the changing experiences within the body, experiences that only the patient can describe. The nurse does not give the patient anything, but rather draws out from within the patient the experience of the everyday challenges and dilemmas of mental illness.

Nursing – when it acts as the educative instrument that Hildegard Peplau defined – will draw forth the person's knowledge of his relationship to these distant atomic and racial selves. The inquisitive process of nursing – through which the person is educated – aims not for any final answers to the person's human predicament but merely to establish where he is at this point on the life path, what sense does he make of experience at this point in time and how can such sense-making help him to make progress? If you think this sounds rather philosophical, you would be right. However, such philosophical uncertainty has great value in practice. In Bertrand Russell's view philosophy was to be:

> studied, not for the sake of any definite answers to its questions, since no definite answers can, as a rule, be known to be true, but rather for the sake of the questions themselves; because these questions enlarge our conception of what is possible, enrich our intellectual imagination, and diminish the dogmatic assurance which closes the mind against speculation [39].

The most elegant nursing interventions involve asking questions: the most central of which is 'What (exactly) is going on here?' The extensive repertoire of questions that we might use to facilitate the person's examination of his situation has only one proper objective: to further his relationship with himself, his world and all those within it, and to extend his appreciation of the meanings he constructs around and about these interacting relationships.

Peplau described a patient with depression who said: 'I'm ugly. I'm repulsive' [40]. The nurses tried to reassure her and she slashed her face because they could not grasp the importance of her recurring statement – 'I am ugly'. Peplau suggested that the nurses might have opened up a discussion by asking:

'When did you first notice this?'
'What is the evidence for that comment?'
'Who told you that?'
'What did you think of yourself when you were little?'
'Give me an example.'

Peplau's aim in pursuing this respectful form of questioning was 'to encourage the patient to begin to feel some doubt in the 100% reliability of her view, seeing this as a product of her past experience, not a part of herself' [41].

This example of the 'extraordinary' nature of questioning and story-telling in psychiatric nursing is all the more remarkable in view of its age. Peplau presented this paper in 1964, a full decade before Aaron Beck published his 'cognitive model' of psychotherapy.

Caring and discovery

Peplau's curiosity might be called a 'discovery-based' form of caring: helping the person clarify who he is, where he came from and how he might 'make himself up' through his manipulation of beliefs, thoughts, feelings, etc. This is to be distinguished from the kind of care that is built around the forcible insertion of 'therapy' into the nursing context.

Since the 1960s nurses in the UK have been fascinated with becoming 'therapists', intent upon treating people, in the belief that caring is somehow inadequate. As a result, many people – both nurses and those in their care – have lost sight of the true meaning of **care**, which I have tried to explicate here. Too much therapy and not enough care may unsettle the person further. The American survivor Rae Unzicker described her recent experience thus: 'To be a mental patient is to participate in stupid groups that call themselves therapy. Music isn't music, it's therapy; volleyball isn't a sport, it's therapy; sewing is therapy; washing dishes is therapy. Even the air you breathe is therapy, and that's called the milieu. [42]'

The inappropriate translation of 'life' into therapy can become doubly problematic if the principles for growth and recovery governing the person do not also support the staff. Recently, when running a workshop with psychiatric nurses on the care of people with severe depression, the group suggested that the client (*sic*) should keep a daily diary of thoughts and feelings as a means of reflecting, therapeutically, on the experience of depression. Everyone in the group, of 30 or so nurses, supported the use of this approach. I was curious to know how many in the group kept diaries of their own thoughts and feelings. The answer was none. I wondered what that meant. I wondered if by becoming 'therapists', who encouraged processes like diary-based reflection, these nurses had, unwittingly, distanced themselves from their clients.

Powering-up [43]

I have a hunch that there is no need to 'change' people or to 'lessen their distress' through one form of magic or another. People will change only when the conditions are right, but they will be the prime mover in the change process. I recall working with a 72-year-old woman with a history of manic depressive psychosis extending back to her early twenties. She was recognized by family, friends and staff as a shy, yet eager-to-please woman who had a difficulty acknowledging any success openly – indeed she shrank back physically, when success was even suggested. My intervention involved little more than asking her questions, persistently yet carefully, over several weeks. My curiosity helped her to construct a picture of herself haunted by her mother, whose voice and ghostly presence she had often translated into what we called auditory hallucinations and delusional beliefs. Ultimately, she used some of the experiences she had gained in 'letting go' her dying husband – which she had told me about in great detail – to release the restrictive ghost of her mother. She used experiences gained – painfully – in one part of her life to heal another part. I had no idea whether what she reported was 'true' in any absolute sense. That she changed suggested that she had constructed a personal truth, which was valid at least at that point in time. I have often asked myself: What more is there?

I have an abiding interest in people who might be called intractably depressed or 'in psychosis'. The proper focus of nursing such people is to help the person clarify the experience: how their experience 'works'; so that they might 'draw forth' new perspectives – a definition, I think, of real education. We can facilitate such education even when the person is reluctant to name the problem. I have had several experiences of working with women who had been sexually abused in childhood. I would begin by acknowledging, openly, that the woman knew the problem but that there was no need for me to know unless she explicitly wished this. This exchange would mark the starting point for an exploration of this unidentified problem, an experience that belonged to her but which she knew she need not necessarily share directly with me. Counsellors and therapists often expect that the person must openly address the problem if any progress is to be made. This does not match my experience. Indeed, such a requirement may, of itself, be taken as no more than a further form of abuse.

People always own experience, whether or not they can communicate it; or even when their capacity to label and communicate such experiences has deserted them. I repeated earlier Wittgenstein's dictum that 'language is the only reality'. Recently, I read Alan Bennett's diaries, in which he talked of his dementing mother's difficulty in finding words for ordinary situations. When riding in a car she asked her son: 'Do you have one of these?' 'What?' 'One of these … what we're in just now.' 'What … a car?' 'Yes, that's it, do you have a car?' Bennett wisely observed that she knew what she was experiencing but had lost the language to communicate what she knew she wanted to say. He added that he wished Wittgenstein could have been in the back seat.

Many nurses working with people with dementia will have reached similar conclusions. The challenge appears to be not to concern ourselves with the decaying of the physical self – the pathology of dementia – but to focus upon the experiences of confusion and agitation, anger and resentment, which are but some of the human dimensions of this disorder. As Dylan Thomas observed: 'Old age should burn and rave at close of day; rage, rage against the dying of the light'. At least part of our caring for people with dementia should acknowledge that the disorder may, in human terms, be raging against the dying of the light. How we respond to such rage is the challenge for nursing.

I comfort myself, in these concluding pages, with the knowledge that nothing I have said in this chapter – if not in the whole text – is in any way new. It is a truism to suggest that all 'modern' thought is no more than 'footnotes to Aristotle'. If my efforts are interpreted as no more than footnotes to Peplau or Altschul my efforts will not have been in vain. My realization of what might be the 'proper focus of nursing' has, as I have illustrated been recognized by other nurses for generations. The knowledge of the inherent meaningfulness of compassionate caring has also been described by people who are not nurses. The American writer Robert Pirsig wrote 20 years ago: 'When one isn't dominated by feelings of separateness from what he's working on, then one can be said to "care" about what he is doing. That is what caring really is, a feeling of identification with what one's doing. [44]' More recently the American psychiatrist Edward Podvoll described the importance of a compassionate environment for people suffering from more severe mental illness, such as psychosis. Podvoll has defined the ability of staff to 'be fully' with their charges, offering the kind of human support they sorely need. Podvoll suggests that 'basic attendance' 'requires more than just what one knows it requires that one use everything of who one is and how one relates to the world. It involves a genuine nursing of the mind. [45]'

A few years ago I visited the University of Pennsylvania, where, on a huge stained glass mural, I discovered Walt Whitman, the American poet my wife introduced me to over 30 years ago. It was typical of an American university that it should include an untutored nurse among the ranks of the great and the good in their nursing history. Given that men in nursing are rare in the US I was doubly pleased to find Whitman held in such high esteem. This reminded me how Whitman, who cared for both sides in the Civil War, wrote of a dying soldier:

One turns to me his appealing eyes – poor boy! I never knew you,
Yet I think I could not refuse you this moment to die for you, if that would save you. [46]

If we could purchase compassion, how much of our health service budgets would we allocate to the humanity that Whitman personified and Podvoll seeks? It is becoming clear that people who are, or have been, patients value compassion highly; as society becomes more complex, as even mother Earth appears to be under threat, the need to heal all our lives assumes a dreadful urgency. Things are no different today than they have been down the centuries: the plight of the disadvantaged and dispossessed – including those with mental illness – serves as a benchmark for the quality of all our lives.

Therapy in life: therapy through living

I began by suggesting that the mind is a reflection of the business of living and, through living, we reflect the mind. What it means to suffer a disturbance of the mind in the late 20th century may well be more complex than it was in 16th-century Portugal, far less when the Celtic brothers began the art of human caring 1000 years ago. Some things have, however, remained the same and I have tried, in this concluding chapter, to tease out some of these 'eternal truths' [47].

Mental illness affects – but **is not** – the whole person. Recovery must, therefore, address the whole person. True care of the person with mental illness must involve careful attention to bodily needs: certainly medication, but also attention to diet, exercise, physical contact, massage – all of which can promote growth. These dimensions of life and the person also belong within the assessment.

The patient's psychological dimension needs similar care: through effective interpersonal relations the sense of alienation, stigma and isolation may be reduced and the person may uncover hidden psychological resources, which may overcome the fears and self-abasement that characterize serious mental illness.

These lead naturally into the social domain, where relationships with nurses under ordinary life circumstances take prominence and the business of 'healing lives' can begin. These relationships can be powerful and a sense of kinship and bonding brings rewards as well as challenges for the nurses themselves.

Finally, this excursion into 'therapy in life – therapy through living' makes an impact on the spiritual identity of the person – and, by implication, the nurse. The person may begin to develop an awareness of who he is and to appreciate the meaning of distress, which goes far beyond mere personal issues. The American nurse Rosemary Parse has suggested that nursing can deal, in this sense, with the art of 'becoming'; treading the path that Maslow charted to the further reaches of human nature [48].

I admit to holding what might be described as an overoptimistic view of the human condition and of the potential for genuine recovery from mental illness. Such a position seems appropriate, given that people with mental illness already know too much of pessimism. Without the compassion, mutual discovery and optimism I have sketched here, I fear that people may well cope with mental illness, may apparently recover but will acquire no real human lessons from the experience. Without these attitudes I fear that the assessment may become grounded in mechanical measurement of mechanical faults in mechanized people.

I have met many people who changed dramatically following serious physical illness. The confrontation with death encourages many people to become aware of the need to live life minute by minute; to live fully right up to the moment of death. These are lives that have been healed through the challenge of illness. These examples suggest the possibilities also for people 'healing their minds' by becoming aware, in the words of Sheldon Kopp, that: 'This is it; there is nothing else'. This also reminds me of Alan Watts's rephrasing of the Zen adage: 'One is more likely to achieve enlightenment by peeling potatoes than by meditating on the Buddha' [49]. Our lives – embracing relationships, work, challenges, disasters, hustle and bustle, activity and rest – have the capacity to wound us but also a capacity for repair. Often the recipe for spiritual repair is under our very noses, if not in the kitchen sink. Some extraordinary life problems may well have ordinary solutions. Assessment may help us to discover these eternal truths.

Through interpersonal relations with effective nurses some people may experience the true meaning of 'taking care' [50]. This experience may be like their original experience of mental illness: something of which they have true knowledge; but which often can be beyond words. True care might begin the development of their true selves; a process that they will continue in their own everyday lives through their own version of 'taking care'.

People with mental illness have taught me that 'we cannot turn the clock back; there is no going back. The aim of all our strivings may be to help the person express what she experiences and then to learn how to find her own faith, through doing what needs to be done [51].'

And now I am back where I started: the story of our reflection on ourselves and how, through the power of stories, we might learn how to live life fully. If psychiatric nursing is ever to acquire a 'mental health' dimension, the nursing assessment needs to explore (fully) how people live their lives. The difficulty in grasping the 'wholeness' of the mind and its intangible relationship with our lives, was described by Deng Ming Dao, who suggested:

When admiring a painting
Don't examine the paint
When meeting the artist
Don't look at the brush. [52]

Searching for an explanation of what nursing is and how it is done by deconstructing it is like analysing the paint in a picture. In art we fumble for an understanding of the idea that the painting conveys. We shall never know the essence of art or life, or indeed of nursing, as long as we observe it like viewer and object. The essential value of life, and indeed of nursing, can only be comprehended by merging fully into the flow of life so that one can become fully a part of it. By losing ourselves in our relationships with the people 'in our care' and in the stories they tell us, we may come to appreciate the point of their illness, if not also of their lives. The stories of nurses and of nursing may, by implication, become enriched in the process.

Let this be the resting place for my soliloquy on assessing the whole person. Maybe we shall find ourselves – and something of the person – by getting lost in the stories that are woven between us and through us.

NOTES

1. McKenna, H. (1994) *Nursing Theories and Quality of Care*, Avebury, Aldershot.
2. Taken from Lao Tzu (1993) *Tao Te Ching*, (trans. Man-Ho Kwok and M. Palmer), Element Books, Shaftesbury.
3. Flanagan, O. J. (1989) *The Science of the Mind*, MIT Press, London.
4. Nolan, P. (1993) *The History of Mental Health Nursing*, Chapman & Hall, London.
5. Barker, P. (1990) The conceptual basis of mental health nursing. *Nurse Education Today*, **10**, 339–48.
6. Rippiere, V. and Williams R. (eds) (1995) *Wounded Healers: Workers' Experiences of Depression*, John Wiley, London.
7. Bennett, G. (1987) *The Wound and the Doctor*, Secker & Warburg, London.
8. Sullivan, H. S. (1953) *The Interpersonal Theory of Psychiatry*, W. W. Norton, New York.
9. Nolan, P. (1993) *The History of Mental Health Nursing*, Chapman & Hall, London.
10. Barker, P. and Jackson, S. (1996) Seriously misguided. *Nursing Times*, **92**(34), 56–8.
11. This is, of course, a convention. Truth may be eternal, but there is no single truth.
12. Barker, P. (1996) The logic of experience: developing appropriate care through effective collaboration. *Australian and New Zealand Journal of Mental Health Nursing*, **5**, 3–12.
13. Partington, A. (ed.) (1992) *Oxford Dictionary of Quotations*, Oxford University Press, Oxford.
14. Parse, R. R. (1995) *Illuminations: The Human Becoming Theory in Practice and Research*, National League for Nursing, New York.
15. Frame, J. (1980) *Faces in the Water*, Women's Press, London.
16. Van Blise, M. (1995) Everything I learned I learned from patients! *Journal of Psychosocial Nursing*, **33**, 18–25.
17. Barker, P. (1996) The logic of experience: developing appropriate care through effective collaboration. *Australian and New Zealand Journal of Mental Health Nursing*, **5**, 3–12.
18. Frankl, V. E. (1973) *Psychotherapy and Existentialism: Selected Papers on Logotherapy* , Pelican, Harmondsworth.
19. Sullivan, H. S. (1953) *The Interpersonal Theory of Psychiatry*, W. W. Norton, New York.
20. American Nurses Association (1980) *Nursing: A Social Policy Statement*, American Nurses Association, Kansas City, MO.
21. I am indebted to my colleague Dr Irene Whitehill for this personal reference.
22. Barker, P. (1996) Chaos and the way of Zen: psychiatric nursing and the certainty principle. *Journal of Psychiatric and Mental Health Nursing*, in press.
23. Barker, P. (1989) The nursing care of people experiencing affective disorder: a review of the literature. *Journal of Advanced Nursing*, **14**, 618–29.
24. Barker, P. (1990) The conceptual basis of mental health nursing. *Nurse Education Today*, **10**, 339–48.
25. O'Toole, A. W. and Welt, S. R. (eds) (1994) *Hildegard E. Peplau: Selected Works – Interpersonal Theory in Nursing*, Macmillan, Basingstoke.
26. Barker, P. (1992) *Severe Depression: A Practitioner's Guide*, Chapman & Hall, London.

27. Peplau, H. E. (1969) Psychotherapeutic strategies. *Perspectives in Psychiatric Care*, **6**, 264–70.
28. Barker, P. (1989) Reflections on the philosophy of caring in mental health. *International Journal of Nursing Studies*, **26**(2), 131–41.
29. The actual framing of this neologism was made by a Greek scholar at the University of St Andrews. I regret that I cannot more specifically honour his contribution.
30. Peck, M. S. (1980) *The Road Less Travelled*, Rider, London.
31. Barker, P. (1996) The logic of experience: developing appropriate care through effective collaboration. *Australian and New Zealand Journal of Mental Health Nursing*, **5**, 3–12.
32. Peplau, H. E. Personal communication.
33. Schwartz, M. S. and Shockley, E. L. (1956) *The Nurse and the Mental Patient: A Study in Interpersonal Relations*, Russell Sage Foundation, New York.
34. *Ibid.*
35. Barnes, E. (1968) *Psychosocial Nursing*, Tavistock Publications, London.
36. Altschul, A. T. (1972) *Patient–Nurse Interaction: A Study of Interactive Patterns on Acute Psychiatric Wards*, Churchill Livingstone, Edinburgh.
37. O'Toole, A. W. and Welt, S. R. (eds) (1994) *Hildegard E. Peplau: Selected Works – Interpersonal Theory in Nursing*, Macmillan, Basingstoke, p. 101.
38. Parse, R. R. (1995) *Illuminations: The Human Becoming Theory in Practice and Research*, National League for Nursing, New York.
39. Russell, B. (1912) *The Problems of Philosophy*, Williams & Norgate (Home University Library), London, p. 249.
40. Peplau, H. E. (1994) General applications of theory and techniques of psychotherapy in nursing situations, in *H. E. Peplau: Selected Works*, (eds A. W. O'Toole and S. R. Welt), Macmillan, London.
41. *Ibid.*
42. Unzicker, R. (1992) To be a mental patient, in *Psychopoetry II. Changes*, **10**, 226–7.
43. Parse, R. R. (1995) *Illuminations: The Human Becoming Theory in Practice and Research*, National League for Nursing, New York.
44. Pirsig, R. (1974) *Zen and the Art of Motorcycle Maintenance*, Corgi, London.
45. Podvoll, E. (1990) *The Seduction of Madness: A Compassionate Approach to Recovery at Home*, Century, London.
46. Whitman, W. (1993) *Walt Whitman: Selected Poems*, Bloomsbury Poetry Classics, London.
47. Kopp, S. (1974) *If You Meet the Buddha on the Road – Kill Him!*, Sheldon Press, London.
48. Maslow, A. (1971) *Farther Reaches of Human Nature*, Viking Press, New York.
49. Watts, A. (1957) *The Way of Zen*, Thames & Hudson, London.
50. Smail, D. (1987) *Taking Care: An Alternative to Therapy*, J. M. Dent, London.
51. Barker, P. (1992) *Severe Depression:a Practitioner's Guide*, Chapman & Hall, London.
52. Dao, D. M. (1992) *365 Tao: Daily Meditations*, Harper, San Francisco, CA.

Appendix A: The development of assessment instruments

Phil Barker and Bill Reynolds

INTRODUCTION

Assessment 'instruments' have been mentioned throughout the text. There are many reasons why one instrument is chosen over the many others available. The reasons offered often say more about the priorities of the user than the instrument itself. We may, for example, observe that the instrument:

- is easy to use;
- requires little prior knowledge or training;
- can be scored 'in a few minutes'.

In addition to the apparent ease, simplicity and cost-efficiency, people often choose one instrument for the simple reason that they know of no other.

In Appendix B a range of assessment instruments is reviewed briefly in an effort to help the reader make more informed choices. Most of the assessment instruments reviewed have been developed from research projects, where their 'usefulness' has been analysed using standard procedures. Special attention is paid to the reliability and validity of instruments, where this is known, as well as considering the 'effort' required to use the measure in the standard clinical environment.

Here an introduction to the process of analysing assessment instruments is provided. We aim to describe briefly how the utility of any assessment instrument is established: how we go about deciding 'how good' is any assessment instrument. These processes equate to the 'road tests' that are used to evaluate new cars, or the test of any new product, when they are described in consumer magazines.

We shall use one measure – the Reynolds Empathy Scale (RES) – to illustrate the process of developing, and testing the utility of, an assessment instrument. Although the RES was developed as part of a nursing research programme, its usefulness as a clinical nursing assessment has also been established. It represents, therefore, one example of a 'useful' assessment method for clinical and research purposes. It is included here as an example of an assessment scale developed by a nurse researcher with a recommended value in nursing practice.

THE REYNOLDS EMPATHY SCALE

The RES comprises 12 items [1]. The scale was designed to measure the extent to which nurses express 'empathic behaviour' within the context of their interaction with the client (*sic*). The items on the scale are:

1. Attempts to explore and clarify feelings
2. Leads, directs and diverts
3. Responds to feelings
4. Ignores verbal and non-verbal communication
5. Explores personal meanings of feelings
6. Judgemental and opinionated
7. Responds to feelings and meaning
8. Interrupts and seems in a hurry
9. Provides the client with direction
10. Fails to focus on solutions/does not answer direct questions/lacks genuineness
11. Appropriate voice tone, sounds relaxed
12. Inappropriate voice tone, sounds curt.

The item pool

The first stage in developing any assessment instrument involves identifying what should be assessed. In developing a measure of 'empathy' the researcher needed to ask: 'What aspects of human interaction might illustrate the concept of empathy?' These 'aspects of human interaction' would represent the 'item pool': the statements or questions that would provide the basis for developing the scale.

The initial item pool was developed from a number of sources. The author drew on his experience of studying nurse–client relationships; the views of different professionals were solicited; and clients' descriptions of interpersonal conditions that they perceived as 'helpful' were also included. From these various contributions, common themes were isolated to comprise the 'item pool'.

A Likert scale was developed for the purpose of scoring the instrument [2]. This allowed the individual nurse's attitudes and behaviours to be rated, to the extent that they were 'present' or 'absent'. This 'empathic' behaviour and/or expressed attitude of the nurse could, as a result, be expressed as a series of numbers, providing the opportunity to obtain an overall score. By using this form of scaling, it would be possible to identify specific 'strengths' and 'weaknesses' in 'empathic behaviour' as well as providing an overall score that might distinguish 'high' from 'low' empathy nurses.

To score each item a seven-point Likert scale was developed. Completion of the scale required the respondents to choose one of seven statements that reflected best their perceptions of themselves, or another person. The points on the Likert scale were:

- Always like
- Nearly always like
- Frequently like
- Quite often like
- Occasionally like
- Seldom like
- Never like.

Some items on the Empathy Scale measured the 'relative presence' of empathy: e.g. item 5: 'Explores personal meanings of feelings'. These were scored from 6 for 'Always like' to 0 for 'Never like'.

Other items measured the 'relative absence' of empathy: e.g. item 8: 'Interrupts and seems in a hurry'. For these items the scoring procedure was reversed: 6 = 'Never like'; 0 = 'Always like'.

Use of this scaling allowed more precise information to be obtained about the respondent's degree of agreement or disagreement with the statements supplied. This is the major advantage of Likert scales over a simple agree/disagree score [3]. Many assessment scales use a five-point, rather than a seven-point scale [4]. The conventional five-point Likert scales allows for a middle, undecided response. However, this has the disadvantage of allowing an acquiescent response, where the person completing the scale may agree, reluctantly, to one rating in the absence of options [5]. The seven-point Likert scale also allows a middle response, but the greater number of points reduces the likelihood of the acquiescent response.

Users' understanding of scale items

The success of any assessment instrument depends greatly on being applied correctly. Following the development of the Likert scale, a user's manual was prepared to guide the scoring of the empathy instrument. The manual consisted of:

- scoring instructions;
- detailed operational definitions of each item;
- clinical examples of each item on the empathy scale.

The operational definition and clinical examples were developed by the researcher, selected from audiotaped records of clinical interviews conducted by registered nurses, who had been supervised during clinical work by the researcher's colleagues.

The clinical examples of items on the empathy scale were intended not to be a comprehensive list but to guide users' understanding of scale items. Specifying in detail how ratings were to be made increased the likelihood that different raters would give similar scores in given situations.

Reliability and validity of the scale

To gauge the usefulness of any assessment instrument two key questions need to be asked. To what extent does the instrument:

- measure what it claims to measure (validity);
- measure consistently (reliability)?

An instrument may be valid but unreliable, or *vice versa*. A watch that runs 2 minutes fast is reliable but invalid – the time is always wrong by 2 minutes [6].

An instrument which claimed to measure 'empathy' but which did not provide the user with a 'useful' measure of 'empathic behaviour' would be invalid. If different raters produced different scores when assessing the same situation the instrument would be unreliable.

Different forms of validity

The development and testing of the empathy scale involved examining the scale for reliability and validity. Validity is reported first because that represents the sequence of investigations. The initial investigations of the scale included the following tests of validity:

- face validity;
- content validity;
- concurrent validity.

Face validity

Face validity is concerned with establishing the extent to which it is reasonable to assume that the scale measures what it is supposed to measure. The RES items were examined independently by a panel of six independent experts in Rogerian theory, five from nursing and one from clinical psychology. All used Rogerian theory in either their clinical work, education or research. The expert panel adopted two approaches to establish face validity.

- They identified items on an existing scale – Empathy Construct Rating Scale (ECRS) [7] – which were similar to items on the RES. A majority of the expert panel paired 75% of the items on the ECRS with items on the RES. These pairings were analysed using a statistical test called Kappa statistic. This revealed that the probability of these pairings being a chance occurrence was very low ($p < 0.0001$). This suggested that the ECRS and the RES were measuring similar constructs.
- The expert panel also commented on whether the items on the empathy scale were indicators of empathy. Each member of the panel agreed that all items on the scale were indicators of empathy.

These results of these two approaches established the face validity of the empathy instrument.

Content validity

The expert panel proposed changes to the wording of some of the scale items and some of the operational definitions. Following the incorporation of these changes it was concluded that the instrument represented adequately the full range of questions that could be asked about empathy. Agreement had now been reached between the researcher and the expert panel on the content of the scale.

Concurrent validity

The RES is not the first such scale to be developed. A common approach to establishing concurrent validity is, therefore, to measure the extent to which the new instrument (RES) correlates with an existing empathy scale. Such an approach is only appropriate if the existing scale is valid and is a different kind of measure from the new scale. The ECRS had been shown to be a valid measure and was different from the new scale. The ECRS was used, therefore, as a comparison to establish the concurrent validity of the RES.

A total of 34 registered nurses were invited to rate themselves on the RES and the ECRS under similar circumstances. The relationship between the subjects' scores on the two scales was compared using a statistical test called the Pearson product moment coefficient (Pearson's r). The results of this comparison showed a high degree of correlation between the nurses' ratings on the two scales. (The computed correlation coefficient was 0.85; $p < 0.001$.)

Reliability of the empathy scale

Reliability is usually defined as the ability of an instrument to yield consistent results [8] or the extent to which measurement error is minimized [9]. The reliability of the RES involved the investigation of:

- test–retest reliability;

- internal consistency among items on the scale;
- the internal discrimination of scale items;
- inter-rater reliability.

Test–retest reliability

Test–retest reliability involves the administration of the scale twice to the same subjects. The repeat administration should be after a period of time sufficient to allow the subjects to forget the original scores made but not so long that a natural change in the scores could be expected to occur.

A total of 32 registered nurses scored themselves on the scale twice over a 2–4 week period. The test–retest reliability was established by correlating the two sets of data using the Pearson product moment coefficient. The results showed that there was little difference between the two sets of ratings over the time period. (The correlation coefficient was 0.90; $p < 0.001$.)

The 2–4 week time period was considered appropriate since the construct being measured (self-reported state empathy) was not expected to change greatly across time. Previous research had shown that self-reported state empathy did not change significantly among measures when subjects are not receiving empathy education [10]. None of the 32 nurses was receiving empathy education at the time of testing.

The internal reliability of scale items

Internal reliability, or consistency, is concerned with the homogeneity of the scale: to what extent are all the items measuring the same 'thing'? There are several ways of measuring internal reliability. The method chosen here involved observed correlations between items on the scale.

A total of 103 registered nurses were asked to score themselves on the RES. Use of a specific statistical procedure (Cronbach's alpha) showed that the correlation between items on the scale was high: similarities in the scores on different items suggesting that all items were measuring the same 'thing' – i.e. 'empathy'. (The correlation coefficient was 0.90.) If any item had shown a low correlation with the other items, the researcher would have considered removing this item. In the circumstances, all items on the scale were retained.

The internal discrimination of the empathy scale

The RES was also designed to distinguish between people with high and low 'empathy' scores. This is a vital question since, according to Rogerian theory, 'high empathizers' would attempt consistently to 'explore and clarify feelings' (item 1 on the scale), but would not consistently 'divert a person from areas of concern' (item 2 on the scale). If those items failed to distinguish 'high' from 'low' empathizers, they could be considered to be unreliable indicators of empathy.

The internal discrimination of the scale was assessed by examining the scores of the 103 nurses using a statistical test called Phi coefficient. The top third and the bottom third of the scores for each item and the total scores for the instrument were retained for analysis. Phi was calculated by correlating the top and bottom scores for each item with the top and bottom scores for the entire instrument.

This test addressed the question: 'Is there an association between individual scale items and overall scores?' The results (Phi values) suggested that all items in the scale distinguished high empathy scorers from low empathy scorers.

Inter-rater reliability

Inter-rater reliability measures the extent to which two people using the scale in the same situation will produce similar ratings. The RES was developed within a study where trained raters scored audio-tape recordings of nurses' counselling work. Consequently, it was necessary to test the reliability between raters. Using the RES three raters scored several taped nurse–client verbal interactions simultaneously and independently. The resulting records were used to establish the degree of inter-rater reliability.

All raters had received training in use of the scale. The purpose of the observations, the operational definitions of the individual items on the RES, and the seven-point Likert scale, were examined and discussed to achieve mutual understanding. When a common understanding of the 12 scale items existed among raters, they were invited to rate independently an audiotaped record of a nurse–client counselling interview. The degree of agreement between raters was measured by using the formula: Number of agreements/Number of agreements plus disagreements. Initially the degree of agreement between the raters was low (25–33%). Following further discussions between the raters and the researcher, the raters assessed a further set of recordings. The degree of inter-rater reliability had now risen to between 67% and 92%. This suggested that different raters were measuring the same phenomena to much the same degree.

CONCLUSION

We have outlined briefly the process commonly employed to judge the reliability and validity of an assessment instrument. By subjecting the instrument to these tests a judgement on its relative 'usefulness' can be made: to what extent is the instrument fit for the purpose for which it was designed? This brief summary shows how the RES was tested, and found to be a useful means of measuring the construct 'empathy'.

NOTES

1. For further details of the Reynolds Empathy Scale contact Bill Reynolds at the Department of Continuing Education, University of Stirling, Highland Campus, Raigmore Hospital, Inverness.
2. Oppenheim, A. (1992) *Questionnaire Design, Interviewing and Attitude Measurement*, Pinter Publishing, London.
3. *Ibid.*
4. *Ibid.*
5. Polgar, C. and Thomas, S. (1988) *Introduction to Research in Health Sciences*, Churchill Livingstone, Edinburgh.
6. Cormack, D. F. S. (1983) *Psychiatric Nursing Described*, Churchill Livingstone, Edinburgh.
7. La Monica, E. (1981) Construct validity of an empathy instrument. *Research in Nursing and Health*, **4**, 389–400.
8. Treece, E. and Treece, J. (1982) *Elements of Research in Nursing*, C. V. Mosby, St Louis, MO.
9. Polit, D. and Hungler, B. (1983) *Nursing Research: Principles and Methods*, J. B. Lippincott, Philadelphia, PA.
10. Reynolds, W. (1986) A study of empathy in student nurses. MPhil thesis, Dundee College of Technology.

Appendix B: Psychosocial assessment instruments – a selective bibliography

THE TOOL BOX

Psychiatric nurses are expected to assess the people in their care for a variety of reasons. These range from purely clinical assessment through clinical audit to research inquiry. The need to identify the nature and scale of the person's problems of living was a prevailing concern throughout this book. In many nursing situations, these aims will be achieved best through the qualitative inquiry of interviewing and other collaborative 'narrative' methods.

Increasingly, nurses are expected to 'quantify' the person-in-care's problems and to evaluate the effects of nursing – and other – interventions. A number of assessment instruments have been described briefly in the chapters in Part Two. The assessment instruments summarized here may assist nurses further to fulfil these expectations for clinical measurement and evaluation. Some of these methods may also be worthy of consideration by nurses considering undertaking clinical nursing research or audit projects.

The selection of assessment instruments included here are akin to 'tools' in a tool box. Each instrument was designed for a specific purpose; and some tools are fit only for that purpose. Other tools may, however, be useful across a wide range of situations. I expect that most readers will use this short bibliography to help them decide which tool might best suit their needs. I expect also that other readers might marry the information here to their experience and knowledge, thereby allowing them to assess the people in their care more 'creatively'

Note: I have chosen not to recommend any of the following instruments. All the methods included have been developed within research studies. Some instruments are 'robust', in terms of their reliability and validity, whereas others may only be 'popular' – perhaps because of their ease of administration or attractiveness to people-in-care. I summarize the key features and obvious strengths and weaknesses of each instrument. I leave the individual reader to exercise her judgement of the utility of any method.

BECK DEPRESSION INVENTORY (BDI)

Beck, A. T., Ward, C. H., Mendelson, M. *et al.* (1961) An inventory for measuring depression. *Archives of General Psychiatry*, **4**, 561–71.

This scale measures the severity of depressive states. The factors associated with depression measured are: self debasement, vegetative depression, inhibition-fatigability, hopelessness-suicidal wishes.

Method: The scale involves 21 items, each of which is self-rated using a four-point scale (0–3) each arranged in order of increasing severity.

Item example:

0= I don't feel disappointed in myself
1= I am disappointed in myself
2= I am disgusted with myself
3= I hate myself.

The questions and accompanying ratings may be read out to the person in the form of an interview, in the case of more severe depressive states or where the person has reading difficulties (see note below on validity). The person is usually asked to use the previous 3–7 days as a time frame for the self-report. The scale can be completed in 10 minutes.

Reliability and validity: Good levels of reliability (test–retest and split-half) have been reported. Generally the BDI is assumed to have good levels of validity, since it is based on a clinical theory of depression. Doubts have been expressed, however, about the cognitive bias of items in the scale, and only moderate correlations have been reported between the BDI and the Hamilton Depression Scale. Where the person is suffering from a severe depressive state the validity of the BDI is doubtful; however this criticism would apply to all self-rating scales. Doubt has also been expressed about the BDI's validity as a screening instrument for depression.

Comments: This is a widely used scale, which has become more popular as Beck's cognitive therapy for depression has become more widespread. It provides a useful – and simple – means of monitoring the effects of treatment. Short-term studies have suggested, however, that the Hamilton Depression Scale is more sensitive to change over time.

BRIEF PSYCHIATRIC RATING SCALE (BPRS)

Lukoff, D., Neuchterlein, K. H. and Ventura, J. (1986) Manual for the Expanded Brief Psychiatric Rating Scale (BPRS). *Schizophrenia Bulletin*, **12**, 594–602.

This scale measures the presence of a range of phenomena associated with various forms of mental illness: anxiety and depression; loss of energy; thought disturbance; hostility and suspiciousness, etc.

Method: The scale is applied following a semi-structured interview, supported by observation by the rater and information provided by staff and family. The scale measures 18 symptoms (21 in an expanded version) using a seven-point rating scale signifying varying levels of presence or absence: 1 = 'Not present'; 7 = 'Extremely severe'.

The scale takes 20–30 minutes to complete and is based on the presentation of the person over the past 2 weeks. The scale generates a total score as well as individual factor scores.

Item examples: The rater/interviewer is looking for discrete symptoms of mental illness, e.g.:

- the degree to which speech is confused, disorganized or disconnected;
- reported perceptual experiences in the absence of external stimuli;
- reported behaviours which are odd or unusual.

Reliability and validity: The BPRS is often used as a measure of the overall 'psychotic state', with the total scale indicative of severity. Five discrete factors have been validated through factor analysis: thought disorder (items 4, 12 and 15); emotional withdrawal (items 3, 13 and 16); anxiety and depression (items 3, 5 and 9); aggressiveness (items 10, 11 and 14); and agitation (items 6 and 17). A number of reliability studies have been undertaken and, overall, the inter-rater reliability has been found to be acceptable.

Comments: The BPRS is one of the most widely used scales internationally and has been found to be valid both in research and clinical practice. The scale tends to focus on more severe symptoms, such as those present in psychotic disorders. Although published sample questions and operational definitions help promote validity and reliability, training and practice in the use of the scale are recommended.

CLINICAL ANXIETY SCALE (CAS)

Snaith, R. P., Baugh, S. J., Clayden, A. D. *et al.* (1982) The Clinical Anxiety Scale: an instrument derived from the Hamilton Anxiety Scale. *British Journal of Psychiatry*, **141**, 518–23.

This interview-based measure is a shorter version of the Hamilton Anxiety Scale (see below).

Method: The person is rated by a clinician, who gauges how the person has been feeling 'over the past 2 days, including today', using the following six areas: psychic tension; ability to relax; startle response; worrying; apprehension; restlessness.

No specific questions are recommended but the clinician is guided by detailed criteria for scoring each area.

Item example: 'Restlessness'.

4: The client is unable to keep still for more than a few minutes and engages in restless pacing or other purposeless activity
3: As above, but he/she is able to keep still for an hour or so at a time
2: There is a feeling of 'needing to be on the move' which causes some, but not severe, distress
1: Slight experience of restlessness which causes no distress
0: Absence of restlessness.

Reliability and validity: The content validity of the CAS is ensured since it is based on the previously validated Hamilton Anxiety Scale: only items that correlated significantly were included in the CAS (correlations from 0.44–0.76). Reliability data has not yet been published.

Comments: The CAS scores can be graded within four ranges (recovered/absent; mild; moderate; severe). The authors suggest that these may be used to gauge need for treatment. A 'panic attacks' item has been added: the score for this item is not computed as part of the overall CAS score.

GENERAL HEALTH QUESTIONNAIRE (GHQ)

Goldberg, D. and Williams, P. (1988) *A User's Guide to the General Health Questionnaire*, NFER-Nelson, Windsor.

This scale measures general 'well-being' and the presence of 'mental illness'.

Method: This scale is available in a number of formats. Originally designed to include 60 items, shorter versions are now available comprising 30, 28, 20 and 12 items.

The scale measures subjective experience during periods of stress, illness or general 'strain'. The scale is a self-report questionnaire, usually completed over the previous week. Each item is rated using a four-point rating scale, the ratings being phrased slightly differently according to the question. Four factors were identified: social dysfunction; somatization; anxiety; and depression.

Item example: Have you recently: felt constantly under strain?

- Not at all
- No more than usual
- Rather more than usual
- Much more than usual.

Reliability and validity: Validity and reliability have been shown through several studies to be consistently very good.

Comments: The GHQ is useful for clinicians in identifying reduced well-being and possible mental health problems in individuals, and for researchers in screening the frequency of mental illness in large populations. In both situations the scale may be used to measure change over time. The scoring is, however, varied depending on the purpose of the assessment. Similarly, the cut-off point for determining psychiatric 'caseness' varies with the population, scoring method and version used. Intending users of the GHQ need to take these complexities into account when considering its possible application.

HAMILTON ANXIETY SCALE (HAS)

Hamilton, M. (1969) Diagnosis and rating of anxiety. *British Journal of Psychiatry*, **Special pub. 3**, 76–9. See also Maier, W., Buller, R., Philipp, M. and Heuser, I. (1988) The Hamilton Anxiety Scale. *Journal of Affective Disorders*, **5**, 163–70.

This scale provides a measure of the severity of anxiety as a psychiatric disorder.

Method: The scale is applied by a clinician through a semi-structured interview which focuses on the person's experience of anxiety only, over the past 2–3 days. The scale includes 14 items, each of which is rated using a five-point scale (0–4).

Reliability and validity: Inter-rater reliability has been reported as 'adequate' (Kendall concordance test 0.80). The scale was designed for use only with people experiencing anxiety, but it has also been shown to be valid for people with depression with anxiety features.

Comments: This scale has been described as one of the most commonly used observer rating scales for anxiety. The scale may be used to distinguish generalized anxiety from panic attacks.

HOSPITAL ANXIETY AND DEPRESSION SCALE (HADS)

Zigmond, A. S. and Snaith, R. P. (1983) The Hospital Anxiety and Depression Scale. *Acta Psychiatrica Scandinavica*, **67**, 361–70.

This self-report questionnaire was designed to detect anxiety and depression when used in general hospital out-patient departments.

Method: The scale comprises 14 items, seven each for anxiety and depression. Although identified as a 'hospital' scale, it is appropriate for community-based assessment.

Each item is rated on a four-point scale (0–3) which identifies the relative presence of the item identified. The scale is completed by underlining the response that most accurately suggests the person's state over the preceding 7 days.

Item example: 'Worrying thoughts go through my mind'

- A great deal of the time
- A lot of the time
- From time to time but not often
- Only occasionally.

The ratings (0–3) are arranged at the left-hand side of the questionnaire for completion by the clinician. These distinguish between anxiety (A) and depression (D) factors.

Reliability and validity: The scale is easy to complete and acceptable to patients, conferring a good level of face validity. Concurrent validity for both anxiety (0.54) and depression (0.79) is good: these were obtained by comparison with interviews blind to the results of the scale. Internal consistency measures also found significant associations (0.41–0.76 for anxiety; 0.30–0.60 for depression). Reliability data has not yet been reported.

Comments: The HADS is a valid scale for the assessment of anxiety and depression in outpatient settings, and may also be valid for other patient groups providing that a supplementary brief interview is conducted.

INVENTORY FOR DEPRESSIVE SYMPTOMATOLOGY (IDS)

Rush, A. J., Giles, D. E., Schlesser, M. A. *et al.* (1986) The Inventory for Depressive Symptomatology (IDS): preliminary findings. *Psychiatry Research*, **18**, 65–87.

The IDS provides a measure of signs and symptoms of depression. The instrument is available in two forms: a self-report questionnaire for completion by the patient (the IDS-SR) and a clinician rating scale (the IDS-C). The IDS measures 'mood', 'anxiety', 'weight', 'sleep' and 'atypical features'.

Method: Each version of the IDS comprises 30 items. In the self-report measure the patient circles the response that most closely represents their feelings over the past week. In the clinician rating the rater judges the response 'that best describes the client' over the preceding week. Both versions employ a four-point scale (0–3). The higher the score, the more severe the depression is assumed to be.

Item example (self-report): 16. View of myself

0: I see myself as equally worthwhile and deserving as other people.
1: I am more self-blaming than usual.
2: I largely believe that I cause problems for others.
3: I think almost constantly about major and minor defects in myself.

There are four items for weight (increase or decrease in appetite; both rated over the past 2 weeks). Since only an increase or a decrease is possible, only 28 items are included in the total rating, which is achieved by adding all the circled responses.

Reliability and validity: The reliability of both versions has been assessed by item–whole correlation and coefficient alpha, both of which are acceptable. Test–retest reliability has not yet been reported. Concurrent validity of the IDS was reported through a significant association with the Beck Depression Inventory (see above). A factor analysis also identified the four factors expected thereby providing a measure of construct validity.

Comments: The IDS is a useful measure of depressive symptomatology, which was designed for use in both inpatient and community clinic settings. Normative data is available that suggests the possibility of distinguishing between 'endogenous' and 'non-endogenous' forms of depression.

INSTRUMENTAL AND EXPRESSIVE FUNCTIONS OF SOCIAL SUPPORT (IEFSS)

Ensel, W. M. and Woelfel, J. (1986) Measuring the instrumental and expressive functions of social support, in *Social Support, Life Events and Depression*, (eds N. Lin, A. Dean and W. Ensel), Academic Press, New York.

This scale assesses the function and emotional content of the person's social relationships.

Method: The person is asked to rate a list of 28 problems by noting 'how often' they have been 'bothered by each problem' over the previous 6 months. A five-point scale is used to rate each item (1 = Most or all of the time; 5 = Never). The scale covers five main areas: demands; money; companionship; marital conflict; communication.

Item example: How often have you been bothered by:

- too many demands on your time?
- conflicts with people who are close to you?

Reliability and validity: The reliability and validity are judged to be good: Cronbach's alpha (total scale) 0.93.

Comments: This is an efficient assessment of social support: the completion time is approximately 10 minutes. The emphasis on the function and emotional content of relationships distinguishes it from other scales, which emphasize the size of the person's network.

MANIA SCALE

Bech, P., Bolwig, T. G., Kramp, P. and Rafaelson, O. J. (1979) The Bech–Rafaelson Mania Scale and the Hamilton Depression Scale. *Acta Psychiatrica Scandinavica*, **49**, 248–56. See also Bech, P. (1993) *Rating Scales for Psychopathology, Health Status, and Quality of Life. A Compendium on Documentation in Accordance with the DSM-III-R and WHO Systems*, Springer-Verlag, Berlin.

This scale measures mood changes in people diagnosed as suffering from manic depressive psychosis.

Method: The scale measures the severity of and changes in mania. The scale is administered by a clinician using a semi-structured interview focused on the past 2–3 days. The scale includes 11 items, each of which is rated using operational criteria on a five-point scale (0–4).

Reliability and validity: Both validity and reliability are generally considered to be adequate. Analyses of internal and external validity indicate the presence of a general dimension for mania. Cronbach's alpha has been reported – 0.93.

Comments: This scale was developed from an earlier scale, which was administered by nurses. Studies indicate that it is sensitive to changes occurring during treatment. It is therefore particularly appropriate for use as a therapeutic evaluation instrument.

MOBILITY INVENTORY FOR AGORAPHOBIA

Chambless, D. L., Caputo, G. C., Jasin, S. E. and Gracely, E. J. (1985) The Mobility Inventory for Agoraphobia. *Behaviour Research and Therapy*, **23**, 35–44.

This self-report questionnaire is focused on the patterns of avoidance behaviour associated with agoraphobia.

Method: The Inventory comprises 29 items. The 28th item is a frequency count of panic attacks over the past week and the final item provides a rating of panic intensity. All other items (27) address avoidance behaviours, which are rated using a five-point scale (1–5). The person may also use midpoint ratings (e.g. 3.5).

Two ratings are required: when the person is accompanied by a 'trusted companion' and when alone.

Item example: 'Rate your amount of avoidance ....using the following scale:'

1 = Never avoid
2 = Rarely avoid
3 = Avoid about half the time
4 = Avoid most of the time
5 = Always avoid

Places	**When accompanied**	**When alone**
1. Theatre		
2. Supermarkets		
....		

Reliability and validity: Significant validity correlations have been reported for the inventory following comparison with other validated measures of agoraphobic avoidance (Kinney, P. J. and Williams, S. L. (1988) Accuracy of fear inventories and self-efficacy scales in predicting agoraphobic behaviour. *Behaviour Research and Therapy*, **26**, 513–18). The test–retest reliability and individual item reliability are also good.

PADUA INVENTORY

Sanavio, E. (1988) Obsessions and compulsions: the Padua Inventory. *Behaviour Research and Therapy*, **26**, 169–77.

This self-report scale rates the relative presence of common obsessional thoughts and compulsive behaviours.

Method: The Inventory comprises 60 items, each of which is negatively phrased: 'I feel I have to remember completely unimportant numbers'. Each item is rated on a five-point scale (0–4) in terms of their frequency of occurrence. The scale comprises four factors: I = impaired control over mental activities; II = becoming contaminated; III = checking behaviours; IV = urges and worries of losing control.

Item example: 'At certain moments I am tempted to tear off my clothes in public'

0 = Not at all
1 = A little
2 = Quite a lot
3 = A lot
4 = Very much.

Completion of the scale takes approximately 10 minutes. The total score is computed by adding the individual ratings (maximum 240).

Reliability and validity: Internal consistency and stability of scores over time are good (correlations between 0.78 and 0.94). Good concurrent validity (0.70) has been measured by comparison with other established measures of obsessive compulsive behaviour.

Comments: This inventory is easy to use and provides a valuable means of assessing severity pre- and postintervention.

PERCEIVED SUPPORT NETWORK INVENTORY (PSNI)

Oritt, E. J., Paul, S. C. and Behran, J. A. (1985) The perceived support network inventory. *American Journal of Community Psychology*, **13**, 565–81.

This scale measures the availability and quality of social support available to the person assessed.

Method: The person is asked to identify up to 12 people to whom they would go for help in a time of crisis. An identical set of six questions is asked for each of the following areas: initiation of support seeking; availability; satisfaction; multidimensionality; reciprocity; network conflict.

Each set of questions is answered for each person identified, using a seven-point scale: 1 (Almost always) to 7 (Almost never). Subscale scores are averaged for each item. The questions can be completed in about 1 minute for each person identified.

Item examples:

- During times of stress I seek out this person for support or help (initiation).
- This person receives support from me during times of stress for him/her (reciprocity).

Reliability and validity: Good validity and reliability have been reported. Test–retest 0.88.

Comments: This is a useful measure of the presence and strength of the person's supportive relationships.

POSITIVE AND NEGATIVE SYNDROME SCALE (PANSS)

Kay, S. R., Opler, L. A. and Lindenmayer, J. P. (1988) Reliability and validity of the positive and negative syndrome scale for schizophrenics. *Psychiatry Research*, **23**, 99–110. See also Kay, S. R. (1991) Positive and Negative Syndromes in Schizophrenia: Assessment and Research, Brunner-Mazel, New York.

This scale is a development of the Brief Psychiatric Rating Scale (see above) containing many of the items from that scale.

Method: This 30-item scale is applied by a clinician through a semi-structured interview which takes approximately 50 minutes to complete. Approximately seven items address negative symptoms and seven positive symptoms. The remaining 16 items are focused on measures of 'general psychopathology'. Some items are based on assessment within the interview; others include observations from 'significant others'.

Each item is rated using a Likert scale (0–6), which assesses severity.

Reliability and validity: The scale has been subject to factor analysis. Reliability and validity are generally considered to be adequate.

Comments: A wide range of scales have been published that purport to measure positive and negative symptoms in schizophrenia. The PANSS is probably more useful, given its inclusion of a broad 'psychopathology' section. Although time-consuming, it is more cost-effective than structured psychiatric interviews.

PROGRESS EVALUATION SCALE (PES)

Ihilevich, D., Gleser, G. C., Gritter, G. W. *et al.* (1981) Measuring program outcome: the progress evaluation scales. *Evaluation Review*, **5**, 451–77.

This scale measures functional psychosocial performance by focusing on severe deficits. Versions are available for adults, adolescents, children and developmentally disabled people.

Method: The scale comprises seven scales: family interaction; occupation; getting along with others; feelings and mood; use of free time; problems; attitude toward self. Each scale is rated on a five-point scale: 1 (Most pathologic) to 5 (Healthiest). The scale may be completed by either a clinician, the individual concerned or a family member. No total score is computed.

Item examples 'Takes care of own basic needs but must have help with everyday plans and activities' (Family interaction scale: rating =2).

Reliability and validity: This scale possesses good validity and reliability (inter-rater reliability 0.49–0.86; test–retest reliability 0.54–0.75).

Comments: This scale provides a comprehensive assessment of psychosocial functioning. It can be completed in a few minutes, quite unobtrusively, and is particularly useful in community settings to guide both clinical programmes and policy planning.

QUALITY OF LIFE (QOL)

Olson, D. H. and Barnes, H. L. (1982) Quality of life, in *Family Inventories: Inventories Used in a National Survey of Families Across the Family Cycle*, (eds D. H. Olson, H. I. McCubbin, H. Barnes *et al.*), Family Social Science, University of Minnesota, St Paul, MN.

This scale measures the subjective experience of quality of life through estimates of personal satisfaction.

Method: The adult scale comprises 40 items and the adolescent scale 25 items: 19 are common to both scales. The person rates satisfaction with each item using a five-point scale (1 = Dissatisfied; 5 = Extremely satisfied). The scale takes approximately 10 minutes to complete.

Item example: 'How satisfied are you with':

• your job security (adult)
• your current school situation (adolescent)
• your current housing arrangement (both forms)?

Reliability and validity: Good validity and reliability have been reported. Cronbach's alpha 0.92 (parent), 0.86 (adolescent). Test–retest 0.65.

Comments: The assessment of 'quality of life' is a difficult area. This is generally accepted to be a useful measure, encompassing many of the key experiences of adults and adolescents.

QUALITY OF LIFE SCALE (QLS)

Heinrichs, D. W., Hanlon, T. E. and Carpenter, W. T. (1984) The quality of life scale: an instrument for rating the schizophrenic deficit syndrome. *Schizophrenia Bulletin*, **10**, 388–98.

This scale measures the person's capability to perform and manage appropriate social roles.

Method: The scale measures three main areas: interpersonal relations; occupational role; and richness of personal experience. The scale comprises 21 items, each of which is rated on a seven-point scale (0 = Low; 6 = High) with every other item described. The scale is completed by a clinician through a semi-structured interview and results in a total score representing the person's presentation over the preceding month. The scale is time-consuming, however, taking up to 45 minutes to complete.

Item example: 'Rate the degree to which the person actively avoids social interaction due to discomfort or disinterest'.

Reliability and validity: This scale possess good reports for both validity and reliability. The 'intraclass correlations' (0.58–0.98) for each of the 21 items have been reported.

Comments: This scale assesses deficits and impaired functioning in non-hospitalized people with a diagnosis of schizophrenia. The scale has the added advantage of usefulness in evaluating programmes aimed at promoting adaptive functioning in the natural community.

QUALITY OF LIFE SELF-ASSESSMENT SCALE (QLS-100)

Skantze, K., Malm, U., Dencker, S. J. *et al.* (1992) Comparison of quality of life to standard of living in schizophrenic patients. *British Journal of Psychiatry*, **161**, 797–801.

This scale was designed specifically to assess quality of life in psychiatric patients.

Method: This 100-item scale grew out of rehabilitation work and aims to assess changes in quality of life and, to some extent, a measure of the quality of care. The items are grouped in 11 sections: housing; environment; knowledge/education; contacts; dependence; inner experiences; mental health; physical health; leisure; work; and religion. Each item within each section is assessed in terms of 'satisfactory' or 'unsatisfactory' function and is focused on self-reports of satisfaction.

Reliability and validity: This is a pragmatic scale focused on subjective accounts of well-being and satisfaction. However studies have shown that repeated measures of ANOVA differentiate levels of satisfaction across the 11 domains. Test–retest reliability has been shown to be adequate.

Comments: This scale derives from earlier measures which involved checklists or observational rating scales. The scale is based on substantial work with patients (*sic*) and family members, which adds greatly to its 'validity'. The focus on self-report is a strong feature, given recognition that staff and patients (*sic*) have very different perceptions of quality of life.

SELF-EFFICACY SCALE

Sherer, M., Maddux, J. E., Mercandante, B. *et al.* (1982) The self-efficacy scale: construction and validation. *Psychological Reports*, **51**, 663–71.
  This scale measures general self-efficacy and social self-efficacy.

Method: The scale comprises 30 items: 17 address general self-efficacy, six address social self-efficacy and eight filter items make the purpose of the test more ambiguous. Each item is rated on an A (Disagree strongly) to E (Agree strongly) scale. The scale takes approximately 10 minutes to complete.

Item examples:

- 'One of my problems is that I cannot get down to work when I should.'
- 'I have acquired my friends through my personal abilities at making friends.'

Reliability and validity: The scale has good reliability and validity estimates: general self-efficacy – Cronbach's alpha 0.86; social self-efficacy – 0.71.

Comments: This scale measures the person's tendency to attribute success to personal skill (or other personal quality) rather than to chance or 'fate'. It has particular usefulness in evaluating outcomes of psychotherapeutic programmes.

SELF-ESTEEM SCALE

Rosenberg, M. (1965) *The Measurement of Self-esteem*, Princeton University Press, Princeton, NJ.

  This scale measures self-esteem.

Method: The scale comprises ten items, which are rated using a four-point scale (Strongly agree–Strongly disagree). The items alternate between positively and negatively worded items.

Item examples:

- 'I am able to do things as well as most other people.'
- 'I feel I do not have much to be proud of.'

Reliability and validity: Reliability and validity are generally considered to be good. Cronbach's alpha 0.86–0.89.

Comments: This scale is easily administered. It is particularly appropriate for adolescents. The scores correlate highly with measures of depression and anxiety.

SYMPTOM DISTRESS CHECKLIST 90-R (SCL90R)

Derogatis, L. R. (1992) *SCL-90-R: Administration, Scoring and Procedures Manual – II*, Clinical Psychometrics Research, Towson, MD.
  This scale measures the level of psychiatric distress.

Method: The scale comprises 90 items, each of which is rated on a five-point scale (0 = Not at all; 4 = Extremely). Nine factors are included: somatization; obsessive-compulsiveness; interpersonal sensitivity; depression; anxiety; hostility; phobic anxiety; paranoid ideation; psychoticism. The person is rated on his experience over the preceding 7 days.

Item examples:

- 'feeling tense or keyed up'
- 'thoughts of ending your life'
- 'hearing voices that other people do not hear'.

Reliability and validity: Both are considered to be adequate: Cronbach's alpha 0.77–0.90; test–retest reliability 0.55–0.90.

Comments: The scale is used for both research and clinical purposes. It takes approximately 15 minutes to complete. Scores for each of the nine dimensions can be calculated, as well as three global scores.

SYMPTOMS OF STRESS INVENTORY (SOS)

Thompson, E. A. and Leckie, M. (1989) Interpretation manual for symptoms of stress inventory. Unpublished manuscript, University of Washington Stress Management Program, Seattle, WA.

  This scale measures the experience of stress across ten discrete factor areas, usually over the preceding week, but other time frames are possible. The scale takes approximately 10 minutes to complete.

Method: This self-report scale comprises 94 items, which reflect physical, psychological and behavioural responses to stress. The ten factors represented are: peripheral manifestations; cardiopulmonary; central neurologic; gastrointestinal; muscular; habit patterns; depression; anxiety/fear; emotional irritability; cognitive disorganization. Each item is rated on a five-point scale (0 = Never; 4 = Very frequently), providing a total and subscale score.

Item examples:

- Have you ever been bothered by cold hands or feet?
- Does it seem that little things get on your nerves?
- Have you noticed excessive tension, stiffness, soreness, or cramping of the muscles in your neck?

Reliability and validity: The validity and reliability of this scale are generally considered to be good (subscale Cronbach's alpha 0.62–0.91; test–retest reliability 0.47–0.86).

Comments: This scale provides a comprehensive measure of stress related symptoms. The scale is particularly useful in planning focused interventions and in evaluating outcomes of treatment.

Index

Page numbers in **bold** refer to figures, page numbers in *italic* refer to tables or notes at end of chapters.